Multifunctional Hydrogels for Biomedical Applications

Multifunctional Hydrogels for Biomedical Applications

Edited by

Ricardo A. Pires
Iva Pashkuleva
Rui L. Reis

WILEY-VCH

Editors

Dr. Ricardo A. Pires
University of Minho
3B's Research Group
Parque de Ciência e Tecnologia
Zona Industrial da Gandra
4805-017 Barco, Guimarães
Portugal

Dr. Iva Pashkuleva
University of Minho
3B's Research Group
Parque de Ciência e Tecnol
4805-017 Barco, Guimarães
Portugal

Prof. Rui L. Reis
University of Minho
3B's Research Group
Parque de Ciência e Tecnologia
4805-017 Barco, Guimarães
Portugal

Cover Image: © NANOCLUSTERING/Getty Images

Library of Congress Card No.: applied for

British Library Cataloguing-in-Publication Data
A catalogue record for this book is available from the British Library.

Bibliographic information published by the Deutsche Nationalbibliothek The Deutsche Nationalbibliothek lists this publication in the Deutsche Nationalbibliografie; detailed bibliographic data are available on the Internet at <http://dnb.d-nb.de>.

Print ISBN: 978-3-527-34716-2
ePDF ISBN: 978-3-527-82581-3
ePub ISBN: 978-3-527-82583-7
oBook ISBN: 978-3-527-82582-0

Typesetting Straive, Chennai, India
Printing and Binding CPI Group (UK) Ltd, Croydon, CR0 4YY

Printed on acid-free paper

C099347_030522

Contents

Preface

Hydrogels have a long history as biomaterials that address different clinical needs: substitutes of human tissues affected by disease or accidents, scaffolds for tissue engineering, carriers for cells and/or bioactive molecules, are some examples of the hydrogels' biomedical applications. These diverse applications require development of specific and often multifunctional systems that meet a set of characteristics imposed by the nature of the injured tissue and present bioactivities that are important for clinical outcomes. Contemporary approaches address these needs using different natural and synthetic materials that encode bioinformation themselves or are further modified to confer bioactivity. The responsiveness and adaptiveness of the hydrogels are other assets targeted by current developments. During the last decade, we have witnessed tremendous advances not only in terms of materials' design and synthesis but also in terms of methods used to process these materials. In this context, the present book gives an overview of some of the recent progress in the development of multifunctional hydrogels from different perspectives: chemistry, materials science and engineering, biology, nanotechnology and bioengineering, and medical aspects are discussed in the light of different biomedical applications. The book also presents critical opinions on future developments and expected breakthroughs in the interconnected fields of biomaterials, tissue engineering, and regenerative medicine.

Since a major goal was to provide a comprehensive matter that is useful for readers with different backgrounds and academic or professional qualifications, we gathered contributions from experts who have been teaching, developing, and using different types of hydrogels. The diverse contributions provide balanced and up to date content that we hope will be a valuable resource not only for experienced researchers working in the field of hydrogels, but also for the novices who are interested to learn more about these materials. We aimed to encourage our contributors to develop new ideas rather than to simply present facts and thus, several pioneering and inspiring efforts from different groups are in the origins of the book.

We hope that the readers will enjoy the book and keep it as a companion in their research endeavors.

1

Extracellular Matrix Hydrogels from Decellularized Tissues for Biological and Biomedical Applications

Brendan C. Jones[1,2], *Nicola Elvassore*[1], *Paolo De Coppi*[1,2], *and Giovanni G. Giobbe*[1]

[1] *University College London, Great Ormond Street Institute of Child Health, Stem Cell and Regenerative Medicine Section, Developmental Biology and Cancer Research and Teaching Department, 20 Guilford St, London WC1N 1DZ, UK*
[2] *Great Ormond Street Hospital, Department of Specialist Neonatal and Paediatric Surgery, Great Ormond Street, London WC1N 3JH, UK*

1.1 Introduction to Hydrogels

1.1.1 Definition and Use of Hydrogels in Biomedical Applications

A hydrogel is a hydrophilic three-dimensional (3D) network composed of polymer units that is capable of absorbing large amounts of water relative to the dry weight of the component polymers [1–3]. Interaction between polymer units and a gelation stimulus in a hydrated environment, which in the context of biomedical applications may include physiologic liquids rather than pure water, results in formation of the 3D network. Since pioneering work by Wichterle and Lim [4], hydrogels have been used in numerous biological and biomedical applications including tissue engineering, drug delivery, cell culture, and as biosensors, hemostatic agents, and self-healing materials [1, 3]. Their widespread and growing use is due to numerous advantageous characteristics, such as tunable mechanical properties, ability to add functional groups to polymers that may act as ligands or be responsive to external stimuli, cytocompatibility, and low toxicity [1].

Hydrogels have received particular attention in cell culture and tissue engineering applications. Specific advantages of hydrogels in this field include the ability to encapsulate cells, proven biocompatibility and cytocompatibility, the potential to mimic physiologic environments, and act as cell and drug delivery vehicles [3, 5, 6]. In the context of these applications, some practical problems related with the use of hydrogels remain: the hydrogels are often difficult to handle, relatively fragile, hard to sterilize once gelation has occurred, and many are not currently produced using Good Manufacturing Protocol (GMP) grade processes limiting their translation into human patients [3, 5].

Multifunctional Hydrogels for Biomedical Applications, First Edition.
Edited by Ricardo A. Pires, Iva Pashkuleva, and Rui L. Reis.

1.1.2 Classification and Properties of Hydrogels

There are numerous methods to classify and describe hydrogels, many of which are discussed in detail elsewhere in this book, and are summarized in Table 1.1 [1, 3, 5–7]. The variables most relevant when considering biomedical applications of hydrogels are the nature of the forces holding the network together (response), the source of the polymers, and the cross-linking stimulus. The network of a reversible hydrogel is held together by molecular entanglements and/or secondary forces (ionic, hydrogen, or hydrophobic bonding), which can be reversed by changes in physical conditions. By contrast, permanent hydrogels are held together by covalent cross-linking [3]. Polymers may be naturally occurring, synthetic, or a hybrid natural-synthetic copolymer and may be tunable, allowing variation of mechanical

Table 1.1 Classification of hydrogels.

Classification variable	Subtypes
Response	Physical/reversible *Ionotropic hydrogel* *Polyelectrolyte complexes* Permanent/chemical *Copolymerization of polymer and cross-linking molecule* *Cross-linking of water-soluble polymers*
Cross-linking stimulus	pH Temperature Light/laser Chemical and ionic Magnetic field
Source of polymers	Synthetic Natural Hybrid
Macromolecular structure of polymers	Linear polymers Block copolymers Graft copolymers
Mix of polymers	Homopolymeric Copolymeric Multipolymer interpenetrating networks (IPNs)
Degradability	Degrading Nondegrading

Source: Adapted from Chai et al. [1], Hoffman [3], Giobbe et al. [5], Holloway et al. [6], and Capeling et al. [7].

properties. The stimulus to initiate cross-linking may be a defined range or change in temperature, pH, light, magnetic field, or ion strength/chemical composition of solution, or the addition of a specific cross-linking molecule [1, 2].

Temperature is a useful trigger of the gelation in the context of biological applications. When polymer units and water (or physiologic liquid) are mixed, the polymer network will take on water to swell, followed by gelation in a definable temperature range for a given hydrogel [1, 2, 5]. The lower bound of this range is termed the lower critical solution temperature (LCST) – above the LCST phase separation and gelation occurs, while below the LCST the system is miscible in all proportions – with transition from gel to sol or sol to gel states related to changes in Gibbs free energy [1, 3]. This property can be extremely useful in biological applications. For example, a hydrogel may be in solution at room temperature but undergo gelation at 37 °C.

The amount of water in a hydrogel is termed total bound water, composed of primary bound water (the first water to enter the 3D network and hydrate the most polar groups) and secondary bound water (which is bound to hydrophobic groups exposed by initial swelling), and the proportion of water in a hydrogel is called the volume fraction of water. Osmotic force will draw water into the network toward infinite dilution until an equilibrium is reached with the opposing force of elastic retraction by the network (equilibrium swelling theory) [1, 3]. When equilibrium is reached, water exists in the spaces in the hydrogel between polymers (pores), which are usually inhomogeneous in size, distribution, and connectedness in a given gel. These variables, in combination with solute size, shape, polarity, and solute–matrix interactions, determine the permeation of a solute through a hydrogel [3].

Properties of hydrogels can be studied using a multitude of techniques including histology, immunostaining, electron microscopy, and proteomics by liquid chromatography–tandem mass spectrometry (LC–TMS). Additionally, turbidity (measured by spectrophotometry) is commonly used to determine gelation kinetics, while atomic force microscopy and rheometric techniques are used to study the mechanical properties of hydrogels, for example, storage (G′) and loss (G″) moduli [3, 5, 8].

Finally, any hydrogel under consideration for use in biomedical or biological applications must be cytocompatible. Whenever a hydrogel is modified (polymer type, polymer concentration, change in functional groups, etc.), it must be proven to be cytocompatible or it cannot be used *in vitro* or in clinical applications.

1.1.2.1 Synthetic Hydrogels

Synthetic hydrogels are composed of polymers that have been chemically synthesized and are not found in nature. Examples include poly(ethylene glycol) (PEG), poly(lactic acid) (PLA), poly(*co*-glycolic acid) (PGA), and poly(vinyl alcohol) [2]. A brief summary of advantages and disadvantages of this broad range of hydrogels will be presented here but is more comprehensively discussed elsewhere in this book.

Potential advantages in the use of synthetic hydrogels for biomedical applications are several. They have well-defined molecular composition and architecture, can be manufactured with low batch-to-batch variability, and avoid the use of xenogeneic material in production process [1, 6]. The monomers are uniform and modular, leading to a relatively predictable relationship between composition and physicochemical properties when polymerized [9]. Therefore, the concentration of monomers can be varied, or the monomers can have functional units added rationally to alter the mechanical and biological signally properties of the resulting hydrogel. These features allow synthetic hydrogels to be easily tuned for specific circumstances [6, 8, 9].

There are several important disadvantages of synthetic hydrogels in biological contexts. Many synthetic hydrogels are covalently cross-linked and resistant to enzymatic degradation (due to lack of proteolytic sensitive domains), such that these gels behave as linear elastic networks. This is of particular relevance in cell culture contexts as these networks can accumulate substantial compressive forces that are then transmitted to encapsulated cells [9, 10]. Furthermore, the breaking of covalent bonds is irreversible, meaning that permanent synthetic hydrogels cannot "self-heal" like reversible gels [9]. Despite the ability to tune synthetic gels, in most products, this occurs as a bulk property of the hydrogel; that is, there is minimal spatial control over variation in mechanical properties. However, recent innovation in the functionalizing of synthetic gels with photosensitive functional groups may allow for improved spatial control of mechanical properties, which could be used to study symmetry breaking and other aspects of stem cell and niche biology [9, 11, 12]. Perhaps the most important disadvantage of synthetic hydrogels in biological applications is the lack of biological ligands to interact directly with cell surface receptors, such as integrins [2, 9]. However, several groups have taken advantage of this fact to study the influence of microenvironment on cell behavior or have functionalized the hydrogel to overcome this barrier [8–10].

PEG is a commonly used synthetic hydrogel for biomedical applications because of its modular macrostructure (e.g. 4 or 8 arm PEG) and ability for functional groups to be added, as recently described by Urciuolo et al. [12]. Gjorevski et al. [10] used 8-arm PEG to study the effect of matrix stiffness on the culture of murine intestinal stem cells (mISCs). First, they demonstrated that functionalizing of PEG with 1 mM of cell adhesion peptide arginylglycylaspartic acid (RGD) on vinylsulfone facilitated mISC survival, expansion, and passaging with comparable expression to Matrigel® of intestinal stem cell (ISC) marker leucine-rich repeat-containing G-protein coupled receptor 5 (Lgr5). The stiffness of the PEG–RGD was then varied that resulted in the optimal expansion of Lgr5-expressing mISC at 1.3 kPa with concomitant nuclear translocation of yes-associated protein 1 (YAP). Furthermore, at lower stiffness (190 Pa), the mISC-containing epithelium-only organoids were shown to bud and differentiate. Human ISC and colorectal cancer organoids were also shown to be viable in PEG–RGD [10]. In a similar strategy, Cruz-Acuña et al. [8] used 4-arm PEG with a maleimide group on each terminus functionalized with 2 mM RGD and cross-linked with protease-degradable peptide GPQ-W to culture human embryonic stem cell (hESC) and induced pluripotent stem cell (hiPSC) derived intestinal organoids, which contain both mesenchymal cells and epithelial cells, with morphology and protein expression (immunofluorescence) and RNA expression (real-time polymerase chain reaction [PCR]) similar to culture in Matrigel. Amongst other findings, this hydrogel was used as a delivery vehicle with *in situ* polymerization that facilitated engraftment of the organoids in a mouse model of colon epithelial injury [8].

1.1.2.2 Natural Hydrogels

Natural hydrogels are composed of polymer chains that are naturally occurring or where the subunits do not need to be chemically synthesized in laboratory or commercial settings. The polymer network is composed of peptides and/or polysaccharides and may be homopolymeric or contain a mixture of polymers [1]. However, recent work has utilized DNA to produce tunable hydrogels, opening another category of natural polymers for use [13]. Commonly used examples are presented in this book and include gelatin, collagen I, hyaluronic acid, chitosan, alginate, dextran, cellulose, and agarose [2]. Extracellular matrix-derived hydrogels (ECM), including Matrigel, are a subset of natural hydrogels [9].

Natural hydrogels are already extensively used in laboratory and clinical applications. Gelatin, Matrigel, and collagen I are routinely used in cell culture. Gelatin is produced from the partial hydrolysis of animal collagens, retaining the cell-binding motifs (including RGD) and matrix metalloprotease (MMP)-sensitive degradation sites of the original proteins [1]. This inherent cell-binding activity and protease-mediated degradability result in gelatin being commonly used as a substrate in 2D cell culture without further modification. However, modified gelatin has been used in more complex applications. For example, methacrylated gelatin has been used as an injectable vehicle for human endothelial cells into the subcutaneous space of immunodeficient mice, followed by *in situ* polymerization using ultraviolet (UV) light [14].

Similarly, Matrigel can be used as a substrate for 2D cell culture, and it is currently accepted as the gold standard for 3D cell and organoid culture to which other hydrogels are compared in this context. Matrigel is a laminin-rich mixture of ECM proteins secreted by the Engelbreth–Holm–Swarm mouse sarcoma cell line. It is a proprietary product known to contain key components of the basement membrane, including laminin-1, collagen IV, and nidogen-1, as well as heparan sulfate and numerous growth factors [8, 9]. Matrigel has been used in seminal papers published on epithelium-only [15] and mesenchyme-containing organoids [6], amongst innumerable other works.

While Matrigel is the current gold standard for most 3D cell culture, it is also an example of the limitations of natural hydrogels. There is significant batch-to-batch variability in protein and growth factor composition, it is not chemically defined, not easily tunable (beyond simple dilution), it is xenogeneic, and expensive [6, 7]. However, the most important limitation, in terms of clinical translation, is the fact that Matrigel is derived from a sarcoma cell line.

Homopolymeric natural hydrogels can support 3D cell culture. Mouse small intestinal epithelium-only organoids were encapsulated in collagen I hydrogel (0.75 mg/ml), allowed to gelate in a ring shape, then the ring detached and cultured floating in media [16]. This method allowed the organoids to fuse together into a tube with a continuous lumen and cause contraction of the gel ring, demonstrating the ability of a simple defined ECM-mimetic hydrogel to support structurally complex cell culture [16]. Others have shown that growth factors and adhesive cues can be added to simple natural hydrogels with positive effects on organoid growth, while exhibiting minimal batch-to-batch variability [6].

However, not all natural hydrogels are inherently biologically active. For example, alginate, a polysaccharide derived from algae, is biologically inert and lacks inherent cell recognition molecules. The Spence lab has demonstrated that 1% alginate, cross-linked with calcium ions, can be used to differentiate hiPSC-derived intestinal organoids, albeit with yields <50% of that in Matrigel [7]. The mesenchymal cells of the hiPSC-derived organoids did not penetrate into the alginate and, importantly, epithelium-only intestinal organoids did not proliferate in the alginate and lost polarity, suggesting that the basement membrane secreted by the mesenchymal cells was crucial in the absence of such signals from the hydrogel itself. However, in contrast to Matrigel, alginate is cheap (US$0.44 vs. US$300 per 10 ml) and U.S. Food and Drug Administration (FDA) approved for clinical use in humans already (see Section 1.4), making it worthy of further study for translational purposes [7, 17].

DNA-based hydrogels have recently been investigated, aiming to take advantage of several fundamental features of nuclei acids that could be useful in hydrogels [13]. These features include the modular structure of DNA, ability to control the changes in the macromolecular structure of DNA (for example, strand displacement), and the existence of sequence-specific DNA-cleaving technologies. This potentially allows for rational predesign of the hydrogel matrix. Yue et al. [13] demonstrated reversible control of shape and stiffness in a DNA-based hydrogel using oligonucleotide sequences as triggers. Furthermore, they showed the ability for the hydrogels to be loaded with doxorubicin and control its release using the same triggers.

1.2 Key Features and Functions of the Extracellular Matrix in Homeostasis and Development

Considering both the broad categories and specific examples described above, some important themes emerge with regard to biomedical applications of hydrogels:

1. Mechanical properties of hydrogels are important but not sufficient to sustain cells in culture.
2. At least some of the signaling essential for successful cell culture is derived from cell–matrix interactions.
3. Mimicry of the native organ microenvironment is important for *in vitro* cell culture to recapitulate *in vivo* cell behavior.
4. GMP-grade processes need to be available for the manufacture of any hydrogel intended for translation to clinical applications in humans.

The ECM comprises "structural" ECM proteins, such as collagens, glycoproteins, and proteoglycans, and a vast array of ECM-associated proteins, including ECM-modifying enzymes, ECM-bound growth factors, and ligands for cell surface receptors [18]. The structural "matrisome" is estimated to comprise ~300 proteins, not including ECM-associated proteins, and is highly conserved across mammalian species.

Collagens are essential to strength in almost all forms of ECM and are composed of the basic repeating unit "glycine-X-Y," where X is usually proline and Y is 4-hydroxyproline. Glycoproteins serve multiple functions in the ECM, including interactions that facilitate the assembly of structural proteins like collagen, as well as the display of motifs for cell signaling and adhesion [19]. Glycoproteins where a substantial proportion of the molecular mass is made from glycosaminoglycans (GAGs) are called proteoglycans. Proteoglycans and glycoproteins of particular relevance to this chapter include perlecan (also called heparan sulfate proteoglycan 2) and laminins, which are core components of basement membrane, and fibronectin, which binds integrins [5, 10, 19]. GAGs on proteoglycans and glycoproteins are highly polar, acting to sequester cations and water, and have many binding sites for growth factors and matrix-bound extracellular vesicles [20]. In fact, this binding allows the ECM to act as a reservoir for growth factor that can be released during ECM remodeling or be presented as ligands in their bound state [21]. This is perhaps one of the most important functional aspects of the ECM in development and homeostasis. The ECM can be remodeled by numerous classes of proteases, such as MMPs and elastases, which can restructure collagens, liberate growth factors and matrix-bound extracellular vesicles, and produce cryptic peptides that may be further sources of local signals to cells [20, 21]. Examples of common cell surface receptors for ECM proteins include integrins, which bind to RGD motifs and laminin, and dystroglycan, which binds laminin and perlecan. Cell surface receptors provide the links between the ECM and the cytoskeleton, transmitting physical signals for cell shape, polarity, and motility, and between the ECM and the nucleus, altering gene expression [18, 19]. An example of such signaling with importance to ECM hydrogels is the negative regulation of transforming growth factor-β (TGF-β) signaling following laminin binding by epithelial cells [18]. In fact, the signaling functions of ECM adhesion receptors are likely as complex as soluble growth factor signals but are yet to be studied in the same depth. The interested reader is referred to an excellent review by Hynes and Naba for further details [19].

Together, the ECM and associated proteins not only give physical structure to tissues and organs but also critical inputs to cells by controlling cell shape, survival, proliferation, differentiation, migration, and polarity. This is true during organogenesis and development, normal homeostasis, and is increasingly recognized as important in disease states [6, 18, 19]. That is, the ECM is a critical component of the cellular microenvironment, which, in addition to the above-mentioned functions, also includes paracrine, endocrine, and neural signals [18, 19]. However, it is clear that cells secrete ECM and this leads to the important theory of "dynamic reciprocity," which is the concept of tissue architecture as a cause of tissue specific functions but also a consequence to tissue-specific cell activity. Put another way, the ECM provides biophysical and soluble cues that influence cell morphology and phenotype, and in turn cells modify the secretion of ECM products in response to these cues [18, 22].

These fundamental roles for ECM in biology have spurred intense research into the derivation and use of ECM-based hydrogels from the decellularization of organs, including as a mechanism for increasing the biomimicry of *in vitro* cell culture with the aim of increasing complexity of cell culture models [5, 6]. In Sections 1.3 give an overview of methods of production and the published work using ECM hydrogels derived from several different organs.

1.3 Extracellular Matrix-Based Hydrogels Derived from Decellularization of Organs

1.3.1 Production of ECM Hydrogels

ECM hydrogels have been produced from several organs. While the detail of published protocols varies widely, the principal steps of most methods are [20] as follows:

1. Removal of cellular components and nucleic acids from the organ (decellularization)
2. Solubilization of protein components (digestion)
3. Restoration of physiologic pH and electrolyte concentration (neutralization)
4. Gelation under appropriate conditions

Approaches to decellularization can be broadly classified as perfusion or immersion techniques. Perfusion-based protocols take advantage of the vascular network and/or the lumen of the organ itself to deliver the decellularizing agents into an intact organ. The distribution of solution recapitulates blood flow in the tissue by utilizing the native vasculature. This technique has been shown to produce scaffolds that retain the macroscopic and ultrastructure of the original organ in esophagus [23, 24], intestine [25], heart [26], trachea [27], lung [28], liver [29], and kidney [30]. By contrast, immersion-based protocols bathe the tissue in the decellularization agent, which usually requires the tissue to be cut into volumes small enough for the agent to penetrate by diffusion. To aid this process, immersion-based protocols usually occur in agitation and with regular changes of decellularization solution. While this process does not preserve whole-organ level structure, it maintains ECM components in appropriate ratios and is capable of retaining the native ultrastructure in the fragments of tissue [5].

Whether by immersion or perfusion, decellularization is usually based on supplying a combination of hypotonic solutions (e.g. de-ionized water), detergents, and enzymes, collectively known as detergent-enzymatic treatment (DET) (Table 1.2). DET may be preceded by freezing and thawing cycles, which can be used to mechanically disrupt cells through the changes in volume of water between phases. DET protocols take advantage of the post-assembly modifications of ECM, for example disulfide bonding, transglutaminase-mediated cross-linking, and the actions of lysyl oxidases and hydroxylases, which render the ECM relatively insoluble in detergents such as deoxycholate [5, 25]. Established DET processes have been shown to preserve glycoproteins, proteoglycans, GAGs, and growth factors, as well as the structural

Table 1.2 Example reagents used in decellularization protocols.

Detergents	Sodium deoxycholic acid (SDC)
	Sodium dodecyl sulfate (SDS)
	Triton X-100
	3-[(3-Cholamidopropyl)dimethylammonio]-1-propanesulfonate (CHAPS)
	Polyoxyethylene [20] sorbitan monolaurate (Tween 20)
Enzymes	DNase
	Trypsin
	Dispase
Other	Ethylenediaminetetraacetic acid (EDTA)
	Peracetic acid
	Chloroform
	Methanol
	Ethanol

proteins, retaining the biochemical complexity of the tissue of origin in appropriate stoichiometric ratios [5, 20, 25, 31].

It is important to remember that inherent in these protocols is a trade-off between complete removal of cellular proteins and nucleic acids vs. the retention of ECM proteins and ECM-associated proteins (including ECM-bound growth factors). The optimal balance between retention of the diversity of ECM components and complete removal of cellular components is not clear. There is evidence that incomplete removal of cellular components may elicit an adverse inflammatory response to decellularized scaffolds [22]. However, future work may demonstrate that preservation of matrix supersedes the complete removal of cellular components, or vice versa, and the protocol chosen will depend on the intended application of the decellularized material.

Following decellularization, the ECM is lyophilized and milled to allow solubilization by pepsin-mediated digestion. Two commonly used methods are the Freytes method (0.1 M hydrochloric acid + pepsin) and the Voytik–Harbin method (0.5 M acetic acid + pepsin). Utilizing pepsin-based digestion is particularly useful for xenogeneic ECM as it cleaves the telopeptide of collagen, which is the main antigenic component [32]. Changing the duration of digestion produces pre-gels that contain different profiles of cryptic peptides, theoretically allowing tailoring of the hydrogel at this stage of production to optimize it for a given application [20]. During digestion, there is the desired fragmentation of larger structural ECM proteins, but also some depletion of growth factors compared to intact decellularized scaffolds and native tissues. The extent to which this affects the bioactivity of the final ECM hydrogel is not known [20, 33]. Neutralization is simply performed with small volumes of high-molarity hydrochloric acid (HCl) or sodium hydroxide (NaOH) to restore physiologic pH and the combination of the digested ECM with an appropriate volume of solution with physiologic salt concentration. Once neutralized, the hydrogel is ready for use with cells.

ECM hydrogel gelation is an entropy-driven self-assembly process, the kinetics of which are governed predominately by collagen [20]. However, ECM hydrogels from decellularized organs have been shown to have distinct matrix assembly kinetics and fiber morphologies, compared to purified collagen I hydrogels. These differences depend on proteoglycans (e.g. decorin), GAGs (e.g. heparan sulfates), fibronectin, and minor collagens, which are known to act as nucleation sites for collagen fibrillogenesis, again demonstrating the importance of their conservation during production of the hydrogel. Gelation occurs by reformation of bonds and entanglements at physiologic temperature [20, 34].

An example protocol from our group utilizes 4% sodium deoxycholate, purified and deionized water, DNase-I for decellularization of porcine small intestinal mucosa-submucosa (pSIS), digestion using the Freytes method (1 mg/ml pepsin in 0.1 M HCl), and neutralization with 10× Dulbecco's modified eagle medium (DMEM)/F12 and 10 M NaOH. The final hydrogel is used while working on ice to encapsulate cells before thermally induced gelation at 37 °C [5]. An alternative process involves homogenization by physical disruption in high salt buffer; use of dispase to cleave fibronectin, collagen IV, and collagen I; a urea extraction step for further solubilization; and centrifugation and removal of insoluble remnants. The resulting extract undergoes gelation at 37 °C or by lowering the pH to 4 with acetic acid. This is included for completeness, as it is based on the method used to produce Matrigel [20].

1.3.2 Characterization of ECM Hydrogels

As introduced in the opening Section 1.1.2 of the chapter, ECM hydrogels can be characterized in a multitude of ways, including ultrastructure, mechanical properties, and biochemical composition. The ultrastructure of ECM hydrogels is influenced by tissue of origin, protein and GAG concentration, and processing and gelation methods. Light, confocal, and electron microscopy is used to interrogate gel ultrastructure, including pore size and fiber architecture, with scanning electron microscopy usually demonstrating a loosely organized nanofibrous scaffold with interconnecting pores [35].

Rheometry and turbidimetric assays are the main methods to assess gelation and mechanical properties of ECM hydrogels, but other methods include atomic force microscopy, indentation, and compression testing. Turbidimetric assays can be used to describe gelation kinetics such as time to initiation of gelation (lag phase), time to 50% turbidity, and describe the curve of gelation (sigmoidal, exponential) [20]. Rheology gives more granular detail regarding pre-gel viscosity and storage and loss moduli of the final gel. Viscosity of ECM pre-gel, rate of gelation, and storage modulus of final gel tend to be positively correlated with protein concentration. The solid-like behavior of the final gel is confirmed on oscillatory rheology when the storage modulus is independent of frequency and is greater than the loss modulus by an order of magnitude. Using these methods, it has been shown that ECM hydrogels, as other gels, exhibit viscoelastic behavior with similarity to embryonic tissues [7, 20].

The biochemical composition of ECM hydrogels can be evaluated in most detail using paired LC–TMS [5], while commercially available kits can be used to easily measure residual nucleic acid content or specific matrix components, such as collagens or GAGs. Proteomic profiling of decellularized ECM in this manner has been done for numerous organs and has shown that biochemical composition may vary by source organ, but only subtly between tissues of the same embryonic germ layer [5, 20].

As the examples below demonstrate the diversity of tissue of origin, processing, and preparation methods that allow ECM hydrogels to be tuned in a near-infinite way. However, any such changes require the resulting gel to be treated as a novel gel and tested accordingly prior to use. For example, it has been shown that hydrogels derived from dermis have ultrastructural differences depending on whether they undergo temperature-dependent or pH-dependent gelation [36]. Furthermore, when considering the subsequent examples and their biological applications, it is crucial to remember that cells (encapsulated in the gel or recruited from the recipient animal) interacting with the ECM hydrogel will remodel it and eventually replace it with *de novo* matrix. Therefore, it is likely that each application will require an "individualized" gel. For example, in one setting it may be the aim that the gel provides sustained support for the cells and is replaced slowly, while in another the ECM hydrogel may be tuned to allow ECM signaling molecules to be released from the gel and diffuse into the surrounding tissue.

1.3.3 Pancreatic ECM-Derived Hydrogels

Diseases of the endocrine and exocrine pancreas are major causes of mortality and morbidity worldwide. Pancreatic ECM-derived hydrogels may be useful in the study of islet cell biology and further development of islet cell transplantation as a human therapy, as 3D culture methods have shown promising effects on beta-cell survival and functionality, with basement membrane proteins in particular having a crucial role *in vitro* and *in vivo* [37, 38]. However, the pancreas presents two unique challenges to the production of a pancreas ECM hydrogel. Namely, the fat content and the presence of proteases in the native pancreas could inhibit the formation of a stable gel or further digest the ECM during decellularization and digestion phases, respectively.

Gaetani et al. [39] utilized readily available porcine pancreas in a study to optimize a protocol for the production of a pancreas ECM hydrogel by immersion–agitation DET and Freytes digestion. They examined a range of concentrations of sodium dodecyl sulfate (0.1%, 0.5%, 1% SDS) and Triton X-100 as the detergent, but also examined the effect of adding a synthetic serine protease inhibitor (0.1 mM Gabexate) to the protocol, aiming to mitigate the effect of pancreatic proteases on the gel. Interestingly, they demonstrated that successful gelation (no residual liquid phase) only occurred in 1% Triton X-100 groups, both with and without Gabexate, and that laminins were not detectable at the conclusion of any of the SDS protocols. At a molecular level, addition of Gabexate improved the sulfated-GAG (sGAG), basement membrane, and matricellular protein content of the gel. The 6 mg/ml hydrogel produced by 1% Triton X-100 with Gabexate supported 3D cell culture of rat insulinoma cells to 10 days, which were able to secret insulin in response to glucose stimulation. However, the gel was not used to passage cells, culture human cells, or in any *in vivo* experiments [39].

In a major work, Sackett et al. [40] were the first to demonstrate the production of an ECM hydrogel from decellularization of human pancreas. Importantly, they showed that reproducibly successful gelation only occurred when utilizing a homogenization and centrifugation protocol to de-lipidise the pancreas prior to decellularization with sodium deoxycholic acid (SDC). Fat content decreased from 38% in native pancreas to 14% in the SDC only protocol, which was further reduced to 4% when the homogenization step was added. Furthermore, this study was the first to demonstrate preservation of laminins in decellularized pancreatic scaffold or hydrogel. The hydrogel was able to sustain 2D culture of rat insulinoma cells, human umbilical vein endothelial cells (HUVECs), and expansion culture of hiPSCs and H9 and H1 hESC lines. The hydrogel performed well in 3D culture of ESC-derived pancreatic progenitors and islet-like cell clusters, demonstrating similar numbers of PDX1, Ki-67, and Caspase-3 positive cells compared to standard suspension cultures. With a view to future clinical application, the hydrogel could be injected subcutaneously into humanized immunodeficient mice with successful *in situ* gelation and minimal host inflammatory response [40].

1.3.4 ECM Hydrogels Derived from Liver

The development of high-fidelity *in vitro* systems to study human liver development, disease, and function has proven challenging. Primary hepatocytes and sinusoidal endothelial cells lose maturity in plastic-adherent or pure collagen-based culture [41, 42], iPSC-derived hepatocytes show a relatively immature phenotype, and immortal cell lines are inappropriate for translational applications [22, 43]. As a result, many groups have developed strategies utilizing hepatic ECM in cell culture models attempting to overcome these issues. For example, it has been shown that a solution of porcine hepatic ECM contained >40 liver-derived growth factors and supplementation of culture media with this solution improved albumin gene expression and secretion in porcine iPSC-derived hepatocytes [33].

ECM hydrogels have been successfully produced from the livers of several species, including rat [44], pig [32, 33], sheep [43], and human [45, 46]. Depending on the protocol and species, lyophilized hepatic ECM has 75%–100% sGAG and 60% total collagen content of native liver [33, 43, 45], with 18 mg of powder produced per 1 g wet weight of porcine liver [32]. Gelation has been successful with protein concentrations varying from 3 to 10 mg/ml [32, 43]. Cytocompatibility of hepatic ECM hydrogels has been shown with a range of cell lines, including human hepatocellular carcinoma (HCC) and hepatoblastoma (HepG2) cells [43, 46], and porcine [33] and human [45] iPSC-derived hepatocytes.

Saheli et al. [43] cocultured human HCCs with HUVECs and mesenchymal stem cells (MSCs) to examine the effect of 3D culture and a sheep liver-derived ECM hydrogel on *in vitro* hepatocyte maturity. Three-dimensional liver organoids cultured in hepatic ECM hydrogel demonstrated the most mature cellular phenotype by RT-PCR and secretion of albumin, α_1 antitrypsin, and urea, compared to all other conditions (HCC only 2D culture, 3D organoid culture in collagen, 2D culture supplemented with solubilized ECM, hydrogel-free 2D culture). Alpha-fetoprotein, cytochromes 3A4 and 3A7 expression approximated native adult human liver, and while albumin and tyrosine aminotransferase did not reach native liver levels, their expression was greatest in 3D ECM hydrogel culture.

Most iPSC-hepatocyte differentiation protocols, including seminal work by Taniguchi's group [47], use laminin-rich Matrigel as the culture substrate. However, laminin is not a major component of liver ECM, and such protocols have generated human iPSC-hepatocytes with maturity similar to fetal hepatocytes [45, 47]. Jaramillo et al. [45] studied the effect of adult human liver-derived hydrogel on iPSC-hepatocyte differentiation. In comparison to Matrigel, iPSC differentiated entirely on ECM hydrogel showed upregulation of albumin, most major cytochromes (CYP3A4, CYP2B6, CYP2D6), and hepatic nuclear and transcription factors (forkhead box A [FOXA1], FOXA2, hematopoietically expressed homeobox [HHEX], hepatic leukemia factor [HLF], hepatocyte nuclear factor [HNF4α], luteinizing hormone receptor [LHR1], polysaccharide biosynthesis domain containing [PBDC1]). Furthermore, the expression of these markers was highest when iPSCs were differentiated on ECM from the induction of definitive endoderm, compared to switching to ECM hydrogel later in the protocol, and markers of hepatoblast differentiation (e.g. HNF6) appeared earlier and were upregulated in the ECM protocol compared to Matrigel. Functionally, ECM-differentiated iPSC-hepatocytes demonstrated intracellular glycogen storage, bile canaliculi formation, cytosolic albumin expression, and secretion of albumin into the media. Importantly, levels of albumin secretion and CYP3A4 activity were comparable to human neonatal hepatocytes, but still lower than human adult hepatocytes [45].

1.3.5 Lung ECM Hydrogels

Early studies into the decellularization of lung tissue focused on obtaining intact acellular lung scaffolds for repopulation with lung epithelial and vascular endothelial cells for whole organ tissue engineering [28, 48, 49]. While successful removal of DNA and cellular components was achieved, this was usually at the expense of complexity of the remaining ECM, with as little as 15% fibronectin, 40% elastin, and <10% sGAG content remaining (compared to native lung levels) at the conclusion of protocols using CHAPS [48, 49]. The result was somewhat improved with a change to SDC/Triton X-100 in a later study by the same group [48].

The first group to produce a lung ECM hydrogel was Pouliot et al. [50]. They decellularized porcine lung by perfusion DET via trachea and pulmonary artery using 0.1% Triton X-100 and 2% SDC. After 48 hours of digestion, the pre-gel elastin content was reduced by 60% compared to native lung levels, but collagen content and sGAG content were reduced by 40% and 50%, respectively. The resulting hydrogel was shown to be cytocompatible with human bone marrow mesenchymal stem cells (BM-MSCs) *in vitro* and increased the engraftment of rat BM-MSC by 2.5× (compared to saline vehicle) when injected intratracheally in an elastase-induced rat model of emphysema [50].

Recently, a group from Groningen reported the production of ECM hydrogels from human lungs, including donor lungs unsuitable for transplantation and lungs affected by chronic obstructive pulmonary disease (COPD) and idiopathic pulmonary fibrosis (IPF) [51]. The protocol used was complicated – homogenization in a blender, 3 hours in 0.05% trypsin, then 24 hours each of 6 M NaCl, 70% ethanol, 1% SDS, 1% Triton X-100, 1% SDC, and finally DNase. While characterization of the hydrogels was very limited and they were not used with cells *in vitro* or *in vivo*, the stiffness of native lung and hydrogel from lungs affected by IPF was significantly greater than normal and COPD-affected lungs and their respective hydrogels [51]. This suggests the potential value of using hydrogels from diseased organs for modeling *in vitro*.

1.3.6 Hydrogels Derived from Decellularized Colon

Most studies of decellularized colon have focused on intact scaffolds in colorectal neoplasia [52, 53] or using other hydrogels to deliver cells into the lumen of the colon [54, 55]. Decellularized human colorectal carcinoma scaffolds have been demonstrated to polarize macrophages to an anti-inflammatory M2 phenotype and that this phenotype promotes invasion through basement membrane *in vitro*, while scaffolds from normal colon did not [53]. In mouse models of colonic mucosal injury, ECM-based hydrogels, fibrin glue, and gelatin have been used as delivery vehicles for organoids with successful engraftment in the recipient animal [54, 55].

Keane et al. [56] performed a detailed analysis of a novel hydrogel derived from decellularized porcine colon. Following delipidization 2 : 1 chloroform: methanol and graded ethanol baths, the decellularization protocol utilized 0.02% trypsin/0.05% EDTA and 4% SDC, and the lyophilized powder was then digested using the Freytes method. By immunostaining, laminin was largely absent and fibronectin signal was much reduced. sGAG concentration was reduced by ~1/3 and hyaluronic acid by about 75%. Interestingly, basic fibroblast growth factor (bFGF) and vascular endothelial growth factor (VEGF) were retained after decellularization, albeit at much reduced concentrations. Stable gels were formed at 4 and 8 mg/ml, with a positive correlation between concentration and maximum storage modulus. Intestinal epithelial cells were compatible with the hydrogel with minimal cell death seen at 24 hours. In further experiments, supplementation of media with soluble porcine colon ECM promoted M2-like phenotype in mouse macrophages *in vitro*, similar to most reports, but in contrast to Pinto et al., perhaps suggesting interspecies difference [53, 56]. The M2 macrophage phenotype was also seen after implantation of the colon hydrogel in a rat abdominal wall defect model [56].

Romero-López et al. [57] generated a hydrogel by decellularization of human colorectal cancer metastases to the liver. The hydrogel derived from metastases had a threefold higher stiffness compared to hydrogel from normal colon and on LC–TMS contained higher amounts of collagen IV, VI, XIV, fibrillin, emilin, vitronectin, and laminin-γ1. Interestingly, fibronectin, versican, thrombospondin-2, periostin, tenascin, and several other laminin subunits were only detectable in tumor ECM hydrogel. However, it is important to note that the decellularization protocols differed significantly in the detergent used – 1% SDS for tumor and, 2% SDC for normal colon. In terms of disease modeling, SW620 colon tumor cells grew faster in tumor hydrogel and demonstrated an increase in glycolysis compared to normal colon hydrogel. Furthermore, when endothelial cells were cultured in the tumor hydrogel, they formed vessels mimicking tumor vasculature with high variability in vessel diameter and fractal dimension of the network [57].

1.3.7 ECM-Derived Hydrogels from Small Intestine

Acellular pSIS-based products have been in commercial use since the 1990s and have become an accepted and routine part of mechanical reconstruction in most surgical disciplines including cardiovascular surgery, otorhinolaryngology, and abdominal surgery [58]. The regulatory acceptance and established clinical use of pSIS products make it an attractive option to derive hydrogels for clinical translation.

The effect of a pSIS hydrogel on tissue regeneration was studied in a dextran sodium sulfate model of colitis [59]. When delivered to the rodents by enema, the acellular hydrogel adhered to injured colonic mucosa and resulted in a reduction in clinical and histologic severity of the disease, with corresponding improvement in colonic epithelial barrier function. This occurred in the setting of reduced numbers of pro-inflammatory macrophages in the colon following pSIS hydrogel treatment [59].

Initial investigations into small intestine submucosa (SIS) hydrogels suggested that collagen and sGAG content are similar to the decellularized scaffold and contain at least some intact growth factors [20, 34]. A recent study by our group reported a deep characterization of a pSIS hydrogel and its potential for human organoid culture and regenerative medicine [5]. The hydrogel was prepared by dicing pSIS, immersion-agitation decellularization using 4% SDC and DNase, lyophilization, milling, and digestion by the Freytes method, before neutralization with 10X DMEM-F12 and 10 M sodium hydroxide (Figure 1.1). This protocol allowed for effective removal of cellular material and nucleic acid from the tissue but preserved concentrations of elastin and GAGs and an (expected) increase in total collagen concentration, compared to native tissue. Successful gelation of the pSIS hydrogel was observed at 6, 8, and 10 mg/ml with storage and loss moduli by temperature ramping oscillatory rheology and elastic modulus by nanoindentation showing that 6 mg/ml pSIS hydrogel and Matrigel had similar mechanical profiles [5].

Deep characterization of the proteomic profile of the pSIS hydrogel was undertaken with LC-TMS. The most abundant proteins included several types of fibrillar (types 1, 2, 3, 5, 6), fibril-associated (types 12, 14, 21), and sheet-forming (type IV) collagens. Interestingly, on comparison to the publicly available map of the *human* proteome, the set of ECM proteins identified in the pSIS gel showed a high degree

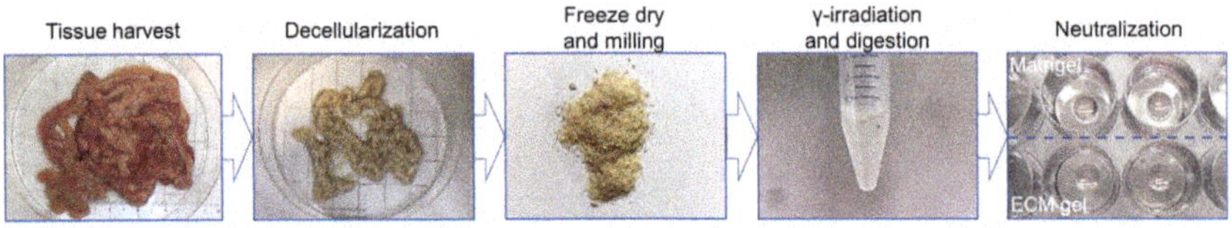

Figure 1.1 Example process for ECM hydrogel preparation. The gelation preparation protocol consists of decellularization of the SI mucosa/submucosa, freeze-drying, milling into a fine powder, γ-irradiation for sterilization, Freytes method digestion for 72 hours, and neutralization to a physiological pH and salinity. The hydrogel undergoes temperature-dependent gelation at 37 °C. Source: Giobbe et al. [5]/Figure 1a/Springer Nature/Attribution 4.0 International (CC BY 4.0).

of similarity to the group of tissues of endodermal origin by principal component analysis (PCA) and hierarchical clustering analyses (Figure 1.2). Indeed, when the pSIS gel was used to culture organoids in 3D, multiple human endodermal organs were supported, including gastric, intestinal, ductal hepatic, fetal intestinal, fetal hepatic, and fetal pancreatic, with comparable performance to culture in Matrigel. For example, human small intestine (SI) organoids culture in pSIS hydrogel showed morphology and protein expression of stem, crypt, and villus markers similar to culture in Matrigel for up to four passages, and fetal SI organoids could be passaged to single cells in pSIS hydrogel with successful *de novo* organoid formation. Furthermore, human ductal and fetal hepatocytes showed similar levels of phenotype-specific markers whether cultured in basement membrane extract or pSIS hydrogel and produced similar levels of albumin [5].

Analysis of the transcriptome of human SI organoids by bulk RNA-Seq demonstrated upregulation of OLFM4, SMOC2, and lysozyme (LYZ) in pSIS hydrogel but similar levels of LGR5, BMI1, and LRIG1 (stem and transit amplifying [TA] cell markers). Villus domain markers Ezrin (EZR), VIL1, MUC12, MUC13, MUC17, and MUC20 were upregulated in Matrigel; FABP1, MUC1, MUC3A, MUC5B were similar between the two conditions; while chromogranin A (CHGA) was the only differentiated cell marker overexpressed in pSIS hydrogel-cultured organoids. Together, this suggests a higher fraction of crypt cells in human SI organoids cultured in pSIS hydrogel compared to Matrigel. Interestingly, ECM-specific proteins detected on proteomic analysis of the decellularized pSIS were found to be overexpressed in Matrigel-cultured organoids, leading us to speculate that human SI organoids may need to produce their own intestine-specific ECM to compensate when cultured in Matrigel [5].

From a regenerative medicine standpoint, we were able to use the pSIS hydrogel for successful *in vivo* transplant of human fetal pancreatic and mouse SI organoids with preserved morphology and marker expression at eight weeks. Importantly, all reagents used in generating the hydrogel are already commercially available at GMP-grade and we demonstrated that while the highly antigenic galactose-α1,3-galactose (α-Gal) was present in whole decellularized tissue but was absent in final gel. These points underscore the potential utility of this hydrogel to

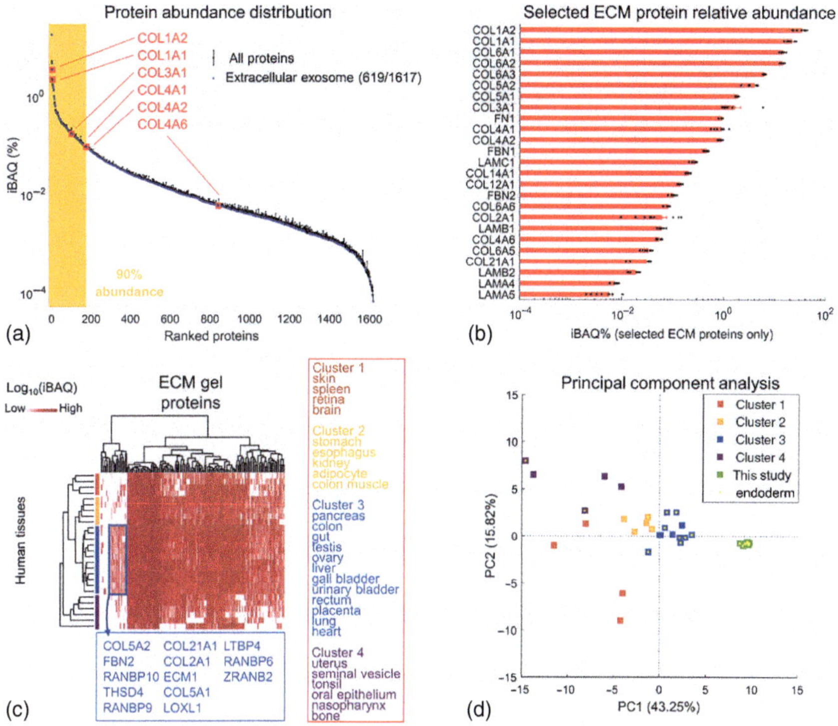

Figure 1.2 pSIS ECM proteomic analysis. (a) Protein abundance range, with 619 (on 1617 total) proteins mapped to GO-CC:0070062~extracellular exosomes highlighted. Yellow-shaded area represents the range covering 90% of total protein abundance. Example collagens also highlighted. (b) Relative abundance of selected ECM proteins. (c) Hierarchical clustering analysis of mass spectrometry native human tissue data from a draft map of the human proteome, conducted for proteins in our data mapped to GO-CC:0031012~ECM. Four main clusters are identified whose color-coded tissues are shown on the right. A small group of proteins especially expressed in cluster 3 is highlighted. (d) Principal component analysis (PCA) of data from native human tissue reported in (c) and from decellularized pSIS. Tissues and samples having endodermal origin are also highlighted. Source: Giobbe et al. [5].

deliver cell-based therapeutics in humans and suggests there may be less of a need for organ-specific cell–hydrogel combinations than first thought [5, 60].

1.3.8 Cellular Responses to ECM Hydrogels

As discussed, *in vitro* methods of evaluating cellular responses to ECM hydrogels include supplementing the media with solubilized ECM, 2D culture on ECM hydrogel substrate, and 3D culture with cells encapsulated in ECM hydrogel. Cellular response can be assessed in terms of survival, proliferation and differentiation capacity, and the preservation or *in vitro* rescue of tissue-specific functions. In these regards, ECM hydrogels have shown impressive abilities across numerous cell types and sources of ECM, including cross-species and interorgan compatibility, likely related to the conservation of the matrisome across mammals [5, 19, 20].

Current experience with *in vivo* applications of ECM scaffolds and hydrogels has shown several important beneficial components of the host response including [5, 20, 22, 56, 58, 59, 61]:

- Promotion of angiogenesis
- Modulation of the immune response, including M2-like macrophage activation and Th2-type T-cell response, which favor tissue regeneration
- Stem cell recruitment
- Promotion of innervation

While the mechanisms underlying these responses are beginning to be elucidated in the setting of decellularized ECM scaffolds, they have not been studied in depth for ECM-derived hydrogels. As discussed earlier, there is evidence that bulk mechanical properties of ECM hydrogels can influence cell behavior but questions regarding the effect of alterations to ECM proteins, matrix-bound nano-vesicles, and growth factors during solubilization and gelation are only beginning to be addressed [20, 22, 62]. For example, in our study of pSIS hydrogel, LC–TMS revealed 619 proteins in the decellularized material known to be from extracellular exosomes [5].

1.4 Commercially Available Products

Possible physical forms of hydrogels used in biomedical applications include solid/molded (e.g. contact lenses), pressed powders, microparticles, coatings, membranes and sheets, and encapsulated semi-solids [3].

Natural hydrogels have been in clinical use for decades with proven safety and efficacy. Commercially available alginate and gelatin-based dressings are particularly useful in burns and wound management, maintaining a favorable moist environment, having hemostatic effects, allowing diffusion of nutrients and gases, while also acting as a barrier to microorganisms [2, 17].

As mentioned earlier, pSIS-based products are in regular therapeutic use in humans. Most common commercially available pSIS products are based on laminated sheets fabricated into appropriate shapes for the clinical application of interest. Products include Surgisis®, Biodesign®, and Durasis® (Cook Medical). For example, CorMatrix® make a range of cardiovascular implants from pSIS, which have been used in congenital cardiac and vascular reconstruction, pericardial reconstruction, and valve replacement [58].

By contrast, ECM hydrogels from decellularized organs have yet to be introduced into regular clinical practice. A Phase I clinical trial was recently completed using porcine myocardial ECM hydrogel (Ventrigel®, Ventrix Inc.) injected into the infarcted area of patients with evidence of left ventricular remodeling following ST segment elevation myocardial infarction. The trial showed Ventrigel to be safe and well tolerated, and patients had some improvement in six-minute walk test and New York Heart Association symptom class [63]. The study was not designed to assess efficacy of the treatment but does pave the way for further clinical trials.

References

1 Chai, Q., Jiao, Y., and Yu, X. (2017). Hydrogels for biomedical applications: their characteristics and the mechanisms behind them. *Gels* 3 (1): 6.
2 Feksa, L.R., Troian, E.A., Muller, C.D. et al. (2018). Hydrogels for biomedical applications. In: *Nanostructures for the Engineering of Cells, Tissues and Organs* (ed. A. Grumezescu), 403–438. Elsevier.
3 Hoffman, A.S. (2012). Hydrogels for biomedical applications. *Adv. Drug Delivery Rev.* 64: 18–23.
4 Wichterle, O. and Lím, D. (1960). Hydrophilic gels for biological use. *Nature* 185 (4706): 117–118.
5 Giobbe, G.G., Crowley, C., Luni, C. et al. (2019). Extracellular matrix hydrogel derived from decellularized tissues enables endodermal organoid culture. *Nat. Commun.* 10 (1): 5658.
6 Holloway, E.M., Capeling, M.M., and Spence, J.R. (2019). Biologically inspired approaches to enhance human organoid complexity. *Development* 146 (8): dev166173.
7 Capeling, M.M., Czerwinski, M., Huang, S. et al. (2019). Nonadhesive alginate hydrogels support growth of pluripotent stem cell-derived intestinal organoids. *Stem Cell Rep.* 12 (2): 381–394.
8 Cruz-Acuna, R., Quiros, M., Farkas, A.E. et al. (2017). Synthetic hydrogels for human intestinal organoid generation and colonic wound repair. *Nat. Cell Biol.* 19 (11): 1326–1335.
9 Blondel, D. and Lutolf, M.P. (2019). Bioinspired hydrogels for 3D organoid culture. *Chimia (Aarau)* 73 (1): 81–85.
10 Gjorevski, N., Sachs, N., Manfrin, A. et al. (2016). Designer matrices for intestinal stem cell and organoid culture. *Nature* 539 (7630): 560–564.
11 Sato, T. and Clevers, H. (2013). Growing self-organizing mini-guts from a single intestinal stem cell: mechanism and applications. *Science* 340 (6137): 1190–1194.
12 Urciuolo, A., Poli, I., Brandolino, L. et al. (2020). Intravital three-dimensional bioprinting. *Nat. Biomed. Eng.* 4 (9): 901–915.
13 Yue, L., Wang, S., Wulf, V., and Willner, I. (2019). Stiffness-switchable DNA-based constitutional dynamic network hydrogels for self-healing and matrix-guided controlled chemical processes. *Nat. Commun.* 10 (1): 4774.
14 Lin, R.Z., Chen, Y.C., Moreno-Luna, R. et al. (2013). Transdermal regulation of vascular network bioengineering using a photopolymerizable methacrylated gelatin hydrogel. *Biomaterials* 34 (28): 6785–6796.
15 Sato, T., Vries, R.G., Snippert, H.J. et al. (2009). Single Lgr5 stem cells build crypt-villus structures in vitro without a mesenchymal niche. *Nature* 459 (7244): 262–265.
16 Sachs, N., Tsukamoto, Y., Kujala, P. et al. (2017). Intestinal epithelial organoids fuse to form self-organizing tubes in floating collagen gels. *Development* 144 (6): 1107–1112.
17 Calo, E. and Khutoryanskiy, V.V. (2015). Biomedical applications of hydrogels: a review of patents and commercial products. *Eur. Polym. J.* 65: 252–267.

18 Nelson, C.M. and Bissell, M.J. (2006). Of extracellular matrix, scaffolds, and signaling: tissue architecture regulates development, homeostasis, and cancer. *Annu. Rev. Cell Dev. Biol.* 22: 287–309.

19 Hynes, R.O. and Naba, A. (2012). Overview of the matrisome – an inventory of extracellular matrix constituents and functions. *Cold Spring Harbor Perspect. Biol.* 4 (1): a004903.

20 Saldin, L.T., Cramer, M.C., Velankar, S.S. et al. (2017). Extracellular matrix hydrogels from decellularized tissues: structure and function. *Acta Biomater.* 49: 1–15.

21 Hynes, R.O. (2009). The extracellular matrix: not just pretty fibrils. *Science* 326 (5957): 1216–1219.

22 Hussey, G.S., Cramer, M.C., and Badylak, S.F. (2018). Extracellular matrix bioscaffolds for building gastrointestinal tissue. *Cell. Mol. Gastroenterol. Hepatol.* 5 (1): 1–13.

23 Urbani, L., Camilli, C., Phylactopoulos, D.E. et al. (2018). Multi-stage bioengineering of a layered oesophagus with in vitro expanded muscle and epithelial adult progenitors. *Nat. Commun.* 9 (1): 4286.

24 Urbani, L., Maghsoudlou, P., Milan, A. et al. (2017). Long-term cryopreservation of decellularised oesophagi for tissue engineering clinical application. *PLoS One* 12 (6): e0179341.

25 Totonelli, G., Maghsoudlou, P., Garriboli, M. et al. (2012). A rat decellularized small bowel scaffold that preserves villus-crypt architecture for intestinal regeneration. *Biomaterials* 33 (12): 3401–3410.

26 Ott, H.C., Matthiesen, T.S., Goh, S.K. et al. (2008). Perfusion-decellularized matrix: using nature's platform to engineer a bioartificial heart. *Nat. Med.* 14 (2): 213–221.

27 Baiguera, S., Jungebluth, P., Burns, A. et al. (2010). Tissue engineered human tracheas for in vivo implantation. *Biomaterials* 31 (34): 8931–8938.

28 Ott, H.C., Clippinger, B., Conrad, C. et al. (2010). Regeneration and orthotopic transplantation of a bioartificial lung. *Nat. Med.* 16 (8): 927–933.

29 Uygun, B.E., Soto-Gutierrez, A., Yagi, H. et al. (2010). Organ reengineering through development of a transplantable recellularized liver graft using decellularized liver matrix. *Nat. Med.* 16 (7): 814–U120.

30 Nakayama, K.H., Batchelder, C.A., Lee, C.I., and Tarantal, A.F. (2010). Decellularized rhesus monkey kidney as a three-dimensional scaffold for renal tissue engineering. *Tissue Eng. Part A* 16 (7): 2207–2216.

31 Giuffrida, P., Curti, M., Al-Akkad, W. et al. (2019). Decellularized human gut as a natural 3D platform for research in intestinal fibrosis. *Inflamm. Bowel Dis.* 25: 1740–1750.

32 Ijima, H., Nakamura, S., Bual, R. et al. (2018). Physical properties of the extracellular matrix of decellularized porcine liver. *Gels* 4 (2): 39.

33 Park, K.M., Hussein, K.H., Hong, S.H. et al. (2016). Decellularized liver extracellular matrix as promising tools for transplantable bioengineered liver promotes hepatic lineage commitments of induced pluripotent stem cells. *Tissue Eng. Part A* 22 (5, 6): 449–460.

34 Brightman, A.O., Rajwa, B.P., Sturgis, J.E. et al. (2000). Time-lapse confocal reflection microscopy of collagen fibrillogenesis and extracellular matrix assembly in vitro. *Biopolymers* 54 (3): 222–234.

35 Freytes, D.O., Martin, J., Velankar, S.S. et al. (2008). Preparation and rheological characterization of a gel form of the porcine urinary bladder matrix. *Biomaterials* 29 (11): 1630–1637.

36 Uriel, S., Labay, E., Francis-Sedlak, M. et al. (2009). Extraction and assembly of tissue-derived gels for cell culture and tissue engineering. *Tissue Eng. Part C Methods* 15 (3): 309–321.

37 Nikolova, G., Jabs, N., Konstantinova, I. et al. (2006). The vascular basement membrane: a niche for insulin gene expression and beta cell proliferation. *Dev. Cell* 10 (3): 397–405.

38 Yap, W.T., Salvay, D.M., Silliman, M.A. et al. (2013). Collagen IV-modified scaffolds improve islet survival and function and reduce time to euglycemia. *Tissue Eng. Part A* 19 (21, 22): 2361–2372.

39 Gaetani, R., Aouad, S., Demaddalena, L.L. et al. (2018). Evaluation of different decellularization protocols on the generation of pancreas-derived hydrogels. *Tissue Eng. Part C Methods* .

40 Sackett, S.D., Tremmel, D.M., Ma, F. et al. (2018). Extracellular matrix scaffold and hydrogel derived from decellularized and delipidized human pancreas. *Sci. Rep.* 8 (1): 10452.

41 Hu, C. and Li, L. (2015). In vitro culture of isolated primary hepatocytes and stem cell-derived hepatocyte-like cells for liver regeneration. *Protein Cell* 6 (8): 562–574.

42 Sellaro, T.L., Ravindra, A.K., Stolz, D.B., and Badylak, S.F. (2007). Maintenance of hepatic sinusoidal endothelial cell phenotype in vitro using organ-specific extracellular matrix scaffolds. *Tissue Eng.* 13 (9): 2301–2310.

43 Saheli, M., Sepantafar, M., Pournasr, B. et al. (2018). Three-dimensional liver-derived extracellular matrix hydrogel promotes liver organoids function. *J. Cell. Biochem.* 119 (6): 4320–4333.

44 Lee, J.S., Shin, J., Park, H.M. et al. (2014). Liver extracellular matrix providing dual functions of two-dimensional substrate coating and three-dimensional injectable hydrogel platform for liver tissue engineering. *Biomacromolecules* 15 (1): 206–218.

45 Jaramillo, M., Yeh, H., Yarmush, M.L., and Uygun, B.E. (2018). Decellularized human liver extracellular matrix (hDLM)-mediated hepatic differentiation of human induced pluripotent stem cells (hIPSCs). *J. Tissue Eng. Regener. Med.* 12 (4): e1962–e1973.

46 Frenguelli, L., Al-Akkad, W., Crowley, C. et al. (2017). Development of human liver extracellular matrix hydrogel for three dimensional cell culture and cell transplantation. *J. Hepatol.* 66 (1): S339.

47 Takebe, T., Sekine, K., Enomura, M. et al. (2013). Vascularized and functional human liver from an iPSC-derived organ bud transplant. *Nature* 499 (7459): 481–484.

48 Calle, E.A., Hill, R.C., Leiby, K.L. et al. (2016). Targeted proteomics effectively quantifies differences between native lung and detergent-decellularized lung extracellular matrices. *Acta Biomater.* 46: 91–100.
49 Petersen, T.H., Calle, E.A., Zhao, L. et al. (2010). Tissue-engineered lungs for in vivo implantation. *Science* 329 (5991): 538–541.
50 Pouliot, R.A., Link, P.A., Mikhaiel, N.S. et al. (2016). Development and characterization of a naturally derived lung extracellular matrix hydrogel. *J. Biomed. Mater. Res. Part A* 104 (8): 1922–1935.
51 de Hilster, R.H.J., Sharma, P.K., Jonker, M.R. et al. (2020). Human lung extracellular matrix hydrogels resemble the stiffness and viscoelasticity of native lung tissue. *Am. J. Physiol. Lung Cell. Mol. Physiol.* 318 (4): L698–L704.
52 Ferreira, L.P., Gaspar, V.M., and Mano, J.F. (2020). Decellularized extracellular matrix for bioengineering physiomimetic 3D in vitro tumor models. *Trends Biotechnol.* 38 (12): 1397–1414.
53 Pinto, M.L., Rios, E., Silva, A.C. et al. (2017). Decellularized human colorectal cancer matrices polarize macrophages towards an anti-inflammatory phenotype promoting cancer cell invasion via CCL18. *Biomaterials* 124: 211–224.
54 Jee, J., Jeong, S.Y., Kim, H.K. et al. (2019). In vivo evaluation of scaffolds compatible for colonoid engraftments onto injured mouse colon epithelium. *FASEB J.* 33 (9): 10116–10125.
55 Yui, S., Nakamura, T., Sato, T. et al. (2012). Functional engraftment of colon epithelium expanded in vitro from a single adult Lgr5(+) stem cell. *Nat. Med.* 18 (4): 618–623.
56 Keane, T.J., Dziki, J., Castelton, A. et al. (2017). Preparation and characterization of a biologic scaffold and hydrogel derived from colonic mucosa. *J. Biomed. Mater. Res. Part B Appl. Biomater.* 105 (2): 291–306.
57 Romero-Lopez, M., Trinh, A.L., Sobrino, A. et al. (2017). Recapitulating the human tumor microenvironment: colon tumor-derived extracellular matrix promotes angiogenesis and tumor cell growth. *Biomaterials* 116: 118–129.
58 Mosala Nezhad, Z., Poncelet, A., de Kerchove, L. et al. (2016). Small intestinal submucosa extracellular matrix (CorMatrix(R)) in cardiovascular surgery: a systematic review. *Interact. Cardiovasc. Thorac. Surg.* 22 (6): 839–850.
59 Keane, T.J., Dziki, J., Sobieski, E. et al. (2017). Restoring mucosal barrier function and modifying macrophage phenotype with an extracellular matrix hydrogel: potential therapy for ulcerative colitis. *J. Crohns Colitis* 11 (3): 360–368.
60 Zhang, Y., He, Y., Bharadwaj, S. et al. (2009). Tissue-specific extracellular matrix coatings for the promotion of cell proliferation and maintenance of cell phenotype. *Biomaterials* 30 (23, 24): 4021–4028.
61 Aachoui, Y. and Ghosh, S.K. (2011). Extracellular matrix from porcine small intestinal submucosa (SIS) as immune adjuvants. *PLoS One* 6 (11): e27083.
62 Huleihel, L., Hussey, G.S., Naranjo, J.D. et al. (2016). Matrix-bound nanovesicles within ECM bioscaffolds. *Sci. Adv.* 2 (6): e1600502.
63 Traverse, J.H., Henry, T.D., Dib, N. et al. (2019). First-in-man study of a cardiac extracellular matrix hydrogel in early and late myocardial infarction patients. *JACC Basic Trans. Sci.* 4 (6): 659–669.

2

Collagen-Based Systems to Mimic the Extracellular Environment

Umber Cheema and Vivek Mudera

UCL Centre for 3D models of Health and Disease, Division of Surgery and Interventional Science, UCL (University College London), Charles Bell House, 43–45 Foley Street, London W1W 7TY, UK

2.1 Cells in Tissues

Barring circulating blood cells and some cells within the bone marrow, most cells in our body are anchorage-dependent. The attachment to other cells or the matrix is mediated through specific cell surface proteins, which are different for cell–cell interactions and for cell–matrix interactions. Cell–cell attachment occurs mainly via transmembrane proteins called cadherins, while cell attachment to the surrounding matrix protein is accomplished via focal adhesions which involve mainly transmembrane adhesion receptors termed integrins. These connections not only "anchor" cells within specific tissues but also play a crucial role in tensional homeostasis and mechanotransduction, as they build a biophysical microenvironment that helps to regulate a multitude of cellular functions. Cells can sense stiffness and mechanical signals received from the matrix, which in turn directly influence cells phenotype and behavior. As an example, cells resident in tissues that are remodelled, for instance following wound healing, can sense this mechanical change and modulate both cell phenotype and signaling. This is a constantly changing environment and an iterative process whereby matrix alters cell phenotype and cells respond by remodeling matrix [1]. 3D collagen gels are particularly good biomimetic materials to reproduce this iterative process as cells can remodel this matrix and generate cell-specific tension. The force generated by different cells to remodel collagen is measurable using specialized sensors in bioreactors to monitor force generation profiles [2].

Tensional homeostasis of tissues and mechanotensegrity are established concepts that are critical to cell survival within any 3D environment and related to the native, *in situ,* tissue architecture [3]. The description of tensegrity within cells has been shown in several studies. Primarily, cells behave as separate, mechanically discrete units with interconnected cytoskeletal filaments. These filaments essentially are "linked" or communicate with external stresses via transmembrane proteins used

Multifunctional Hydrogels for Biomedical Applications, First Edition.
Edited by Ricardo A. Pires, Iva Pashkuleva, and Rui L. Reis.

by cells to attach to the surrounding extracellular matrix (ECM). Second, cells have a determined cytoskeletal "pre-stress." This level of cell stress is specific and has been shown by measuring the force generation by different cells up till the point they reach tensional homeostasis. For example, it has been established that in 3D collagen gels, smooth muscle cells generate almost double the amount of force as compared to skeletal myoblasts (1.8 mN compared to 1 mN) [2]. This is perhaps not surprising given the differences in tissue stiffness and function of smooth muscle compared to skeletal muscle. The final critical aspect of underpinning the function of the tensegrity model within cells is the necessity of cell microtubules that act as compression struts alongside and in a complementary manner with focal adhesions. The relationship between the microtubules and the focal adhesions is crucial as the balance between compression and tension is critical to the tensegrity force balance [3]. To sum up, the biophysical microenvironment of cells is far from biomimetic without attachment to native ECM, which impacts cell tensional homeostasis, the production of artificially induced stress fibers, and results in an imperfect system for mechanotransduction within the cell.

2.2 Collagen in Tissues

Collagen has long been associated with tissues of the musculoskeletal system and connective tissues. Its role in cell-dense organs like the liver and the brain (Figure 2.1) is less critical due to the high cell density and relatively low matrix density. In matrix-rich tissues, including ligament, tendon, skin, cartilage, and bone, collagen plays a crucial role both structurally and in directing cell response. Collagen has a relatively slow turnover. Once this protein is produced by cells, it undergoes cross-linking that stabilizes it and makes challenging the extraction of the native form (non-cross-linked) from animal or human tissues. Due to its critical structural and biofunctional role in different tissues and its structural conservation across species with low immunogenicity, collagen is an ideal biomolecule for the development of 3D biomaterials for tissue engineering and regenerative medicine purposes.

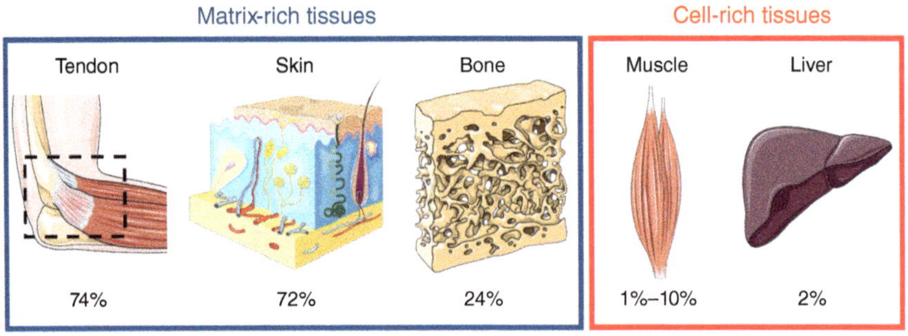

Figure 2.1 The average percentage of collagen type I found in human and bovine tissues [4–7]. Source: Server Medical Art / CC BY 3.0.

2.2.1 Structure of Collagen

Collagen is a helical protein: three polypeptide strands of a repeating arrangement of amino acids essentially wind together to form a right-handed triple helix, which is then stabilized by hydrogen bonds. The repeating amino acid in each strand is glycine-X-Y. Glycine is critical due to its size, which is small enough to allow a tight turn of the collagen molecule. The X-Y amino acids tend to be imino and hydroxylated imino acids. These can include proline-hydroxyproline and lysine-hydroxylysine. The triple helix structure forms the basis of a single collagen molecule also known as tropocollagen. The tropocollagen molecules self-assemble in fibrillar collagens that are staggered with a precise distance of 67 nm, conferring a unique D-band pattern which is easily recognizable when using high magnification electron microscopy. This protein is complex, but biologically very elegantly put together.

The basic triple helix of collagen forms individual monomers, which are around 280 nm long. The ends of these monomers are nonhelical, and cross-linking of monomers occurs to form collagen fibrils. Cross-linking of collagen is either enzymatic or nonenzymatic. The primary enzyme-mediated method utilizes lysyl oxidase. Lysyl oxidase acts on lysine and hydroxylysine to form a divalent, immature cross-link with an opposing amino acid on the triple helix within the telopeptide region [8]. Spontaneously, these cross-links are stabilized to trivalent cross-links that confer mechanical strength of collagen and upon maturation, result in highly cross-linked polymeric collagen. Other form of cross-linking of monomers is via glycation and is driven by oxidative reactions between glucose and collagen. This type of cross-linking is associated with diabetes and aging, where glucose is present at high concentrations and results in the formation of advanced glycation end products (AGEs) [9].

2.2.2 Collagen Sources

Common ways to extract large volumes of collagen from animal tissues involve pepsin treatment, which is an enzymatic method to cleave off the telopeptide ends. The main drawback of this method is the loss of native collagen cross-links. Extraction of intact collagen molecules is possible using a method involving acetic acid. Both methods are used to extract collagen employed to generate 3D hydrogels.

The complexity of collagen conferred by the unique structure makes it virtually impossible to synthesize a material with similar mechanical and biological features. There have been attempts to generate synthetic collagen, and some synthetic analogs showed the formation of fibril-forming units which self-aggregate and form gels. However, specific features such as the D-band register have not yet been achieved [10]. Collagen utilized in a biomimetic manner is only obtained from animals and microorganisms. There are examples where bacteria have been engineered to synthesize collagen, including triple helical proteins; however, more work needs to be done to test these proteins in a robust manner in comparison to animal-derived collagens [11].

2.3 Controlling Collagen Architecture

The cellular and matrix architecture of different tissues is very specific and controlled *in situ*. Recapitulating specific features of tissues is important if we aim to recreate the biomimetic environment of cells in the body and truly capture native cell behavior and response to stimuli and drugs. There are three main feature of collagen architecture, called the 3 "D's" for Direction, Diameter, and Density [12, 13], which are tissue-specific and researchers are actively attempting to engineer (Figure 2.2).

2.3.1 Direction: Collagen Orientation

The orientation of collagen confers very diverse and specific mechanical properties to tissues within the body. Where strength is required along a single axis or direction, collagen fibers are orientated in that direction. An example is the tendon tissue, where all the resident collagen fibers align along a single axis in a parallel array. The specific axis along which the collagen orientates is the load-bearing direction connecting the bone and muscle. In skin, a basket-weave orientation is observed, which confers strength in multiple directions and accommodates the other matrix proteins present in tissue, particularly elastin that renders the tissue elastic. Cornea has collagen fibers that are orientated in layers set at 90° to assure transparency. Bone tissue has a very dense collagen matrix; however, as strength is required in all directions, the collagen is less orientated.

Different methods have been used to control the orientation of collagen fibrils in 3D gels *in vitro*. The oldest technique was proposed by Elsdale and Bard in 1972 and uses gravity-driven fluid flow to orientate the collagen fibrils. This technique can be used to orientate collagen fibrils within collagen gels and has been extended to generate dense, orientated cellular collagen gels [14]. It can be also applied to

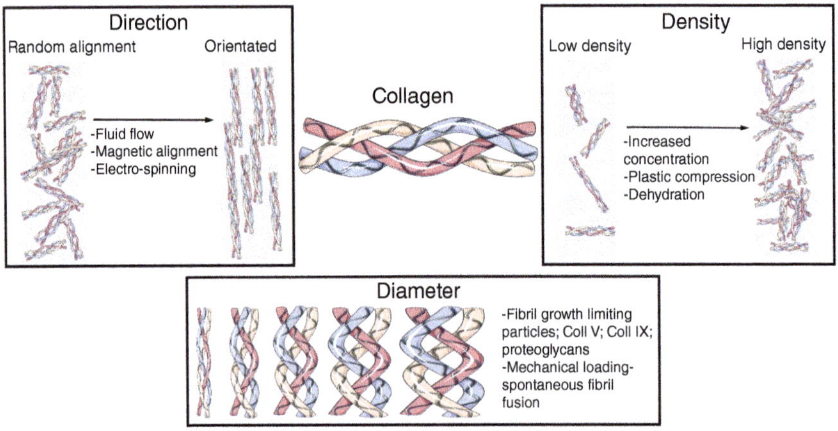

Figure 2.2 Schematic presentation of the collagen 3D's: direction, density, and diameter and some engineering approaches used to control collagen architecture. Source: Server Medical Art / CC BY 3.0.

"set" collagen gels: an orientation is achieved through the disentanglement of fibers driven by the fluid flow [15, 16]. Microfluidic devices have also been used to generate a flow within collagen gels. The width of the channel influences whether flow can induce an orientation: channels with diameter of less than 100 μm induce alignment of collagen fibrils to within 15° of parallel to flow [17]. From an engineering perspective, this requirement limits the size of collagen scaffold/gel that can be produced, rendering this technique appropriate for small-scale models used to study matrix alignment on cell function for example. However, from a regenerative medicine perspective, generation of aligned collagen scaffolds that are 100 μm wide restricts severely the tissues that can be regenerated or engineered.

Collages fibrils have an inherent diamagnetic sensitivity, which can be used to produce aligned collagen fibrils by applying magnetic field [18]. Early work using this method has indicated that some orientation of collagen is possible in thin collagen gels, but there are other factors, e.g. surface interactions, which influence the orientation. Collagen within thicker gels cannot be orientated using magnets. Magnetic beads have been used instead to successfully align collagen within gels. However, this technique is more efficient in combination with fluid flow [19]. It is less restrictive in terms of scaffold size, and larger constructs, relevant for regenerative and tissue engineering purposes, can be generated. There has been significant work on the use of electrospinning to orientate collagen fibers [20]. This method uses a rotating mandrel to orientate the fibers. The collagen is spun along the mandrel to orient it along the axis of curvature. It is effective, precise, and allows to add cells via a separate nozzle to coseed the generated scaffolds with cells. Controlling fibril diameter, however, is not possible using this method.

The importance of matrix, and specifically collagen, alignment is clear, and methods to introduce alignment are not simple. Using physical methods to align the collagen is technically challenging and is currently limited to only one technique. Very effective method for collagen alignment is through the manipulation of cell-generated forces. Cells can remodel collagen as they generate tensional homeostasis of collagen hydrogels. This method is particularly good because different cell types generate different levels of force to remodel, or contract, collagen hydrogels. The cell-specific action can be manipulated to generate force in different planes by leaving parts of the gel tethered and other parts untethered. As this remodeling is cell-generated and cell-type-specific, it will generate the biomimetic stiffness appropriate for cell survival.

2.3.2 Diameter: Collagen Fibril Diameter

The diameter of collagen fibrils is very specific and heavily dependent on the cross-linking of the fibrils (Table 2.1). The fibril diameter of collagen within tissues is critical as it confers distinctive local environment and specific mechanical properties. The range of diameters differs from tissue to tissue and specific location. As an example, significant variation in the diameter of collagen fibrils in the joint and nonjoint regions of median nerves has been found and related to the function compliance of this tissue in specific regions [24]: collagen fibrils are

Table 2.1 Average collagen fibril diameter in multiple tissues.

Tissue	Species	Mean fibril diameter (nm)	References
Tendon-hamstring	Human	144 ± 14	Svensson et al. [21]
Tendon-patellar	Human	100 ± 7.5	Svensson et al. [21]
Bone	Rabbit	63.4 ± 8.6	Tzaphlidou [22]
Skin	Rabbit	90.1 ± 10.2	Tzaphlidou [23]
Liver	Rabbit (Female)	46.2 ± 6	Tzaphlidou [22]
Sciatic nerve-endoneurium	Rat	42.5 ± 1.1	Mason and Phillips [24]
Sciatic nerve-epineurium	Rat	77.0 ± 1.2	Mason and Phillips [24]

thinner in the median nerve at the joint regions, which is likely due to the need for extra compliance in this region. There is, thus, longitudinal heterogeneity of collagen fibril properties and related tensile properties in the median nerve. Data about specific collagen properties in tissues and the heterogenous distribution of these properties throughout tissue are crucial not only to estimate the mechanical properties of tissues but also to develop functional tissue-engineered constructs.

Little effort have been devoted to the engineering of this parameter, because of the lack of information about the mechanism by which it is regulated *in situ*. Generally, it is accepted that the regulation of collagen fibril size is a cell-driven process. There has been significant work on understanding the role of fibril-modifying molecules, which include collagen types V and IX and proteoglycans [25]. The hypothesis is that these proteins "sit" on collagen fibrils to prevent "growth" of the fibril. The mechanisms by which fibrils assemble and adapt to changes in tissues remain elusive, and there is no clear understanding of control mechanisms used to increase fibril size. There is a hypothesis that a cell-independent mechanism may be in play [26]: fibrils spontaneously fuse together when cyclical loading of 3D collagen scaffolds is applied. These results indicate that mechanics can be used to control collagen fibril growth in tissues and similar process can be adopted for engineering collagen fibril size for *in vitro* tissue engineering.

2.3.3 Density: Fibril Packing and Cross-Linking

The density of collagen varies across tissues. *In vitro*, collagen gels or 3D lattices are formed from monomeric, intact collagen fibrils extracted from tissues using acetic acid. When this solution is neutralized and brought to 37 °C, the monomeric collagen rapidly aggregates in its native ¼ staggered manner to produce nanometer diameter fibrils. Over a few hours, these fibrils elongate and "grow" in diameter, entwining to form a loose mesh, termed a hydrogel. This process of *in vitro* fibrillogenesis is not directly engineered, instead the correct environment is provided for self-aggregation of collagen fibrils. Thus, the simple way to control the collagen density is by adjusting the concentration of the extract. However, there is a limitation of the concentration of collagen that can be extracted.

Among the multiple methods to increase the density of collagen scaffolds, is the application of compression to essentially "expel" excess fluid from hyperhydrated collagen hydrogels. This method is effective and rapid [12]. It is particularly pertinent for engineering tissues with high density of collagen, i.e. matrix-rich tissues (Figure 2.1) and 3D solid tumors (the dense matrix is a feature often used to identify the solid tumor prior to surgical intervention). The importance of accurate matrix density has recently been highlighted by comparison of the stiffness of a mammary tumor, that is ~4000 Pa, a low-density collagen hydrogel (2 mg/ml) with stiffness of 330 Pa, and a high-density collagen gel (4 mg/ml) whose stiffness is 1590 Pa [27]. The fact is that we cannot yet replicate easily the density nor the appropriate material properties of different tissue types.

In a summary, different engineering approaches to control each aspect of collagen architecture (density, diameter, and direction) have been developed. However, this natural protein with its unique features and structural complexity requires often a combination of several approaches to achieve biofunctionality.

2.4 Engineering Collagen Scaffolds

2.4.1 Collagen Cross-Linking

Collagen within tissues is cross-linked, thus tissues have much better mechanical properties compared to collagen hydrogels or sponges used in tissue engineering. Chemical cross-linking is the most common approach to improve the mechanical properties of collagen; however, the used chemicals are often cytotoxic and can in some cases render collagen nonbiocompatible. Photochemical cross-linking is another method to cross-link collagen gels and scaffolds and results in a stronger scaffold both in terms of tensile and compressive strength and an increased longevity *in vivo* [28]. For photochemical cross-linking, a photosensitizer needs to be used in conjunction with the correct wavelength of light. Riboflavin in conjunction with ultraviolet light is commonly used because riboflavin is also applied *in vivo* as photosensitizer for the treatment of keratoconus: it stabilizes and cross-links the collagen within the cornea [29]. The mechanism by which it acts is not well defined. However, experimental evidences showed that riboflavin-mediated cross-linked collagen scaffolds are mechanically stronger, with only a slight reduction in cell viability [30]. Collagen cross-linking was achieved by using 0.25 mM riboflavin and exposing collagen scaffolds for 10 minutes to blue light and resulted in mechanical break stress of 0.4 MPa [31], i.e. twofold increase of the strength of the standard 10% density collagen scaffolds.

2.4.2 Diffusion of Nutrients and Oxygen Through Collagen Scaffolds

Tissues have an extensive network of blood vessels to supply cells with glucose and oxygen, as well as to remove metabolic waste products including lactate. When culturing cells in 3D tissue-engineered scaffolds, no inherent vascular network exists. Vascularization either needs to be engineered alongside with the scaffold or cells need to have access to necessary glucose and oxygen in the culture media. This requirement has been extensively described in older research whereby the core of 3D constructs is often found "empty" of cells due to their migration to the periphery of the construct in "search" for nutrients and oxygen.

The use of native ECM components for engineering tissues and 3D culture is not only biomimetic but also confers relatively good perfusive properties when compared to synthetic polymers scaffolds. The glucose diffusion coefficient in collagen gels with high density is between $1.3–1.4 \times 10^{-6}$ cm^2/s [32, 33] and 4.5×10^{-6} cm^2/s [31]. This value is consistent with a reasonably good diffusion of glucose, rendering high survival rate of cells within such scaffolds. However, the use of high cellular densities can result in the formation of gradients of glucose, oxygen, and lactate in 3D tissue-engineered scaffolds. These gradients are cell-density-dependent and cell-specific but can be calculated to estimate the maximum size of a tissue-engineered scaffold [34]. Cells in the core of tissue-engineered scaffolds are exposed to lower levels of nutrients and display a differential response in terms of signaling and cell response [35]. This can be used to manipulate differential cell response signaling: when cells are exposed to lower oxygen levels, angiogenic signaling is increased. This behavior means that angiogenic factors are gradually released from the scaffolds and can "attract" either host vasculature once implanted *in vivo* or can signal to endothelial cells to form basic vascular networks [36].

2.4.3 Proliferation of Cells in 3D

Cell proliferation in 2D has been instrumental to study biological mechanisms *in vitro* and generated valuable information about cells growth, their specific functions, such as deposition of proteins and signaling, and their interactions with other cells. Culturing cells in 2D is relatively quick and easy. However, the growth of cells on stiff, 2D plastic generates unnaturally fast formation of stress fibers and proliferation. There is likely to be an effect of both 2D and 3D geometry on cell proliferation, but also stiffness of the 2D or 3D matrix on/in which cells are cultured. There is a relationship between the stiffness of 3D collagen gels and the proliferation rate of human dermal fibroblasts. Cells cultured in "soft" 3D collagen gels (0.4% collagen, stiffness ~42 kPa) had a doubling time of six days, compared to "stiff" collagen gels (20%, modulus ~1800 kPa), where the doubling time was only two days. The relationship between collagen density and scaffold stiffness is particularly pertinent for this study, as there is a 50-fold increase in both theses parameters, which is a linear relationship [37].

The link between substrate stiffness and cell proliferation is not linear, and it is instead an iterative feedback process where the changing physical microenvironment of cells alters their behavior. This is clearly exemplified in the cellular collagen hydrogel model. Here, cells are embedded in low density, low stiffness collagen hydrogels, and initially there is a very low rate of proliferation [2].

Cells thus remodel the matrix and "stiffen" it in cell-type-specific manner, which is quantifiable. Once the matrix is stiffened, cell proliferation is altered [37]. There is also a level of tensional homeostasis enough for cell turnover and below which cells will not proliferate. These studies generate an understanding on different cell behaviors and how scaffold properties can be used to trigger different cell responses *in vitro*.

2.4.4 Mechanical Stimulation and Bioreactors

Tissues sustain different types of mechanical forces. There is the inherent tensional homeostasis, but there is also the role of external mechanical stimulation. For example, most tissues of the musculoskeletal system are subjected to mechanical loading. Bones are constantly under mechanical loading, as are the tendons, ligaments, cartilage, and skeletal muscle. In cell-rich tissues, heart and lungs, for example, cells are also subjected to mechanical loading and stimulation as these tissues are under constant cyclical mechanical loading regimens. The role of mechanics has been extensively studied and is therefore a feature in successfully engineered tissues. Different bioreactor systems and mechanical loading have been applied to collagen scaffolds. Although it is not easy to directly convert tissue mechanics into mechanical stimulation applied to tissue-engineered constructs, basic patterns for mechanical loading regimens can give insight on cells response (e.g. growth, differentiation, and signaling) toward mechanical stimulation. Work on culturing skeletal myoblasts in 3D collagen scaffolds revealed that application of ramp loading, i.e. applied mechanical load in a slow, unidirectional manner resulted in the upregulation of a specific splice variant of insulin like growth factor (IGF-I), IGF-IEa, which initiates the fusion of single-nuclei myoblasts to form multinucleated myotubes [38]. Within the same study, an application of cyclical loading, i.e. a bidirectional loading regimen, resulted in an upregulation of a different splice variant, IGF-IEb (also known as mechano-growth factor (MGF)) [39]. The upregulation of the IGF-IEb splice variant is associated with the proliferation of mononucleated myoblasts that are required for secondary myotube formation. This study highlights the importance of mechanical loading to cell-specific function and underlying the fact that the use of a biomimetic scaffold, which is mechanically loaded and transmits the load to cells, is critical in tissue engineering. Skeletal muscle is a tissue which is known to atrophy when there is no mechanical stimulation. Consequently, the absence of mechanical stimulation is likely to directly influence skeletal myoblasts and fused skeletal myotubes and fibers. The cells inherently attach to the matrix in which they are cultured, and mechanical loading of the cell-seeded scaffold is transmitted to cells via cell-matrix attachment.

As previously discussed, the linkage of cell surface integrins to both the intracellular cytoskeleton and the surrounding matrix means that these molecules effectively transmit mechanical signals to cells. For any tissue-engineered scaffold, transmission of mechanical stimulation to embedded cells is critical, and the way in which cells attach to any scaffold can influence this transmission.

2.4.5 Growth Factors

It is well documented that components of the ECM can sequester growth factors and that the actions of specific growth factors are dependent on cells type. This reciprocity between these components is critical in tissue formation. For example, the binding of cells to collagen via the $\alpha_1\beta_1$ and $\alpha_1\beta_2$ integrins is critical for vascular endothelial growth factor (VEGF)-induced angiogenesis – as when this binding is prevented by antibodies, there is a significant reduction in angiogenesis. Without the direct adhesion of cells to the surrounding ECM, VEGF is not effective as a growth factor [40]. Another example is the wound healing, which is associated with the release of multiple growth factors bound to the ECM. These factors then aid the process of tissue healing.

2.4.6 Drug-Loaded Scaffolds

During the past four decades, significant differences between a drugs' efficacy *in vitro* using cultures of cells and the efficacy in humans have been reported. Billions of dollars are plugged into new therapeutics developments, which ultimately do not translate from lab (*in vitro*) to humans. This can also be said with regard to animal testing, where drugs which successfully target disease in animal are not translated for targeting human disease. One potential alternative of drug testing is the development of relevant humanized 3D *in vitro* models, which allow testing in a high-throughput manner and have quantifiable and reproduce outcomes. These models also open the way for personalized medicine, where patient-specific organoids or even cancers can be cultured, and then interrogated for response to therapeutic drugs.

Of particular interest is the concept of organ-on-a-chip and body-on-a-chip. The first description of organ-on-a-chip is an engineered lung where alveolar epithelial cells and microvascular endothelial cells were cultured within microfluidic devices [41]. Different cell populations were cultured on opposite sides of the chamber on either collagen gel-coated surfaces (at 3 μg/ml) or on fibronectin-coated surfaces. They formed intact monolayers as media with or without drug was pumped through the device. The importance of using an ECM base, and specifically collagen, should not be underestimated as it provides the basis for a biomimetic environment to ensure cells responses and closely mimic what would happen *in situ*. Recapitulating the features of the biophysical environment remains a key. This technology has now been extended to multiple organ types, but one of the most interesting is the concept of body-on-a-chip, or integrated micro-physiological systems, whereby multiple organ chips are connected in one microfluidic device, and media with or without drug can be passed through multiple organs [42]. This kind of technology helps to build a system where cross-talk between different organs can be studied in a systematic way.

For cancer cultures, the action of drug on spheroids is more biomimetic compared to 2D cultures. Spheroids are essentially clusters of specific phenotype cancer cells. The spheroid grows, and as it does so, matrix is deposited in a haphazard and uncontrolled manner, and at a particular size, the spheroid core becomes necrotic.

Spheroids can be produced by using low adhesion plates, to encourage cells to lift off and spontaneously form spheroids, or by using the hanging drop method, where cells are suspended in a hanging drop and produce their own matrix which eventually forms a stable spheroid. However, spheroids spontaneously form in 3D Matrigel and 3D collagen gels. These can be maintained for long, and using nested cultures it is possible to quantify spheroid invasion from one collagen matrix to the other. The stiffness and orientation of collagen within gels are also remodeled by cancerous cells and can provide insight into cancer cell remodeling of tissues *in situ*.

2.5 Conclusions

The dominance of collagen as a protein of ECM makes it an ideal biomaterial for use in 3D cell culture and tissue engineering. Several processing parameters of collagen materials can be adjusted to mimic different aspects of the biophysical niche of cells. The architecture of different tissues is specific and plays an important role both structurally and functionally, therefore needs to be considered when engineering tissues and scaffolds.

References

1 Grinnell, F. (2000). Fibroblast-collagen-matrix contraction: growth-factor signalling and mechanical loading. *Trends Cell Biol.* https://doi.org/10.1016/S0962-8924(00)01802-X.

2 Cheema, U., Yang, S.-Y., Mudera, V. et al. (2003). 3-D in vitro model of early skeletal muscle development. *Cell Motil. Cytoskeleton* 54: 226–236.

3 Stamenović, D., Wang, N., and Ingber, D.E. (2007). https://doi.org/10.1007/978-1-4020-5062-6_14). Tensegrity architecture and the mammalian cell cytoskeleton. In: *Multiscaling in Molecular and Continuum Mechanics: Interaction of Time and Size from Macro to Nano: Application to Biology, Physics, Material Science, Mechanics, Structural and processing Engineering* (ed. G. Sih), 321–338. Springer.

4 Neuman, R.E. and Logan, M.A. (1950). The determination of collagen and elastin in tissues. *J. Biol. Chem.* 186: 549–556.

5 Bendall, J.R. (1967). Elastin content of various muscles of beef animals. *J. Sci. Food Agric.* 18: 553–558.

6 Dransfield, E. (1977). Intramuscular composition and texture of beef muscles. *J. Sci. Food Agric.* 28: 833–842.

7 Aycock, R. and Seyer, J.M. (1989). Collagens of normal and cirrhotic human liver. *Connect Tissue Res.* 23: 19–31.

8 Eyre, D.R., Weis, M.A., and Wu, J.J. (2008). Advances in collagen cross-link analysis. *Methods* https://doi.org/10.1016/j.ymeth.2008.01.002.

9 Haus, J.M., Carrithers, J.A., Trappe, S.W., and Trappe, T.A. (2007). Collagen, cross-linking, and advanced glycation end products in aging human skeletal muscle. *J. Appl. Physiol.* https://doi.org/10.1152/japplphysiol.00670.2007.

10 Kumar, V.A., Taylor, N.L., Jalan, A.A. et al. (2014). A nanostructured synthetic collagen mimic for hemostasis. *Biomacromolecules* https://doi.org/10.1021/bm500091e.

11 Yu, Z., An, B., Ramshaw, J.A.M., and Brodsky, B. (2014). Bacterial collagen-like proteins that form triple-helical structures. *J. Struct. Biol.* https://doi.org/10.1016/j.jsb.2014.01.003.

12 Brown, R.A., Wiseman, M., Chuo, C.B. et al. (2005). Ultrarapid engineering of biomimetic materials and tissues: fabrication of nano- and microstructures by plastic compression. *Adv. Funct. Mater.* 15: https://doi.org/10.1002/adfm.200500042.

13 Cheema, U., Nazhat, S.N., Alp, B. et al. (2007). Fabricating tissues: analysis of farming versus engineering strategies. *Biotechnol. Bioprocess Eng.* 12: 9–14.

14 Elsdale, T. and Bard, J. (1972). Collagen substrata for studies on cell behavior. *J. Cell Biol.* https://doi.org/10.1083/jcb.54.3.626.

15 Ng, C.P. and Swartz, M.A. (2006). Mechanisms of interstitial flow-induced remodeling of fibroblast-collagen cultures. *Ann. Biomed. Eng.* https://doi.org/10.1007/s10439-005-9067-3.

16 Kureshi, A., Cheema, U., Alekseeva, T. et al. (2010). Alignment hierarchies: engineering architecture from the nanometre to the micrometre scale. *J. R. Soc. Interface* 7: S707–S716.

17 Lee, P., Lin, R., Moon, J., and Lee, L.P. (2006). Microfluidic alignment of collagen fibers for in vitro cell culture. *Biomed. Microdevices* https://doi.org/10.1007/s10544-006-6380-z.

18 Torbet, J. and Ronziere, M.C. (1984). Magnetic alignment of collagen during self-assembly. *Biochem. J.* https://doi.org/10.1042/bj2191057.

19 Guo, C. and Kaufman, L.J. (2007). Flow and magnetic field induced collagen alignment. *Biomaterials* https://doi.org/10.1016/j.biomaterials.2006.10.010.

20 Matthews, J.A., Wnek, G.E., Simpson, D.G., and Bowlin, G.L. (2002). Electrospinning of collagen nanofibers. *Biomacromolecules* https://doi.org/10.1021/bm015533u.

21 Svensson, R.B., Herchenhan, A., Starborg, T. et al. (2017). Evidence of structurally continuous collagen fibrils in tendons. *Acta Biomater.* https://doi.org/10.1016/j.actbio.2017.01.006.

22 Tzaphlidou, M. (2001). Diameter distributions of collagenous tissues in relation to sex. A quantitative ultrastructural study. *Micron* https://doi.org/10.1016/S0968-4328(00)00033-0.

23 Tzaphlidou, M. (2005). The role of collagen in bone structure: an image processing approach. *Micron* https://doi.org/10.1016/j.micron.2005.05.009.

24 Mason, S. and Phillips, J.B. (2011). An ultrastructural and biochemical analysis of collagen in rat peripheral nerves: the relationship between fibril diameter and mechanical properties. *J. Peripher. Nerv. Syst.* https://doi.org/10.1111/j.1529-8027.2011.00352.x.

25 Scott, J.E. (1984). The periphery of the developing collagen fibril. Quantitative relationships with dermatan sulphate and other surface-associated species. *Biochem. J.* https://doi.org/10.1042/bj2180229.

26 Cheema, U., Chuo, C.-B., Sarathchandra, P. et al. (2007). Engineering functional collagen scaffolds: cyclical loading increases material strength and fibril aggregation. *Adv. Funct. Mater.* 17: 2426–2431.

27 Weigelt, B., Ghajar, C.M., and Bissell, M.J. (2014). The need for complex 3D culture models to unravel novel pathways and identify accurate biomarkers in breast cancer. *Adv. Drug Deliv. Rev.* https://doi.org/10.1016/j.addr.2014.01.001.

28 Chan, B.P., Hui, T.Y., Chan, O.C. et al. (2007). Photochemical cross-linking for collagen-based scaffolds: a study on optical properties, mechanical properties, stability, and hematocompatibility. *Tissue Eng.* https://doi.org/10.1089/ten.2006.0004.

29 O, Brart, D.P.S. (2014). Corneal collagen cross-linking: a review. *J. Optometry* https://doi.org/10.1016/j.optom.2013.12.001.

30 Cheema, U., Rong, Z., Kirresh, O. et al. (2011). O_2 diffusion through collagen scaffolds at defined densities: implications for cell survival and angiogenic signalling in tissue models. *IFMBE Proc.* https://doi.org/10.1007/978-3-642-19044-5_4.

31 Cheema, U., Rong, Z., Kirresh, O. et al. (2012). Oxygen diffusion through collagen scaffolds at defined densities: implications for cell survival in tissue models. *J. Tissue Eng. Regen. Med.* 6: 77–84.

32 Wu, D.Q., Zhang, G.L., Shen, C. et al. (2005). Evaluation of diffusion in gel entrapment cell culture within hollow fibers. *World J. Gastroenterol.* https://doi.org/10.3748/wjg.v11.i11.1599.

33 Rong, Z., Cheema, U., and Vadgama, P. (2006). Needle enzyme electrode based glucose diffusive transport measurement in a collagen gel and validation of a simulation model. *Analyst* 131: 816–821.

34 Streeter, I. and Cheema, U. (2011). Oxygen consumption rate of cells in 3D culture: the use of experiment and simulation to measure kinetic parameters and optimise culture conditions. *Analyst* 136: 4013–4019.

35 Cheema, U., Brown, R.A., Alp, B., and MacRobert, A.J. (2008). Spatially defined oxygen gradients and vascular endothelial growth factor expression in an engineered 3D cell model. *Cell. Mol. Life Sci.* 65: 177–186.

36 Pape, J., Magdeldin, T., Ali, M. et al. (2019). Cancer invasion regulates vascular complexity in a three-dimensional biomimetic model. *Eur. J. Cancer* https://doi.org/10.1016/j.ejca.2019.07.005.

37 Hadjipanayi, E., Mudera, V., and Brown, R.A. (2009). Close dependence of fibroblast proliferation on collagen scaffold matrix stiffness. *J. Tissue Eng. Regen. Med.* https://doi.org/10.1002/term.136.

38 Cheema, U., Yang, S., Mudera, V. et al. (2002). Mechanical loading of 3-D muscle constructs. *Eur. Cells Mater.* 4: 16–17.

39 Cheema, U., Brown, R.A., Mudera V. et al. (2005). Mechanical signals and IGF-I gene splicing in vitro in relation to development of skeletal muscle. *J. Cell. Physiol.* 202: 67–75.

40 Senger, D.R., Claffey, K.P., Benes, J.E. et al. (1997). Angiogenesis promoted by vascular endothelial growth factor: regulation through $\alpha_1\beta_1$ and $\alpha_2\beta_1$ integrins. *Proc. Natl. Acad. Sci. U.S.A.* https://doi.org/10.1073/pnas.94.25.13612.

41 Huh, D., Matthews, B.D., Mammoto, A. et al. (2010). Reconstituting organ-level lung functions on a chip. *Science* https://doi.org/10.1126/science.1188302.

42 Edington, C.D., Chen, W.L.K., Geishecker, E. et al. (2018). Interconnected micro-physiological systems for quantitative biology and pharmacology studies. *Sci. Rep.* https://doi.org/10.1038/s41598-018-22749-0.

3

Designing Elastin-Like Recombinamers for Therapeutic and Regenerative Purposes

José Carlos Rodríguez-Cabello, Sara Escalera☆, Diana Juanes-Gusano☆, Mercedes Santos, and Alessandra Girotti

University of Valladolid, BIOFORGE lab (Group for Advanced Materials and Nanobiotechnology) CIBER-BBN, Edificio Lucía, Paseo de Belén 19, Valladolid 47011, Spain

3.1 Introduction

The field of biomedicine relies on the development of advanced systems that mimic the extracellular matrix (ECM) to allow *in vitro* studies of cell–matrix interactions and subsequent implementation *in vivo*. The principal matrices for biomedical applications are hydrogels, which are hydrophilic polymer networks that can absorb a large volume of water in resemblance to natural tissues (see Chapter 1). The materials used to obtain these biomimetic scaffolds include a large variety of synthetic polymers such as polyethylene glycol (PEG) [1], as well as biopolymers, mostly proteins from animal tissues such as collagen [2] (see Chapter 2). Combinations of natural and synthetic polymers have also been tested to improve the properties of hydrogels [3].

Essential characteristics for the development of hydrogels for general biomedical applications include (i) an ability to provide a structural support to the surrounding cells, thus promoting natural and adequate cell growth that helps complete integration of the scaffold into the natural surrounding tissue and provides mechanical stability, (ii) an ability to mimic the ECM topography of tissues, (iii) an ability to mimic the natural environment so that cells can develop their normal functions and help restore damaged tissue, (iv) an ability to absorb and retain large quantities of water while maintaining their structures, thereby maintaining the hydration levels found in most tissues, (v) an ability to modulate their structures to match the shape and the size of defects, (vi) an ability to be easily manipulated, and, particularly, (vii) biocompatibility and biodegradability [4–7]. Depending on the final application, hydrogels for use in regenerative medicine will need specific requirements in order to simulate the tissue to be repaired, such as cell adhesion or growth factors, which could also be included in the scaffold.

☆ equal contribution

Multifunctional Hydrogels for Biomedical Applications, First Edition.
Edited by Ricardo A. Pires, Iva Pashkuleva, and Rui L. Reis.

Although hydrogels have become especially attractive as matrices for tissue engineering, they have also been applied as drug and cell carriers in biomedicine. Indeed, they are promising candidates for the controlled release of active compounds, especially in localized diseases. The advantages of these systems include controlled delivery and release of the drug in time and space, thereby avoiding systemic exposure and lowering toxicity and side effects in healthy tissues [8, 9]. This means that lower amounts of drug are needed as the compounds do not have to overcome hepatic and renal clearance, and; therefore, the number of administrations is also reduced.

Elastin is a fibrous and insoluble protein found in the ECM that provides elasticity and structural integrity to organs and tissues. Indeed, elastin undergoes thousands of elastic deformation and complete recovery cycles while preserving its mechanical properties [10].

The advent of recombinant DNA technology opened a new route to the production of synthetic proteins lacking the disadvantages of chemical synthesis, such as polydispersity or the need to remove organic solvents. A new family of protein-based polymers whose composition is inspired by the primary sequence found in natural elastin has been obtained using this recombinant technology, and the resulting elastin-like polypeptides (ELPs) have been named elastin-like recombinamers (ELRs) to reflect this. ELRs include repetitive sequences comprising the most widely used pentapeptide, VPGXG, (valine–proline–glycine–X–glycine), where the guest residue "X" can be any amino acid except proline. This genetic engineering methodology allows total control over the amino acid sequence, length, and molecular weight and gives rise to monodisperse polymers. In addition, bioactive domains, such as adhesive domains, biological triggers, or degradation sequences, can be also introduced into the amino acid backbone [11, 12].

ELRs show thermoresponsiveness, with an inverse temperature transition (ITT) in aqueous media: below a characteristic temperature known as the transition temperature (Tt), the polymer chains remain soluble in a random coil structure and above this Tt, the ELRs self-assemble and adopt a regular nonrandom structure characterized by the presence of type II β-turns that leads to phase separation (Figure 3.1). Therefore, ELRs can be classified as smart materials that show conformational changes in response to environmental stimuli such as temperature and have gained widespread interest in biomedical applications. ELRs also have other advantages in regard to biomedical applications, such as biocompatibility, bioactivity, and specific and controllable mechanical properties [7, 13].

Hydrogels can be classified depending on their interchain cross-linking as gels formed by physical or "reversible" cross-links and constructs generated by chemical or "irreversible" bonds. In physically cross-linked hydrogels, the polymer chains are maintained together because of molecular entanglements and/or intermolecular forces, including H-bonding and ionic or van der Waals forces. ELRs constructed from different hydrophobic and hydrophilic blocks constitute belong to the so-called "block copolymers," in which the hydrophobic block triggers a conformational change from unimer to "micelle-like" particles above the hydrophobic block transition temperature, with these blocks being found at the core. At higher

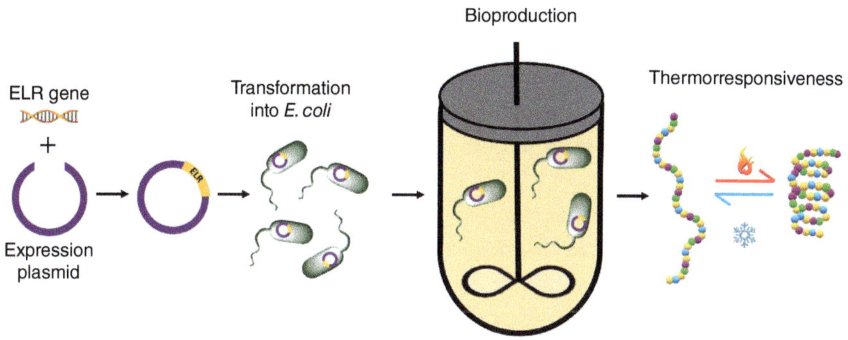

Figure 3.1 Schematic representation of design, bioproduction, and thermoresponsiveness of ELRs.

hydrophilic block transition temperatures, the polar block dehydrates and the micelles aggregate. In this sense, silk-elastin-like corecombinamers (SELRs) have been designed to include the silk fibroin motif (GAGAGS) from *Bombyx mori*. These biopolymers have a secondary structure generated by self-assembling into antiparallel beta-sheet constructs that confer higher stability and mechanical stiffness on the hydrogels [14].

In contrast, ELR-based hydrogels obtained by chemical interchain covalent cross-linking form permanent networks. Such gels can be obtained by chemical bonding between intrinsic groups, such as amines or carboxyls, and adding cross-linkers such as glutaraldehyde [15, 16], carbodiimide-based coupling [17, 18], enzymatic cross-linking [19], or photo-cross-linking [20, 21]. Chemical cross-linking reactions have limitations in terms of long reaction times or toxic byproducts, which means that they are not ideal for clinical applications. Recently, a new strategy based on click methodology involving the Hüisgen reaction has been developed to produce chemical hydrogels under physiological conditions by highly specific and fast click reaction that does not generate toxic byproducts [22, 23].

In this chapter, we will describe the use of ELR-based hydrogels in biomedical applications. ELR-based hydrogels generated from amphiphilic block copolymers and ELRs bearing silk domains will be reviewed. For chemically cross-linked hydrogels, we will focus on those obtained using a click methodology. We will review the most important and recent examples of application of these gels in musculoskeletal, cardiovascular, skin, and neural tissue engineering and regeneration. Advanced drug delivery devices based on ELRs hydrogels will also be reviewed, focusing mainly on cancer therapy.

3.2 ELR-Based Hydrogels in Tissue Engineering

ELR-based hydrogels can be used in the fields of tissue engineering and regenerative medicine to recover, preserve, or enhance biological tissue after damage leading to a loss of functionality. Over the past few years, the use of ELRs has evolved to the construction of scaffolds that mimic the architecture of the native tissue microenvironment. Hydrogels are widely used in regenerative medicine due to the unique network that comprises this scaffold and the large volume of water found inside the structure that is similar to numerous tissues. It is important to note that the aim of such ELR-based scaffolds is to both replace damaged tissues and improve tissue regeneration.

Interchain cross-linking has been used to maintain the internal structure of hydrogel and been shown to have an important impact on the properties of the resulting materials and their applicability in regenerative medicine. Numerous physical and chemical cross-linking methods have been reported for the formation of gels. As mentioned in the introduction, this classification is based on the forces that maintain the structure of the hydrogels. In this sense, amphiphilic block copolymers spontaneously self-assemble to form physical hydrogels and can be cast into constructs with a controlled topography [24, 25]. However, some studies related to tissue engineering can require chemical cross-linking to achieve suitable properties for subsequent use in damaged tissues. A new technique reported recently enables the synthesis of hydrogels via a click chemistry reaction and in the absence of a catalyst [22]. This new methodology represents an important breakthrough for the application of these systems in regenerative medicine as guarantees the cytocompatibility of the product. Briefly, amine groups from lysine residues present in ELRs are chemically modified to have either azide or cyclooctyne groups. The mixing of these functionalized ELRs enables the formation of hydrogels by interchain click chemical cross-linking via the triazole ring formed by these two reactive groups.

Following this methodology, and in an attempt to improve the mechanical properties with an adequate porosity, new click elastin-like hydrogels with adjustable macropores were developed in order to promote cell adhesion, proliferation, and ECM formation within hydrogels. A combined technique known as salt-leaching coupled with gas foaming (SL/GL) was used [26, 27]. In brief, both components of the ELR were dissolved with a porogen with a desired particle size (e.g. $NaHCO_3$ particles). Hydrogels were subsequently immersed in warm acidic solution and the porogen particles leached, giving rise to CO_2 bubbles that provide a high interconnectivity between different pores (Figure 3.2). As a result, macroporous ELR hydrogels with tailored pore size and mechanical properties in the range of a targeted native tissue can be reproducibly obtained, thereby allowing cell migration and depositing ECM into these scaffolds. Furthermore, the swollen polymer network enhances the cell and protein junction and allows cell waste, nutrient, and oxygen exchange.

In order to enhance tissue specificity, the backbone of the ELRs can be modified to incorporate biological cues, namely cell adhesion domains (RGD or REDV), protease sequences or growth factors to help cell attachment and proliferation, ECM degradation, angiogenesis, or regeneration, thus providing an environment suitable for cell survival and adequate tissue growth. As an example, ELR-based hydrogels that can be degraded upon the deposition of ECM by the cells that adhere to and proliferate in these hydrogels have been developed. These hydrogels are based on ELRs bearing

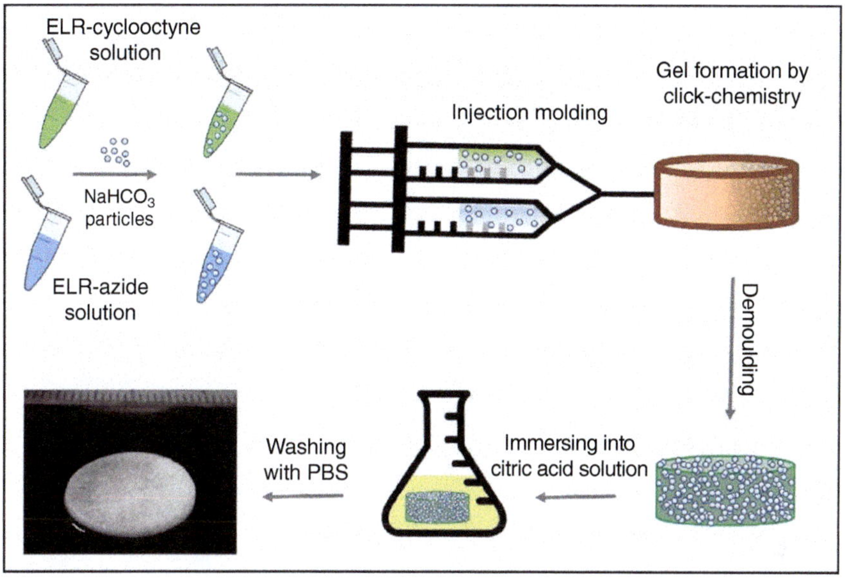

Figure 3.2 Sketch of the procedure followed to obtain the macroporous click–ELR hydrogels. Source: From Fernandez-Colino et al. [26]/Figure2/with permission from Elsevier.

active domains susceptible to cleavage by the enzymes tissue plasminogen activator (tPA) and urokinase plasminogen activator (uPA) in addition to RGD sequences. Their degradation was studied as a function of exposure time to high concentrations of tPA or uPA, and the results showed that the size of the polymer degradation fragments and their relative diffusion rates can be precisely controlled by changing the frequency and location of the protease-cleavable active domains within the protein backbone [28].

Similarly, degradable ELR hydrogels with different proteolytic cleavage kinetics and different network architectures have been constructed by chemical modification of the amine groups from the lysine residues present in ELRs with azide by aqueous diazo transfer, thereby enabling the formation of hydrogels by the bio-orthogonal strain-promoted azide-alkyne cycloaddition reaction (SPAAC). Multiarm PEG cross-linkers were used to control the initial network architecture. Different proteolytic cleavage kinetics was achieved by varying cross-linker functionality and endothelial network formation only occurred in hydrogels that underwent rapid bond cleavage and full disruption of the hydrogel architecture [29]. Another related study demonstrated that controlling the design of the 3D constructs could stimulate programmed cell infiltration via an inside-to-outside pattern (Figure 3.3). These hydrogels were based on ELRs in which two different proteolytic cleavage epitopes of uPA, namely GTAR and DRIR, with different kinetics and sensitivity, were added, in addition to RGD sequences. The degradation of click chemically cross-linked hydrogels was evaluated by measuring the elastic modulus as a function of the exposure time of hydrogels to high concentrations of uPA enzymes. The results showed fast response of the GTAR–ELR hydrogel,

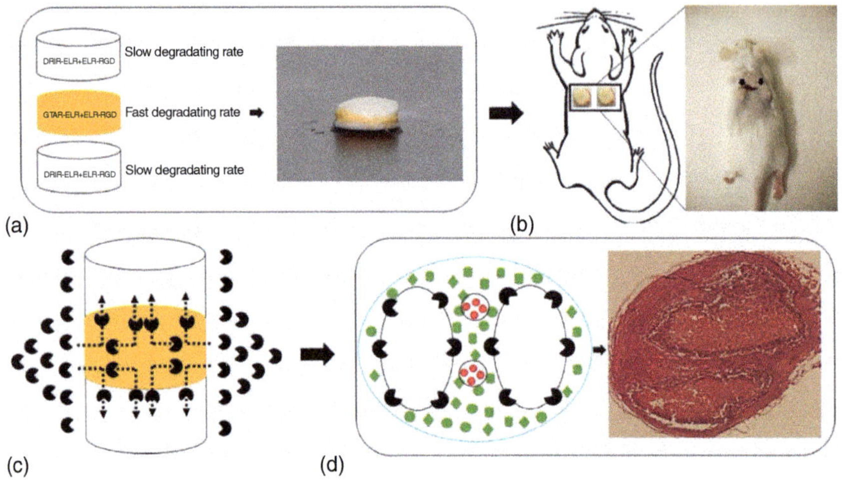

Figure 3.3 Representation of the 3D-structured system with pre-programmed cell invasion. (a) A sandwiched three-layer disc formed by two external layers with a slow degradation rate and a central layer that has a fast degradation rate. (b) This 3D structure was implanted subcutaneously into mice. (c) Cells (the black structures) invaded the central layer of the system first following an inside-to-outside pattern. (d) At six weeks postimplantation, the central layer of the 3D system was completely degraded, with the consequent formation of functional blood vessels (red circles). Source: (a, b, d) Flora et al. [30]/Figure 1a, b, d/with permission from IOPScience.

while DRIR–ELR hydrogels exhibited a slower degradation. A sandwich 3D model construct, with a central layer comprising proteolytic GTAR–ELR (fast degradation) and external layers of DRIR–ELR (slow degradation), allowed spatiotemporal control of cell infiltration when injected intramuscularly into mice. Spatial control was achieved as, on this occasion, the internal layer of the hydrogel was colonized first, following an inside–outside pattern, which contrasts with conventional devices. This behavior is especially important and could be implemented for specific types of tissue regeneration [30].

Although these ELR hydrogels have been widely used in regenerative medicine, in this chapter, we intend to focus on their applications in regeneration of musculoskeletal, cardiovascular, skin, and neural tissues.

3.2.1 Hydrogels in Musculoskeletal Tissue Regeneration

One of the main problems with articular cartilage regeneration is its limited ability to self-heal as a result of its avascularity, low cellularity, and the biomechanical requirements of the joint. ELR-based hydrogels have been used in musculoskeletal tissue regeneration due to their ability to provide structural support, stable mechanical properties, elasticity, and biocompatibility, which make them excellent candidates for this application. Given that wet articular cartilage contains a large quantity of water, the high water content of hydrogels makes them a promising scaffold for cartilage repair applications.

As an example, cytocompatible hydrogels have been prepared via oxidative chain extension of telechelic ELRs that toughen the protein network, thus leading to hard hydrated biomaterials. The introduction of cysteine residues near the N- and C-termini in the protein backbone permits chain extension via oxidative coupling of the thiol functional groups that form disulfide linkages. To enhance the regenerative power of these hydrogels, these ELRs were also endowed with two cell-adhesive RGD peptides genetically fused near the N- and C-termini of the ELR, one on each side. The osteochondral regeneration was demonstrated using human mesenchymal stem cells (hMSCs) and examining the viability and alkaline phosphatase activity associated with bone formation. Examination of the gels after 21 days showed a higher alkaline phosphatase activity in gels in comparison with the control (cells seeded on tissue culture plate in media lacking osteogenic molecules and osteoinductive media) as well as a higher expression of osteocalcin – a protein expressed during osteogenic differentiation and bone mineralization. These results suggested that chain-extended hydrogels are attractive for osteochondral tissue regeneration [31].

Targeting the same application, a new noncovalent bioactive ELR-like hydrogel was developed starting from a diblock copolymer ELR that has a hydrophilic block (containing glutamic acid with a carboxylic group) with a high Tt and a hydrophobic block (containing isoleucine as the guest residue) with a low Tt, as well as RGD cell adhesion sequences. An *in vivo* study in rabbits demonstrated that hydrogels with embedded hMSCs were able to fill the defect, adapting themselves to the surface of the lesion and, at three months posttreatment, the regenerated tissue was well integrated into the surrounding chondral tissue. The regeneration of the osteochondral defect was confirmed by the formation of hyaline cartilage with collagen type II, and the regenerated tissue exhibited excellent mechanical properties that allowed it to withstand high pressures [32].

Another type of injectable hydrogels that include the silk fibroin domain and an elastin domain in the backbone have been developed in order to understand how the gelation properties of hydrogels containing these two components in the same molecule could be improved. An amphiphilic silk-elastin-like corecombinamer (SELR) including two types of elastin-like domains, one hydrophobic and the other one hydrophilic, formed hydrogels. These polymers also contain RGD cell adhesion sequences, which promote specific cell attachment via integrins, thus providing a cell-friendly environment. Mature chondrocytes were embedded within SELR hydrogels in order to evaluate cartilage regeneration, considering that these hydrogels have an adequate interconnected structure, porosity, and permeability. An *ex vivo* bioreactor model was created in an attempt to mimic the cartilage environment. Immunohistochemistry and biochemical assays corroborated the presence of hyaline cartilage (collagen type II) and the absence of unwanted fibrocartilage (collagen type I); therefore, these hydrogels could be a promising candidate for medical regeneration [33].

Self-assembled bioactive ELR-like hydrogel combining two novel ELRs, one consisting of an osteogenic and osteoinductive agent (BMP-2, bone morphogenetic protein, 2) domains and the other containing the RGD cell adhesion motif, has been proposed for bone regeneration. Elastase-sensitive domains (VGVAPG) were also included in both ELRs to improve the enzymatic biodegradability of the biomaterial. A mixture of these two ELR-based polymers (ELR-E-RGD and ELR-E-BMP-2) leads to the formation of a BMP-2-loaded ECM-like hydrogel. For *in vivo* assessment, hMSCs were embedded within this injectable hydrogel and tested in a femoral bone injury of rabbits during three months after posttreatment. The results showed that BMP-2 stimulated osteoblast proliferation and the new formed bone had the same characteristics as normal bone, i.e. this BMP-2-loaded hydrogel has a good osteogenic potential to restore a bone defect. Moreover, scaffold biodegradation occurs concomitantly with bone regeneration, thereby avoiding the need to remove the scaffold after the regeneration [34].

Dynamic covalent chemistry (DCC) can be also applied for the hydrogels' development. The reaction between aldehyde-modified HA (HA-ALD) and hydrazine-modified ELR (ELR-HYD) lead to hydrazone formation and interchain covalent cross-linking. This type of covalent bond is able to form and break reversibly under equilibrium control and thus can be applied to generate tuneable hybrid elastin-like protein-hyaluronic acid (ELR-HA) hydrogels. To evaluate the potential of these hydrogels for cartilage regeneration, neonatal bovine chondrocytes were embedded inside ELP-HA hydrogels with different HA concentrations. The cell phenotype and neocartilage formation were analyzed three weeks postimplantation by studying gene expression (e.g. collagen type II, SOX9, or aggrecan, which are specific markers for chondrocytes), cell proliferation, quantitative biochemical assays (Picogreen, DMMB, and hydroxypoline), and histology. The results showed that a higher HA concentration leads to an increase in gene expression for cartilage-specific markers (collagen type II, SOX9, or aggrecan) and minimized undesirable fibrocartilage phenotype (collagen type I), thus proving that chondrocytes encapsulated within ELP-HA hydrogels induce satisfactory cartilage regeneration [35].

In another recent study, bioactive ELR-based hydrogels for osteochondral reparation were designed to contain two different cell adhesion sequences (RGD and REDV) and an elastase target domain (VGVAPG, human leukocyte elastase I). The hydrogel was formed by click chemical cross-linking, as described previously, by chemical modification of lysine residues to form azide and cyclooctyne groups, respectively, at the different ELR chains. Rabbit mesenchymal stromal cells (rMSCs) were embedded in the hydrogel and applied in an osteochondral lesion created in rabbits and regeneration was observed after four months. The regenerated tissue was integrated with the surrounding tissue, and collagen type I was not produced, thus indicating the absence of fibrocartilage and proving to be a promising system for osteochondral repair [36].

3.2.2 Hydrogels in Cardiovascular Tissue Regeneration

An important approach to enhance vascularization in scaffolds for tissue engineering involves the use of growth factors. Vascular endothelial growth factor (VEGF) is one of the most widely used growth factors for angiogenic processes [37].

Various techniques for loading growth factors within 3D biomaterials to promote biochemical cell signaling have been developed. A cell-compatible single-step synthesis for tethering peptides into the protein backbone of ELP hydrogels is one of the most interesting one. This technique allows a small angiogenic peptide (QK), which mimics the receptor-binding domain of VEGF, to be tethered to ELP hydrogels. The bioactivity of immobilized QK peptides within ELR hydrogels was studied using human umbilical vein endothelial cells (HUVECs). The results showed that an adequate density of QK in the ELR hydrogels enhanced HUVEC proliferation in comparison with cells cultured on ELR hydrogels alone, thus suggesting that QK retained its bioactivity after conjugation [38]. An increase in angiogenic ability was observed both *in vitro* and *in vivo* when using these hydrogels. These recombinamers also contained cell adhesion sequences such as REDV and RGD in their backbone, as well as a proteolytic site (VGVAPG), and it was found that the presence of QK increased capillary formation inside the hydrogels when using a coculture of endothelial and fibroblast cells. The presence of QK peptide inside the hydrogels did not affect their morphological and rheological properties but it did have an effect on cell behavior, inducing an increase in cell proliferation and the formation of endothelial cell clusters. *In vivo* studies demonstrated that QK peptide enhances the formation of prominent functional capillaries at three weeks postinjection [39].

Taking advantage of one of their most important features, namely elasticity, ELR-based hydrogels have been used in cardiovascular regeneration. For instance, metal stents embedded in catalyst-free click ELR hydrogels (ELR–CFCGs) have been developed. Some specific domains, namely cell adhesion sequences (RGD and REDV), were included in the ELRs in order to enhance endothelialization. The stents were embedded in ELR–CFCGs by injection molding, then placed in silicon tubes together with endothelial medium and HUVECs to study dynamic endothelialization. The RGD and REDV sequences induced good cell colonization of the material and the hydrogels exhibited good mechanical stability, as shown by rheological measurements. In addition, a thrombogenicity assay evidenced minimal platelet adhesion and fibrinogen adsorption on the surface of the ELR-embedded stents, thus indicating good hemocompatibility [40].

Tissue-engineered heart valves containing a hybrid component formed by fibrin and an ELR bearing cell adhesion sequences (RGD) have been developed in order to be used in different parts of the valve with the propose of enabling the spatially selective encapsulation of different cell lines, specifically ovine carotid arteries (OCA) and ovine umbilical arteries (OUA). Polymerization of the hybrid hydrogels (fibrinogen and HRGD6-ELR) was initiated using thrombin solution and $CaCl_2$. The valves were cultivated in a bioreactor system for two weeks statically and then for two weeks dynamically. The introduction of the ELR improves the biomechanical characteristics of the valve contributing to the elasticity of the wall and in the leaflets. The mixture of different materials in specific parts of the valves confers specific biomechanical characteristics on these devices, which is an important feature for the biomechanics of heart valves [41].

ELR tubular hydrogels reinforced with poly(lactic acid) nanofibers produced by electrospinning have been used to obtain vascular grafts in a new therapeutic strategy for the regeneration of small-diameter blood vessels. These hydrogels were designed to contain the hydrophobic amino acid sequence $(VPGIG)_n$ in order to mimic the elastic modulus of native tissue at a low-strain region and antithrombogenicity, and with RGD motifs in order to promote cell adhesion. The use of THPP (β-[tris(hydroxymethy)phosphino]propionic acid) as a chemical cross-linker was necessary to obtain these tubular hydrogels. The graft (ELR scaffold) was implanted into rat abdominal aortae for one month and the scaffold supported rapid tissue reconstruction, with no thrombogenicity. As such, these hydrogels could be a promising candidate for blood vessel regeneration [42].

In another strategy, ELR-based hydrogels containing cell adhesion sequences have been formed by click chemistry and used to encapsulate stromal vascular fraction (SVF) – heterogeneous human cells derived from autologous adipose tissue (including mesenchymal and endothelial progenitor cells) and potential tissue regenerative activity. SVF cells can differentiate into different cell types, support neovascularization, replace cells, repair injured tissue, and are able to generate microvessels *in vitro*. These hydrogels were implanted subcutaneously into the back of rats or in perfusion bioreactors in order to study the static and dynamic conditions required to promote vascularization in terms of endothelial cell organization. Although the hydrogels did not degrade, no inflammatory reaction was observed around the grafts. Angiogenesis and host integration of the engineered tissues were demonstrated in this study, thus confirming that these ELR hydrogels could be applied in vascular regeneration [43].

3.2.3 Hydrogels in Skin Tissue Regeneration

All organs and tissues with elastic and resilient properties contain elastin. These properties are coded by the sequence of five amino acids VPGVG. Surprisingly, very few studies have been published in the field of wound healing where the lack of scaffolds elasticity used to date leads to contracted tissues. Several elastin-based materials, such as synthetic tropoelastin, which contains hydrophilic and hydrophobic domains, ELRs, formed using synthetic strategies and recombinant DNA technologies, or an α-elastin-based hydrogel, which was obtained by oxalic acid hydrolysis of elastin, have been designed for wound healing applications. Focusing on ELRs, one of the most important features of recombinant materials is that they can incorporate bioactive sequences [44]. In this sense, various silk fibroin and elastin hydrogels have been proposed for burn treatments. These scaffolds were further cross-linked using genipin, which induced a conformational transition of silk fibroin chains from random coil to β-sheet. *In vitro* studies were then performed to evaluate the possibility that these hydrogels could release a drug, such as the antibacterial agent gentamicin, during the healing process. *In vivo* studies showed that the use of silk fibroin–elastin hydrogels in wounds induced keratinocyte and fibroblast migration from the margins to the wound bed, thus resulting in a completely closed wound covered with new epithelium [45].

Silk-elastin sponges for use in wound healing have been self-assembled from polypeptides with four silk-like blocks (GAGAGS), seven elastin-like blocks (GVGVP), and one modified elastin block containing a lysine substitution. When an aqueous solution of this silk-elastin is applied to a wound, it forms a hydrogel at body temperature and covers the wound due to the ITT of elastin polymers (thermosensitive). These sponges were tested in wounds in pigs (5 days) and in diabetic mice (14 days). The area of tissue formation, in the region where the silk-elastin sponge was placed, was significantly larger than for the control group, thus making this material a perfect candidate for skin regeneration [46].

3.2.4 Hydrogels in Neural Tissue Regeneration

It is very important to develop new materials for the treatment of brain injuries as neural tissue has a very poor regenerative ability. In this regard, a self-assembling peptide (SAP) hydrogel comprising the $RADA_{16}$ domain, a synthetic amphiphilic peptide that self-assembles into fibrils by forming stable beta-sheet structures, and enriched with the lamin-IKVAV motif, which could promote neuronal cell attachment, migration, and neurite spread, was developed. The resulting 3D self-assembled peptide network supports the proliferation and differentiation of neuronal stem cells (NSCs) into neural cells and is promising for repair of the central nervous system [47].

In order to study traumatic brain tissue injury, these scaffolds were tested in rats. A defect of 2 mm in the cortex was filled with $RADA_{16}$–IKVAV peptide hydrogels with and without encapsulated neural stem cells. At three weeks posttransplantation, it was observed that the $RADA_{16}$–IKVAV peptide hydrogel scaffold with NSCs enhance the neurogenic differentiation of implanted cells favoring neurogenesis and regenerating the brain neural tissue [48]. The self-assembling β-peptide hydrogel exhibited a higher stability than α-peptides. Moreover, the mechanical properties and injectability of the β-peptide hydrogel allow its implantation into the body with minimal surgical procedures: the hydrogel has exceptionally rapid and complete shape recovery within seconds. Its biocompatibility was assessed by seeding neuronal progenitor cells (SN4741). These cells attach, spread, and elongate on top of the hydrogels, thus making them a promising environment for the adhesion and proliferation of neuronal cells [49].

Degradable ELR hydrogels with bioactive domains (the integrin-binding RGD motif and protease degradation sites) were generated by cross-linking with an amine-reactive cross-linker, namely tetrakis(hydroxymethyl)phosphonium chloride (THPC). Hydrogel degradability was tuned by varying the network cross-linking density. Maintenance of NPC stemness in hydrogels requires matrix degradation as a new ECM is formed, once the cells are able to adhere and proliferate within these hydrogels. It was observed that NPC proliferation increases with increasing hydrogel degradability. The ability to differentiate into neurons and astrocytes was assessed by immunocytochemistry, and it was found that, in ELR hydrogels with high degradability, cells were able to spread and form cell–cell contacts to promote NPC stemness [50].

3.3 ELR-Based Hydrogels for Drug Delivery

As mentioned earlier, ELR-based hydrogels are promising candidates for the development of advanced drug delivery devices as these hydrogels allow controlled delivery of the therapeutic agent over time and in localized disease, thus decreasing the side effects and amount of drug required. One of the key characteristics of ELRs, namely their thermoresponsive nature, is of particular importance in drug delivery [51].

Among the different classifications of ELR-based framework, we can distinguish between two major groups of hydrogels, namely physically and chemically cross-linked hydrogels. In terms of hydrogel interactions with the drug, they can be classified as adsorbed, chemically bound, or fused to the hydrogel.

3.3.1 Physically Cross-Linked Hydrogels

Physically cross-linked ELR-based hydrogels form a continuous stable framework due to interchain noncovalent interactions predominantly involving hydrogen bonds, ionic interactions, van der Waals forces, or hydrophobic interactions. They are formed by self-gelation and are stable at physiological conditions: the ELR chains are in a random coil conformation (soluble and hydrated) below their Tt, whereas above this temperature a conformational change occurs in their secondary structure and they assemble to form a separate phase. As noted above, recombinant DNA technology allows ELRs to be designed with full control over the amino acid sequence. The ELRs designed to form hydrogels often possess an amphiphilic backbone containing both hydrophilic and hydrophobic blocks with a Tt that is above and below the physiological temperature, respectively. The solubility of the different ELR blocks at physiological conditions determines the formation of a hydrogel upon injection into the body. Consequently, this responsive behavior can be taken advantage for the treatment of diseases such as diabetes or cancer.

Diabetes mellitus type 2 is one of the most common chronic diseases in the world, and it is characterized by a high level of glucose in blood due to a lack of reaction of cells to the presence of insulin, i.e. the cells do not incorporate glucose. In 2015, the International Diabetes Federation estimated that 1 in 11 adults between 20 and 79 years old had diabetes mellitus. Current treatment for this disease is a change in diet and lifestyle and/or a frequent injection of insulin in the severe cases. A promising alternative for its treatment is a construct consisting in glucagon-like peptide 1 (GLP-1) fused to an ELR which formed a depot upon injection, acting as a long circulating carrier for glucose control. In this ELR, the GLP-1 was flanked by protease cleavage sites, giving rise to a so-called protease-operated depot (POD). This POD permitted a controlled release and overcomes the drawback of the short half-life of peptide drugs in a type 2 diabetes mouse model. A single injection of this POD reduced the blood glucose level in mice for up to five days [52, 53].

Recent work in this field includes another potential treatment for type 2 diabetes, which consists in the fusion of fibroblast growing factor 21 (FGF21), that is a metabolic regulator that enhances insulin sensitivity, to a thermally responsive

$[VPGVG]_{60}$ ELR. FGF21 is rapidly degraded *in vivo* and its fusion to ELR that coacervates at body temperature and forms a depot, significantly increases half-life of the growth factor (up to five days) reducing the frequency of injection [54]. Sometimes, diabetes can lead to vascular complications, which can result in mortality because of the progressive blood vessel damage [55]. In this regard, although proinsulin C-peptide is a potential drug against vascular diabetic complications, its efficacy is compromised because of the very short half-life of only about 30 minutes [56]. To overcome this problem, Jung et al. designed an ELR containing nine lysines fused to the C-peptide (K9-C-peptide), which showed a reversible thermal phase behavior and hydrogel formation under physiological conditions. This hydrogel was tested against different proteases and found to undergo slow degradation by blood-circulating proteases, thus resulting in a sustained release of C-peptide. One of the main consequences of chronic hyperglycemia is the vasculopathy caused by the apoptosis of human aortic endothelial cells (HAECs) due to the large quantities of intracellular reactive oxygen species (ROS) and the inhibition of transglutaminase 2 (TGase2), and K9-C-peptide has been shown to inhibit high glucose-induced intracellular ROS generation, TGase2 activation, and, therefore, apoptosis in HAECs [57].

Other strategies based on ELR hydrogels address treatment of complex diseases. According to the World Health Organization, cancer is the second leading cause of death, being responsible for one in six deaths globally and about 9.6 million deaths in 2018. The most common treatments for cancer are chemotherapy, surgery, and radiotherapy. Radiation therapy is widely used to treat tumors because of its limited side effects and comfort for the patient. Brachytherapy is a special type of radiotherapy consisting of the implantation of titanium seeds that encapsulate radioactive isotopes. One of the challenges that researchers are currently trying to overcome is to find a depot for the intratumoral administration of radiotracers to minimize the discomfort of current procedures that require significant surgical skills [58, 59]. A depot comprising ELR conjugated to ^{131}I has been developed to prevent release from the injection site and deiodination of the radiotracer [8]. Some of the advantages of this ELR–radionuclide depot are the low toxicity, high retention of the drug within the tumor for more than a week that causes a delay in the tumor growth, and survival of tumor-bearing mice.

Treatment of glioblastoma, the most common type of brain tumor, is complicated because of the high resistance to chemotherapy, high toxicity, and side effects in normal neural tissue, and the difficulty of most drugs to cross the blood–brain barrier (BBB), thus resulting in a low bioavailability of the drug. To increase the efficiency of glioblastoma treatment, Dragojevic et al. have developed a system comprising an ELR conjugated to a cell-penetrating peptide (CPP) and a doxorubicin-derived prodrug, which accumulates at tumor sites in response to externally applied hyperthermia generated by high-intensity focused ultrasound. This conjugate delivers doxorubicin to the cell cytoplasm and induces apoptosis, thus killing glioblastoma cells [60]. This system can also be used to deliver other small molecules that need to pass the BBB.

Ocular drug delivery is one of the most difficult routes of drug administration due to the different barriers that the eye presents, together with the constant lacrimal turnover and the high water content. Dry eye disease (DED) is one of the most common ocular diseases, affecting between 5% and 35% of the global population [61]. This condition arises due to a chronic lack of moisture at the eye surface and is commonly treated with artificial tear solutions. An alternative therapy for this disease involves administration of the regulatory human tear protein lacritin [62]. To increase the retention time of lacritin at the ocular surface, a lacritin–ELR fusion protein was developed. This fusion protein was able to form a depot upon intralacrimal gland injection and showed an ability to promote secretion in specific lacrimal gland cells. Moreover, *in vivo* studies demonstrated its ability to stimulate tear secretion, and local retention was enhanced sixfold when compared to the soluble drug [63].

One of the unsolved problems in burn patients concerns the exposure, and subsequent infection, in the nosocomial structures. An interesting approach to improve recovery and wound healing involves the antibiotic-loaded ELR hydrogels, which can enhance local concentrations of the drug while acting as a scaffold for wound repair. One example of this approach is the hydrogel developed by Amruthwar and Janorkar, which was obtained by ultrasonication of the $[VPGVG]_{120}$ ELR and exhibited controlled release of a model protein (bovine serum albumin [BSA]) and an antibiotic (doxycycline) [64]. Subsequently, and along similar lines, these authors found that ELR-based hydrogels show a higher elastic modulus than collagen hydrogels. The latter are traditionally employed for wound healing (Chapter 2) but do not show sufficient rigidity and resistance to collagenases [65]. To fulfill the requirements for an ideal scaffold, and following previous studies from the Chaikof group [66, 67], Anderson et al. developed a new composite based on the same ELR $[VPGVG]_{120}$ mixed with a collagen solution and loaded with doxycycline hyclate. Secondary bonding between the ELR and collagen resulted in a smaller swelling ratio compared to collagen hydrogels, thus leading to slower release of the drug. The ELR–collagen composite showed a more gradual release profile and higher antibacterial activity against *Escherichia coli*, *Pseudomonas aeruginosa*, *Streptococcus sanguinis*, and *Staphylococcus aureus* than collagen hydrogels [68]. Recently, this hydrogel was loaded with human bone morphogenetic protein-2 (rhBMP-2) and doxycycline to provide antimicrobial activity and trigger osteogenesis in bone regeneration. In that study, hydrogels with the same composition but different cross-linkings (physical or chemical) were compared, and the authors concluded that there is no significant difference between their mechanical properties, release rate, or bioactivity, thus meaning that the need to use potentially toxic chemical compounds as cross-linkers can be avoided in future studies [69].

Another approach for the construction of physically cross-linked hydrogels is the addition of motifs other than elastin in the sequence. For example, the addition of certain silk fibroin domains of *B. mori* (GAGAGS) to enhance the stability of the ELR gives rise to SELRs. The elastin motifs in SELRs define the cross-linking density and the silk motifs provide mechanical stiffness to the hydrogels [14]. Different SELRs have been created by varying the silk to elastin ratio [70], molecular weight [71], and guest residue (X) in the $(VPGXG)_n$ which determines the elastin sequence [72]. It has been found that gelation is faster for SELRs with increasing silk domains. The higher thermal and chemical stability of SELRs arises from the antiparallel beta-sheet structure in which they tend to self-assemble. This secondary structure provides sites for physical cross-linking, thereby increasing stability in aqueous media and lowering the gelation concentration [73].

SELRs have been exploited in the fields of drug and gene delivery, with the first studies of SELRs for controlled release of active compounds being carried out in the early 2000s. In this study, SELP-47K, which includes four silk units and seven elastin units, one of them with a lysine (K) as guest residue, was constructed. Hydrogels based on this recombinamer were used to deliver and release plasmid DNA. Further work included the *in vitro* and *in vivo* assay of this hydrogel bearing an adenovirus containing green fluorescent protein (GFP) for cancer gene therapy, which was observed to be functional *in vitro* for 28 days, with a high transfection efficiency within the tumor *in vivo* (one to threefold higher than naked DNA) [71].

Different polymers have been assayed for gene therapy, including SELP-815K (eight silk units and seven elastin units, one of them with a lysine (K) as a guest residue), which showed higher gene expression compared to SELP-415K and SELP-47K. It also showed a higher expression in tumors than in nontarget organs such as the liver, thus making it an excellent candidate for gene therapy in head and neck cancer [70]. In subsequent studies, this hydrogel was loaded with an adenovirus containing thymidine kinase 1 to check the efficacy of tumor therapy in conjunction with intraperitoneal ganciclovir and showed an anticancer effect, reducing tumor size with higher adenovirus doses [74]. The high stability of SELRs can become a drawback when faster degradation rates are needed. To overcome this problem, matrix metalloproteinase (MMP) recognition sites were introduced in the SELRs backbone [75]. Degradation of these hydrogels can be controlled by the expression of MMPs, which are overexpressed in different tumors [76]. These hydrogels were tested *in vivo* and showed high efficiency, increasing survival from 29% to 100% over 50 days in a xenograft mouse model of head and neck squamous cell carcinoma [77].

More recent studies include use of these SELP-815K and SELP-47K by taking advantage of their positive charges, which make them able to retain anti-inflammatory and analgesic glycosaminoglycans (GAG) for the treatment of interstitial cystitis or painful bladder syndrome. These SELRs provided a higher delivery rate in comparison with PLGA–PEG–PLGA and Poloxamer 407, other formulations employed for intravesical drug delivery. The SELRs provided a sustained analgesic effect that lasted 24 hours after administration and reduced inflammation [78]. GAG delivery has also been reported for the prophylactic treatment of radiation-induced proctitis using SELP-815K. These hydrogels enhanced the accumulation of GAG in the rectum, thus enhancing therapeutic efficacy and reducing pain in mice [79].

The mucosa is a tissue that covers the outer surfaces of organs, i.e. the surfaces which are in contact with the exterior. As such, the mucosa plays a very important role in regulating the flow of substances such as nutrients, but also acts as a defensive barrier. *Mucosae* are protected by a mucus layer that covers the epithelial cells, thereby contributing to their barrier function but complicating interaction with them, thus making them a particularly challenging target for drug delivery. For this purpose, a mucoadhesive ELR based on self-gelling thermorresponsive blocks that included a domain for interacting with the mucous layer was designed. The mucin-interacting region comprised 144 repetitions of the pentapeptide (VPGKG), which permits electrostatic interactions between the positively charged lysines and the negatively charged mucins. Moreover, the sequence included a hepta peptide – the "T7" peptide – which binds to the transmembrane transferrin receptor present in the gastrointestinal tract (GIT). The authors of this study reported that the T7-ELR molecule enhances interaction in an intestinal endothelium model up to fourfold, without negatively affecting the biocompatibility. In *in vivo* assays, T7-ELR was able to resist the flushing effect of food and remained attached to the walls of the GIT [80].

As stated above, ocular drug delivery is one of the most difficult drug administration routes. As such, Fernández-Colino et al. developed two different recombinamers, namely $[EIS]_2$ and $[EI]_2$, based on the same elastin-like blocks but with and without silk domains, respectively, for timolol maleate delivery against glaucoma. The silk-containing recombinamer showed a strong and irreversible physical interaction, thus resulting in slower release and higher stability and increasing the residence time of the formulation on the eye surface [81].

3.3.2 Chemically Cross-Linked Hydrogels

Covalent bonds between polymer chains are often required to increase the structural stability and mechanical properties of hydrogels. Indeed, different types of chemical cross-linkages have been used to obtain stronger hydrogels. Depending on the used cross-linking strategy, we can distinguish hydrogels formed by high-energy radiation, by chemical reaction of complementary groups, by radical polymerization, and by enzymatic cross-linking.

ELR hydrogels obtained by chemical cross-linkage have been developed for cancer treatment, more specifically to improve brachytherapy application. The material developed for this purpose comprised ELR micelles whose sequence included seven tyrosine subunits $(VPGVG)_{120}(GY)_7$. The micelles were labeled with ^{131}I and formed an *in situ* hydrogel stabilized in two different manners: first, body temperature permitted a fast phase transition of the micelles to form a physically stabilized coacervate; second, the high-energy β emissions of ^{131}I induced the tyrosine-mediated covalent cross-linking that stabilizes the depot. This hydrogel was injected intratumorally and evaluated by comparison of its effect in two orthotopic tumors, namely prostate and pancreatic cancer, in mice. The hydrogel was highly effective, especially for prostate cancer, with over 95% tumor regression and full remission after a 60-day observation period [82].

Chemical cross-linking of hydrogels is often based on the modification of lysines with complementary groups that can give rise to a covalent bond [83]. The sequence $VPGKG(VPGVG)_{16}$-102 was chosen to develop chemically cross-linked hydrogels for intra-articular delivery. β-[Tris(hydroxymethyl)phosphine]propionic acid

(THCC) was utilized as a cross-linker to permit reaction between different lysine residues, and the hydrogels were loaded with Interleunkin-1 (IL-1) and tumor necrosis factor α (TNF-α) inhibitors as a therapy for post-traumatic arthritis, then injected intra-articularly into mice with an articular fracture [84]. Interleukin 1 receptor antagonist (IL-1Ra) and soluble tumor necrosis factor receptor II (sTN-FRII) (U.S. Food and Drug Administration [FDA] approved drugs for rheumatoid arthritis treatment) were detectable in serum for five days after intra-articular injection, and their different molecular weights (17.3 and 150 kDa, respectively) show that a wide range of molecules could be encapsulated for different purposes.

The enzymatically cross-linked hydrogel HELP (human elastin-like polypeptide), developed by Bandiera et al., is based on the most commonly repeated motif in human elastin, namely the hexapeptide VAPGVG, which has an additional alanine that confers a more rigid structure. These authors developed two different hydrogels, HELP (based on the VAPGVG hexapeptides and a cross-linking domain) and HELP1 (with only VAPGVG hexapeptides) [85]. The HELP hydrogel was formed by enzymatic cross-linking with microbial transglutaminase (mTGase) and loaded with eGFP before gelation. The authors wanted to verify whether this hydrogel was able to release the drug in response of the elastolytic activity (associated with many diseases), which they expected because HELP resembles tropoelastin [86]. As such, they treated the hydrogel with different biological systems exhibiting this activity to determine enzymatic degradation of the hydrogel and discovered that the main targets were cross-linking domains, thus permitting release of the active compound and making this hydrogel a promising drug delivery system.

The enzymatically cross-linked hydrogel developed by Dash et al., who created a dual gene delivery system for the treatment of critical limb ischemia (CLI), is also of interest. CLI is an obstruction of arteries that reduces blood flow to the limbs and can lead to amputation. A new gene delivery strategy for treating this condition includes the delivery of proangiogenic compounds to promote angiogenesis within ischemic limbs [87, 88]. The injectable ELR-in-ELR dual delivery system comprised hollow ELR spheres loaded with endothelial nitric oxide synthase (eNOS) plasmid, embedded in an Interleukin-10 (IL-10) plasmid-loaded ELR hydrogel. This hydrogel was formed using mTGase as a cross-linker. The system showed controlled release of the two genes in time and space, thereby reducing inflammation and increasing angiogenesis in both subcutaneous and ischemic mouse models [89].

cELPs, ELRs that include periodic cysteine residues in their structure that permit the formation of reversible disulfide bonds are a special family of hydrogels. These cELPs are halfway between coacervates and chemically cross-linked hydrogels and therefore provide characteristics from both of them, such as intermediate clearance and degradation rates and interesting mechanical properties while avoiding the use of potentially toxic cross-linkers. The cross-linking sites can be tuned by varying the ELR sequence at the genetic level to add cysteine residues, and these sites can also be used to fuse therapeutic proteins or peptides. The hydrgels were prepared by co-injection of cELRs with oxygen peroxide and loaded with either BSA, as a model protein to study release kinetics or with radionuclides for tumor treatment, exhibiting a higher radionuclide retention than previously tested materials

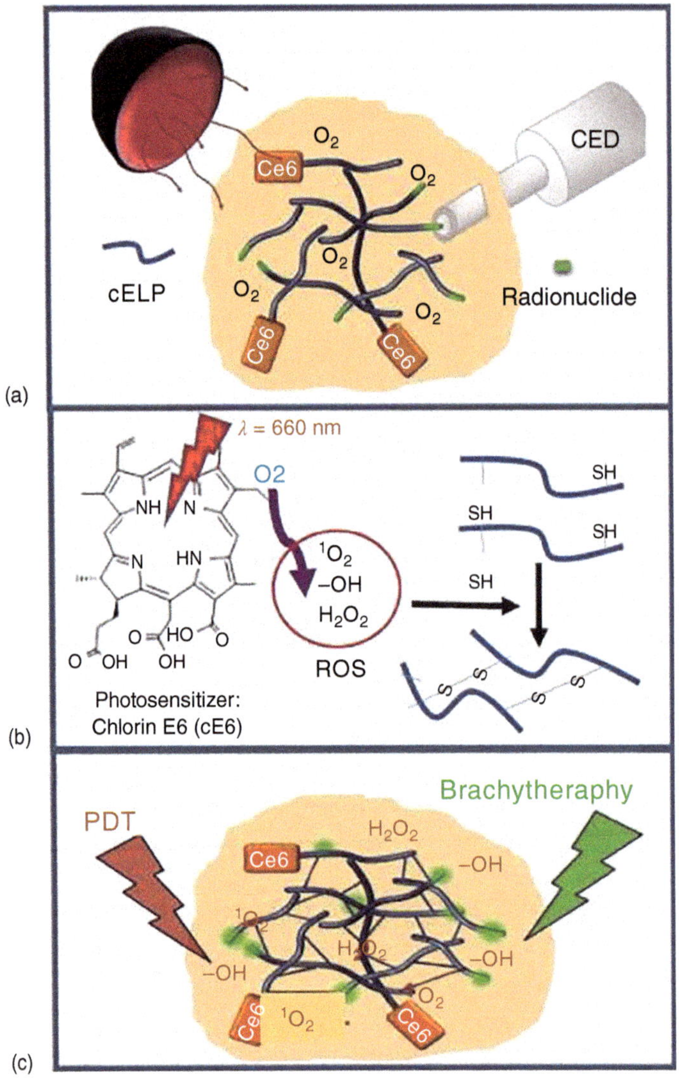

Figure 3.4 Schematic overview of the approach for the development of PRCITD. (a) Soluble cELP loaded with photosensitizer and radionuclide freely distribute in tumor driven by CED (convection enhanced delivery). (b) Photoradiation-generated ROS initiate cELP cross-linking to stabilize the delivery depot; (c) PRCITD simultaneously delivers Ce6 and radionuclide for combination therapy. Source: From Mukerji et al. [92]/with permission of Elsevier.

[90]. Another method for synthesizing cELPs gels involves exposure to ultraviolet (UV) light, which allows formation of a disulfide bond between the thiol groups of the cysteines [91]. These gels show a wide range of applications, such as carriers for brachytherapy [92], antiretroviral therapy [93], or next-generation vaccines [94].

Mukerji et al. have developed photoradiation-controlled intratumoral depots (PRCITD) (Figure 3.4). These involve conjugating ^{125}I-labeled cELPs to a photosensitizer, which produces singlet oxygen molecules when exposed to

660 nm light. These ROS have a double task: they provide an oxidative surrounding that permits cross-linking of the cELPs, and they kill surrounding cells when accumulated in a tumor. When injected intratumorally, convection-enhanced delivery drives the conjugate to diffuse through the tumor. After achieving the desired coverage, 660 nm light is applied and a stable therapeutic depot is formed. These novel hydrogels showed a high stability in subcutaneous tumors and improved retention when compared to controls with no cross-linking [92]. Consequently, different radionuclides and chemotherapeutic rates could be loaded into these hydrogels to treat different types of tumors.

As a proof of concept for antiretroviral therapy, cELPs have been loaded with enfuvirtide, an antiretroviral fusion inhibitor peptide approved by the FDA for the treatment of HIV and mixed with hydrogen peroxide to trigger cross-linking. The mixture was then injected subcutaneously and found to provide controlled release over several hours. One of the main advantages of this system is the increased half-life of the peptide drug in blood of up to eight hours, compared to the naked peptide, which has a half-life of around two hours, thus avoiding the need for regular injections to maintain an effective blood concentration [93]. These hydrogels can be adapted to deliver anti-HIV peptides other than enfuvirtide.

cELPs reportedly show little or no immunogenicity and can be used as a depot for the controlled release of antigen formulations. In this system, tetanus toxoid (Ttd) is mixed with cELPs and hydrogen peroxide and injected subcutaneously to form a depot, which slowly and spontaneously degrades *in vivo*, thus releasing Ttd into the circulation. These processes result in high antibody production, which is an important step toward the design of next-generation vaccines [94].

As stated above, hydrogels can be classified either as physically or chemically cross-linked, although some gels are difficult to classify within these categories. For example, the Heilshorn group recently developed an innovative manner for manufacturing a microstructured ELR hydrogel that permits the controlled release of drugs with different hydrophilicities encapsulated within the same hydrogel [95]. This structure is accomplished by tuning the timing of the chemical cross-linking and physical self-assembly processes during gelation, thus allowing a sequential release that may prove to be very useful for diseases involving complicated signaling pathways (Figure 3.5).

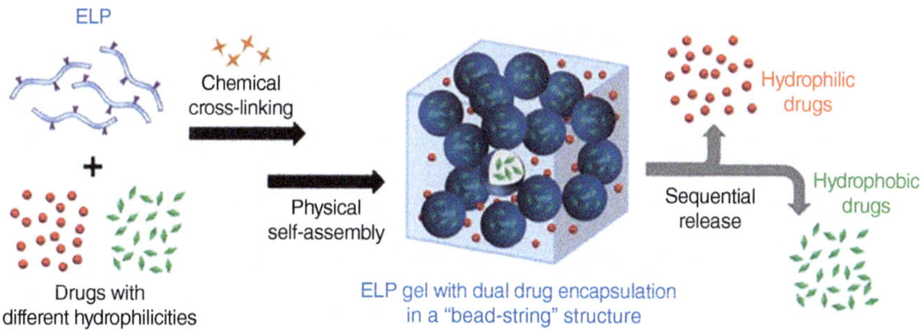

Figure 3.5 Simple, one-pot formation of microstructured ELR hydrogel for dual encapsulation and sequential release of hydrophilic and hydrophobic drugs. Source: From Wang et al. [95]/with permission from American Chemical Society.

3.4 Future Remarks

The prevalent or more suitable matrices for tissue engineering are hydrogels, being the use of proteinaceous biomaterials on the rise. ELRs hydrogels obtained via physical or chemical cross-linking represent advanced systems for applications in the biomedical field. As we have reviewed, these types of ELRs hydrogels have been applied in the most challenging regenerative medicine applications as tissue engineering and as advanced drug delivery devices. We have highlighted their use as scaffolds mimicking ECM suitable for musculoskeletal, cardiovascular, skin, and neural tissue regeneration proving to be good candidates in tissue engineering. They are promising scaffolds to restore the defects achieving satisfactory tissue regeneration becoming future research in *in vivo* experiments. As advanced drug delivery devices, they have proved to be promising systems for diseases such as type 2 diabetes, glaucoma, or ischemia; and an especial focus on cancer therapy has shown their efficacy as they lower the drug concentration in therapy, allow a great versatility in the drugs embedded, and release them at a controlled rate and at the right site. Moreover, the investigations about ELRs are increasing in the last decades, and new designs will lead, given their tuneable nature, to unexplored applications, opening doors to their translation into clinic.

References

1 Engebretson, B. and Sikavitsas, V.I. (2012). Long-term in vivo effect of PEG bone tissue engineering scaffolds. *J. Long-Term Eff. Med. Implants* 22 (3): 211–218.

2 Roberts, J. and Martens, P. (2016). Engineering biosynthetic cell encapsulation systems. In: *Biosynthetic Polymers for Medical Applications* (ed. L. Poole-Warren, P. Martens and R. Green), 205–239. Elsevier.

3 Hoffman, A.S. (2012). Hydrogels for biomedical applications. *Adv. Drug Delivery Rev.* 64: 18–23.

4 Rey, D.F.V. and St-Pierre, J.-P. (2019). Fabrication techniques of tissue engineering scaffolds. In: *Handbook of Tissue Engineering Scaffolds: Volume One* (ed. M. Mozafari, F. Sefat and A. Atala), 109–125. Elsevier.

5 Cabello, J.R., De Torre, I., Cipriani, F., and Poocza, L. (2018). Elastin-like materials for tissue regeneration and repair. In: *Peptides and Proteins as Biomaterials for Tissue Regeneration and Repair* (ed. M.A. Barbosa and M.C.L. Martins), 309–327. Elsevier.

6 Chen, J. and Zou, X. (2019). Self-assemble peptide biomaterials and their biomedical applications. *Bioact. Mater.* 4: 120–131.

7 Ibáñez-Fonseca, A., Flora, T., Acosta, S., and Rodríguez-Cabello, J.C. (2019). Trends in the design and use of elastin-like recombinamers as biomaterials. *Matrix Biol.* 84: 111–126.

8 Liu, W., MacKay, J.A., Dreher, M.R. et al. (2010). Injectable intratumoral depot of thermally responsive polypeptide–radionuclide conjugates delays tumor progression in a mouse model. *J. Controlled Release* 144 (1): 2–9.

9 Liu, W., Mukerji, R., Li, X. et al. (2014). In situ photocontrolled intratumoral depot for combined photodynamic therapy and brachytherapy for solid tumor. *Cancer Res.* 74 (19), Supplement (proceedings AACR Annual Meeting), Abstract nr. 4583. https://doi.org/10.1158/1538-7445.AM2014-4583.

10 Debelle, L., Alix, A.J., Wei, S.M. et al. (1998). The secondary structure and architecture of human elastin. *Eur. J. Biochem.* 258 (2): 533–539.

11 Urry, D.W. (1993). Molecular machines: how motion and other functions of living organisms can result from reversible chemical changes. *Angew. Chem. Int. Ed. Engl.* 32 (6): 819–841.

12 Rodríguez-Cabello, J.C., Martín, L., Girotti, A. et al. (2011). Emerging applications of multifunctional elastin-like recombinamers. *Nanomedicine* 6 (1): 111–122.

13 Girotti, A., Fernández-Colino, A., López, I.M. et al. (2011). Elastin-like recombinamers: biosynthetic strategies and biotechnological applications. *Biotechnol. J.* 6 (10): 1174–1186.

14 Dandu, R., Von Cresce, A., Briber, R. et al. (2009). Silk–elastinlike protein polymer hydrogels: influence of monomer sequence on physicochemical properties. *Polymer* 50 (2): 366–374.

15 Ifkovits, J.L. and Burdick, J.A. (2007). Photopolymerizable and degradable biomaterials for tissue engineering applications. *Tissue Eng.* 13 (10): 2369–2385.

16 Martino, M. and Tamburro, A. (2001). Chemical synthesis of cross-linked poly (KGGVG), an elastin-like biopolymer. *Biopolymers* 59 (1): 29–37.

17 Huang, L., McMillan, R.A., Apkarian, R.P. et al. (2000). Generation of synthetic elastin-mimetic small diameter fibers and fiber networks. *Macromolecules* 33 (8): 2989–2997.

18 Wissink, M., Beernink, R., Pieper, J. et al. (2001). Immobilization of heparin to EDC/NHS-crosslinked collagen. Characterization and in vitro evaluation. *Biomaterials* 22 (2): 151–163.

19 McHale, M.K., Setton, L.A., and Chilkoti, A. (2005). Synthesis and in vitro evaluation of enzymatically cross-linked elastin-like polypeptide gels for cartilaginous tissue repair. *Tissue Eng.* 11 (11, 12): 1768–1779.

20 Annabi, N., Mithieux, S.M., Zorlutuna, P. et al. (2013). Engineered cell-laden human protein-based elastomer. *Biomaterials* 34 (22): 5496–5505.

21 Gaharwar, A.K., Rivera, C., Wu, C.-J. et al. (2013). Photocross linked nanocomposite hydrogels from PEG and silica nanospheres: structural, mechanical and cell adhesion characteristics. *Mater. Sci. Eng. C* 33 (3): 1800–1807.

22 de Torre, I.G., Santos, M., Quintanilla, L. et al. (2014). Elastin-like recombinamer catalyst-free click gels: characterization of poroelastic and intrinsic viscoelastic properties. *Acta Biomater.* 10 (6): 2495–2505.

23 Testera, A.M., Girotti, A., de Torre, I.G. et al. (2015). Biocompatible elastin-like click gels: design, synthesis and characterization. *J. Mater. Sci. Mater. Med.* 26 (2): 105.

24 Martín, L., Alonso, M., Möller, M. et al. (2009). 3D microstructuring of smart bioactive hydrogels based on recombinant elastin-like polymers. *Soft Matter* 5 (8): 1591–1593.

25 Martín, L., Arias, F.J., Alonso, M. et al. (2010). Rapid micropatterning by temperature-triggered reversible gelation of a recombinant smart elastin-like tetrablock-copolymer. *Soft Matter* 6 (6): 1121–1124.

26 Fernandez-Colino, A., Wolf, F., Keijdener, H. et al. (2018). Macroporous click-elastin-like hydrogels for tissue engineering applications. *Mater. Sci. Eng. C* 88: 140–147.

27 Martín, L., Alonso, M., Girotti, A. et al. (2009). Synthesis and characterization of macroporous thermosensitive hydrogels from recombinant elastin-like polymers. *Biomacromolecules* 10 (11): 3015–3022.

28 Straley, K.S. and Heilshorn, S.C. (2009). Dynamic, 3D-pattern formation within enzyme-responsive hydrogels. *Adv. Mater.* 21 (41): 4148–4152.

29 Madl, C.M., Katz, L.M., and Heilshorn, S.C. (2018). Tuning bulk hydrogel degradation by simultaneous control of proteolytic cleavage kinetics and hydrogel network architecture. *ACS Macro Lett.* 7 (11): 1302–1307.

30 Flora, T., de Torre, I.G., Alonso, M., and Rodríguez-Cabello, J.C. (2019). Use of proteolytic sequences with different cleavage kinetics as a way to generate hydrogels with preprogrammed cell-infiltration patterns imparted over their given 3D spatial structure. *Biofabrication* 11 (3): 035008.

31 Glassman, M.J., Avery, R.K., Khademhosseini, A., and Olsen, B.D. (2016). Toughening of thermoresponsive arrested networks of elastin-like polypeptides to engineer cytocompatible tissue scaffolds. *Biomacromolecules* 17 (2): 415–426.

32 Pescador, D., Ibáñez-Fonseca, A., Sánchez-Guijo, F. et al. (2017). Regeneration of hyaline cartilage promoted by xenogeneic mesenchymal stromal cells embedded within elastin-like recombinamer-based bioactive hydrogels. *J. Mater. Sci. Mater. Med.* 28 (8): 115.

33 Cipriani, F., Krüger, M., De Torre, I.G. et al. (2018). Cartilage regeneration in preannealed silk elastin-like co-recombinamers injectable hydrogel embedded with mature chondrocytes in an ex vivo culture platform. *Biomacromolecules* 19 (11): 4333–4347.

34 Coletta, D.J., Ibáñez-Fonseca, A., Missana, L.R. et al. (2017). Bone regeneration mediated by a bioactive and biodegradable extracellular matrix-like hydrogel based on elastin-like recombinamers. *Tissue Eng. A* 23 (23, 24): 1361–1371.

35 Zhu, D., Wang, H., Trinh, P. et al. (2017). Elastin-like protein-hyaluronic acid (ELP-HA) hydrogels with decoupled mechanical and biochemical cues for cartilage regeneration. *Biomaterials* 127: 132–140.

36 Cipriani, F., Ariño Palao, B., Gonzalez de Torre, I. et al. (2019). An elastin-like recombinamer-based bioactive hydrogel embedded with mesenchymal stromal cells as an injectable scaffold for osteochondral repair. *Regen. Biomater.* 6: 335–347.

37 Hoeben, A., Landuyt, B., Highley, M.S. et al. (2004). Vascular endothelial growth factor and angiogenesis. *Pharmacol. Rev.* 56 (4): 549–580.

38 Cai, L., Dinh, C.B., and Heilshorn, S.C. (2014). One-pot synthesis of elastin-like polypeptide hydrogels with grafted VEGF-mimetic peptides. *Biomater. Sci.* 2 (5): 757–765.

39 Flora, T., de Torre, I.G., Alonso, M., and Rodríguez-Cabello, J.C. (2019). Tethering QK peptide to enhance angiogenesis in elastin-like recombinamer (ELR) hydrogels. *J. Mater. Sci. Mater. Med.* 30 (2): 30.

40 de Torre, I.G., Wolf, F., Santos, M. et al. (2015). Elastin-like recombinamer-covered stents: towards a fully biocompatible and non-thrombogenic device for cardiovascular diseases. *Acta Biomater.* 12: 146–155.

41 Weber, M., Gonzalez de Torre, I., Moreira, R. et al. (2015). et al, Multiple-step injection molding for fibrin-based tissue-engineered heart valves. *Tissue Eng. Part C Methods* 21 (8): 832–840.

42 Mahara, A., Kiick, K.L., and Yamaoka, T. (2017). In vivo guided vascular regeneration with a non-porous elastin-like polypeptide hydrogel tubular scaffold. *J. Biomed. Mater. Res. A* 105 (6): 1746–1755.

43 Staubli, S.M., Cerino, G., De Torre, I.G. et al. (2017). Control of angiogenesis and host response by modulating the cell adhesion properties of an elastin-like recombinamer-based hydrogel. *Biomaterials* 135: 30–41.

44 Rodríguez-Cabello, J.C., de Torre, I.G., Ibañez-Fonseca, A., and Alonso, M. (2018). Bioactive scaffolds based on elastin-like materials for wound healing. *Adv. Drug Delivery Rev.* 129: 118–133.

45 Vasconcelos, A., Gomes, A.C., and Cavaco-Paulo, A. (2012). Novel silk fibroin/elastin wound dressings. *Acta Biomater.* 8 (8): 3049–3060.

46 Kawabata, S., Kawai, K., Somamoto, S. et al. (2017). The development of a novel wound healing material, silk-elastin sponge. *J. Biomater. Sci. Polym. Ed.* 28 (18): 2143–2153.

47 Yanlian, Y., Ulung, K., Xiumei, W. et al. (2009). Designer self-assembling peptide nanomaterials. *Nano Today* 4 (2): 193–210.

48 Cheng, T.-Y., Chen, M.-H., Chang, W.-H. et al. (2013). Neural stem cells encapsulated in a functionalized self-assembling peptide hydrogel for brain tissue engineering. *Biomaterials* 34 (8): 2005–2016.

49 Motamed, S., Del Borgo, M., Kulkarni, K. et al. (2016). A self-assembling β-peptide hydrogel for neural tissue engineering. *Soft Matter* 12 (8): 2243–2246.

50 Madl, C.M., LeSavage, B.L., Dewi, R.E. et al. (2017). Maintenance of neural progenitor cell stemness in 3D hydrogels requires matrix remodelling. *Nat. Mater.* 16 (12): 1233.

51 Urry, D.W. (2007). *What Sustains Life?: Consilient Mechanisms for Protein-Based Machines and Materials*. Springer Science & Business Media.

52 Amiram, M., Luginbuhl, K., Li, X. et al. (2013). A depot-forming glucagon-like peptide-1 fusion protein reduces blood glucose for five days with a single injection. *J. Controlled Release* 172 (1): 144–151.

53 Amiram, M., Luginbuhl, K.M., Li, X. et al. (2013). Injectable protease-operated depots of glucagon-like peptide-1 provide extended and tunable glucose control. *Proc. Natl. Acad. Sci. U.S.A.* 110 (8): 2792–2797.

54 Gilroy, C.A., Roberts, S., and Chilkoti, A. (2018). Fusion of fibroblast growth factor 21 to a thermally responsive biopolymer forms an injectable depot with sustained anti-diabetic action. *J. Controlled Release* 277: 154–164.

55 Bhatt, M.P., Lim, Y.-C., and Ha, K.-S. (2014). C-peptide replacement therapy as an emerging strategy for preventing diabetic vasculopathy. *Cardiovasc. Res.* 104 (2): 234–244.

56 Ashby, J.P. and Frier, B.M. (1981). Circulating C-peptide: measurement and clinical application. *Ann. Clin. Biochem.* 18 (3): 125–130.

57 Jung, S.H., Lee, J.Y., Lee, S.H. et al. (2019). Preventive effects of thermosensitive biopolymer-conjugated C-peptide against high glucose-induced endothelial cell dysfunction. *Macromol. Biosci.* 19: 1900129.

58 Bhanabhai, H. and Samant, R. (2013). Pain assessment during conscious sedation for cervical cancer high-dose-rate brachytherapy. *Curr. Oncol.* 20 (4): e307.

59 Holm, H., Juul, N., Pedersen, J. et al. (1983). Transperineal ^{125}iodine seed implantation in prostatic cancer guided by transrectal ultrasonography. *J. Urol.* 130 (2): 283–286.

60 Dragojevic, S., Mackey, R., and Raucher, D. (2019). Evaluation of elastin-like polypeptides for tumor targeted delivery of doxorubicin to glioblastoma. *Molecules* 24 (18): 3242.

61 Friedman, N.J. (2010). Impact of dry eye disease and treatment on quality of life. *Curr. Opin. Ophthalmol.* 21 (4): 310–316.

62 Vijmasi, T., Chen, F.Y., Balasubbu, S. et al. (2014). Topical administration of lacritin is a novel therapy for aqueous-deficient dry eye disease. *Invest. Ophthalmol. Vis. Sci.* 55 (8): 5401–5409.

63 Wang, W., Jashnani, A., Aluri, S.R. et al. (2015). A thermo-responsive protein treatment for dry eyes. *J. Controlled Release* 199: 156–167.

64 Amruthwar, S.S. and Janorkar, A.V. (2012). Preparation and characterization of elastin-like polypeptide scaffolds for local delivery of antibiotics and proteins. *J. Mater. Sci. Mater. Med.* 23 (12): 2903–2912.

65 Ruszczak, Z. and Friess, W. (2003). Collagen as a carrier for on-site delivery of antibacterial drugs. *Adv. Drug Delivery Rev.* 55 (12): 1679–1698.

66 Caves, J.M., Kumar, V.A., Martinez, A.W. et al. (2010). The use of microfiber composites of elastin-like protein matrix reinforced with synthetic collagen in the design of vascular grafts. *Biomaterials* 31 (27): 7175–7182.

67 Caves, J.M., Cui, W., Wen, J. et al. (2011). Elastin-like protein matrix reinforced with collagen microfibers for soft tissue repair. *Biomaterials* 32 (23): 5371–5379.

68 Anderson, T.R., Marquart, M.E., and Janorkar, A.V. (2015). Effective release of a broad spectrum antibiotic from elastin-like polypeptide-collagen composite. *J. Biomed. Mater. Res. A* 103 (2): 782–790.

69 Pal, P., Nguyen, Q.C., Benton, A.H. et al. (2019). Drug-loaded elastin-like polypeptide–collagen hydrogels with high modulus for bone tissue engineering. *Macromol. Biosci.* 19: 1900142.

70 Gustafson, J., Greish, K., Frandsen, J. et al. (2009). Silk-elastinlike recombinant polymers for gene therapy of head and neck cancer: from molecular definition to controlled gene expression. *J. Controlled Release* 140 (3): 256–261.

71 Megeed, Z., Haider, M., Li, D. et al. (2004). In vitro and in vivo evaluation of recombinant silk-elastinlike hydrogels for cancer gene therapy. *J. Controlled Release* 94 (2–3): 433–445.

72 Megeed, Z., Cappello, J., and Ghandehari, H. (2002). Controlled release of plasmid DNA from a genetically engineered silk-elastinlike hydrogel. *Pharm. Res.* 19 (7): 954–959.
73 Fernández-Colino, A., Arias, F.J., Alonso, M., and Rodríguez-Cabello, J.C. (2014). Self-organized ECM-mimetic model based on an amphiphilic multiblock silk-elastin-like corecombinamer with a concomitant dual physical gelation process. *Biomacromolecules* 15 (10): 3781–3793.
74 Greish, K., Frandsen, J., Scharff, S. et al. (2010). Silk-elastinlike protein polymers improve the efficacy of adenovirus thymidine kinase enzyme prodrug therapy of head and neck tumors. *J. Gene Med.* 12 (7): 572–579.
75 Price, R., Poursaid, A., Cappello, J., and Ghandehari, H. (2014). Effect of shear on physicochemical properties of matrix metalloproteinase responsive silk-elastinlike hydrogels. *J. Controlled Release* 195: 92–98.
76 Egeblad, M. and Werb, Z. (2002). New functions for the matrix metalloproteinases in cancer progression. *Nat. Rev. Cancer* 2 (3): 161.
77 Price, R., Poursaid, A., Cappello, J., and Ghandehari, H. (2015). In vivo evaluation of matrix metalloproteinase responsive silk–elastinlike protein polymers for cancer gene therapy. *J. Control. Release* 213: 96–102.
78 Jensen, M.M., Jia, W., Schults, A.J. et al. (2019). Temperature-responsive silk-elastinlike protein polymer enhancement of intravesical drug delivery of a therapeutic glycosaminoglycan for treatment of interstitial cystitis/painful bladder syndrome. *Biomaterials* 217: 119293.
79 Jensen, M.M., Jia, W., Isaacson, K.J. et al. (2017). Silk-elastinlike protein polymers enhance the efficacy of a therapeutic glycosaminoglycan for prophylactic treatment of radiation-induced proctitis. *J. Controlled Release* 263: 46–56.
80 Gonzalez-Obeso, C., Girotti, A., and Rodriguez-Cabello, J.C. (2019). A transferrin receptor-binding mucoadhesive elastin-like recombinamer: in vitro and in vivo characterization. *Acta Biomater.* 88: 241–250.
81 Fernández-Colino, A., Quinteros, D.A., Allemandi, D.A. et al. (2017). Self-assembling elastin-like hydrogels for timolol delivery: development of an ophthalmic formulation against glaucoma. *Mol. Pharm.* 14 (12): 4498–4508.
82 Schaal, J.L., Li, X., Mastria, E. et al. (2016). Injectable polypeptide micelles that form radiation crosslinked hydrogels in situ for intratumoral radiotherapy. *J. Controlled Release* 228: 58–66.
83 Hennink, W.E. and van Nostrum, C.F. (2012). Novel crosslinking methods to design hydrogels. *Adv. Drug Delivery Rev.* 64: 223–236.
84 Kimmerling, K., Furman, B., Mangiapani, D. et al. (2015). Sustained intra-articular delivery of IL-1RA from a thermally-responsive elastin-like polypeptide as a therapy for post-traumatic arthritis. *Eur. Cell. Mater.* 29: 124.
85 Bandiera, A. (2010). Assembly and optimization of expression of synthetic genes derived from the human elastin repeated motif. *Prep. Biochem. Biotechnol.* 40 (3): 198–212.
86 Bandiera, A., Markulin, A., Corich, L. et al. (2013). Stimuli-induced release of compounds from elastin biomimetic matrix. *Biomacromolecules* 15 (1): 416–422.

87 Thomas, D., Fontana, G., Chen, X. et al. (2014). A shape-controlled tuneable microgel platform to modulate angiogenic paracrine responses in stem cells. *Biomaterials* 35 (31): 8757–8766.

88 Cao, R., Bråkenhielm, E., Pawliuk, R. et al. (2003). Angiogenic synergism, vascular stability and improvement of hind-limb ischemia by a combination of PDGF-BB and FGF-2. *Nat. Med.* 9 (5): 604.

89 Dash, B.C., Thomas, D., Monaghan, M. et al. (2015). An injectable elastin-based gene delivery platform for dose-dependent modulation of angiogenesis and inflammation for critical limb ischemia. *Biomaterials* 65: 126–139.

90 Asai, D., Xu, D., Liu, W. et al. (2012). Protein polymer hydrogels by in situ, rapid and reversible self-gelation. *Biomaterials* 33 (21): 5451–5458.

91 Zhang, Y.N., Avery, R.K., Vallmajo-Martin, Q. et al. (2015). A highly elastic and rapidly crosslinkable elastin-like polypeptide-based hydrogel for biomedical applications. *Adv. Funct. Mater.* 25 (30): 4814–4826.

92 Mukerji, R., Schaal, J., Li, X. et al. (2016). Spatiotemporally photoradiation-controlled intratumoral depot for combination of brachytherapy and photodynamic therapy for solid tumor. *Biomaterials* 79: 79–87.

93 Asai, D., Kanamoto, T., Takenaga, M., and Nakashima, H. (2017). In situ depot formation of anti-HIV fusion-inhibitor peptide in recombinant protein polymer hydrogel. *Acta Biomater.* 64: 116–125.

94 Asai, D., Fukuda, T., Morokuma, K. et al. (2019). Injectable polypeptide hydrogel depot system for assessment of the immune response–inducing efficacy of sustained antigen release alone. *Macromol. Biosci.* 19: 1900167.

95 Wang, H., Paul, A., Nguyen, D. et al. (2018). Tunable control of hydrogel microstructure by kinetic competition between self-assembly and crosslinking of elastin-like proteins. *ACS Appl. Mater. Interfaces* 10 (26): 21808–21815.

4

Enzyme-Assisted Hydrogel Formation for Tissue Engineering Applications

Sílvia Pérez-Rafael, Eva Ramon, and Tzanko Tzanov

Universitat Politècnica de Catalunya, Grup de Biotecnologia Molecular i Industrial, Departament Enginyeria Química, Rambla Sant Nebridi 22, Terrassa 08222, Spain

4.1 Introduction

Hydrogels are defined as a three-dimensional (3D) hydrophilic polymeric networks with a stable water-swollen porous structure tailored by cross-linking density [1–3] that governs the encapsulation and controlled release of bioactives, such as drugs [4], growth factors [5, 6], proteins, or genes [7] (Figure 4.1). Their 3D structure provides an excellent cell-mimicking environment, facilitating the cellular proliferation and migration [3, 8]. Moreover, functional scaffolds containing bioactives and/or cells can be self-assembled building up multilayered systems that closely mimic the complexity of body tissues [9, 10]. All these features demonstrate the potential of these materials in the tissue engineering (TE) and regenerative medicine (RM) field as mucoadhesives and bioadhesive [11, 12], wound healing materials [13, 14], bioactive factor delivery vehicles [15, 16], and cell encapsulation systems [16, 17].

As mentioned in Chapter 1, different classifications of hydrogels exist; hydrogels can be classified according to (i) the material source – natural and synthetic polymers, (ii) biodegradability, (iii) structure – homopolymer, copolymer, and interpenetrating network, (iv) charge, and (v) cross-linking method – chemical and physical [18–20]. The applied cross-linking methodology modulates the mechanical strength and stability of the 3D hydrogel constructs (Table 4.1).

In chemically cross-linked hydrogels, nonreversible covalent bonds are formed between the polymer chains, obtaining a "permanent" gel [18]. Generally, this cross-linking is achieved by redox reactions [21], radical polymerization [22], photopolymerization [23], click chemistry [24], Michael addition [25], Schiff's base reactions [26, 27], or enzymes. Chemically cross-linked gels are characterized by high mechanical strength and controllable biodegradability. However, the utilization of toxic catalysts or cross-linkers and harsh conditions may damage the encapsulated proteins, drugs, or cells. In physically cross-linked gels, the 3D matrices are formed by noncovalent interactions between polymer chains driven by crystallization [18, 19], polymerized entanglement, metal coordination [28],

Multifunctional Hydrogels for Biomedical Applications, First Edition.
Edited by Ricardo A. Pires, Iva Pashkuleva, and Rui L. Reis.

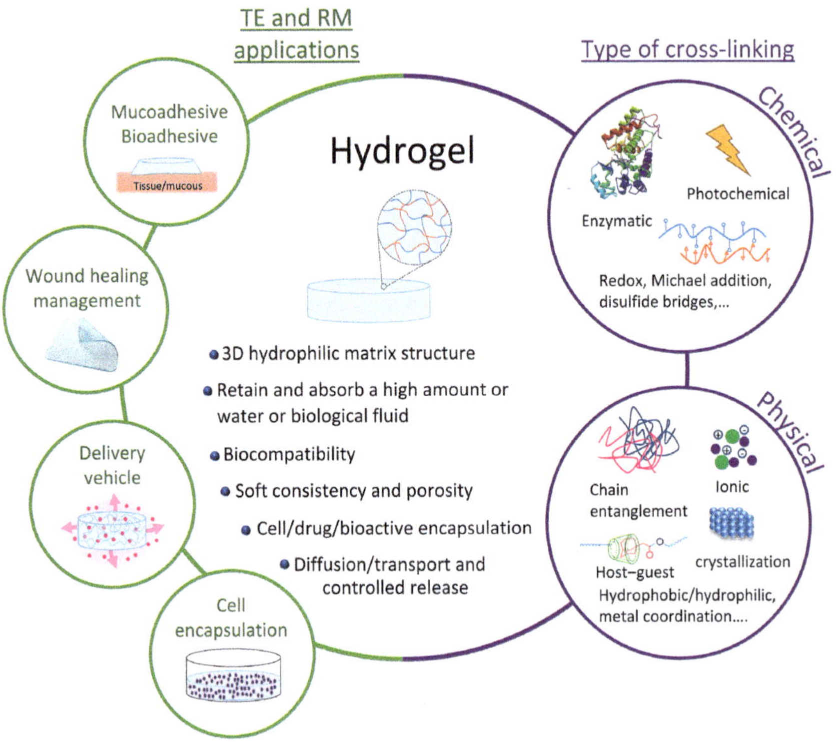

Figure 4.1 Hydrogels characteristics, TE and RM applications, and type of cross-linking methods.

Table 4.1 Type of cross-linking methods and the respective main characteristics, advantages, and limitations of the generated hydrogels.

	Advantages	**Limitations**
Chemical cross-linking		
Photo- and radical polymerization Redox reactions Michael and Schiff's base reactions Click chemistry Enzymatic reactions	Irreversible bonds "Permanent" gel formation High mechanical strength Superior physiological stability	Use of toxic catalysts and cross-linker monomers Harm conditions to encapsulate bioactives and living cells
Physical cross-linking		
Ionic–electrostatic Hydrophobic–hydrophilic Host–guest Crystallization Chain entanglement Hydrogen bonding π–π stacking Metal coordination	Reversible and dynamic bonds Mild conditions Avoid chemical hazard Homogeneous encapsulation of bioactive molecules, drugs, and cells	Poor mechanical properties Low stability *in vivo* and at physiological conditions (ion concentration, pH,...)

π–π stacking [29], hydrogen bonding [30], host–guest [31], hydrophobic–hydrophilic [24], and ionic–electrostatic interactions [32] among others. The reversible and dynamic bonds formed under mild conditions facilitate the *in situ* incorporation of bioactive agents or cells. However, these hydrogels usually have poor mechanical properties for applications where toughness and strength are demanded. Another important issue is that ion concentration or pH changes, associated with different physiological and pathological processes (e.g. inflammation, healing and cancer) may cause hydrogel collapse. The mechanical properties of physically cross-linked networks can be enhanced by a post-gelation chemical cross-linking. Such dual-cross-linking methodology combines the advantages of physical and chemical interactions to generate high strength, self-healing, and shape-memory hydrogels for biomedical applications as tissue scaffolds, actuators, and wearable devices [33–36].

Chemical and physical cross-linking can be prompted by an enzymatic reaction. Enzymes efficiently catalyze the formation and transformation of biomolecules through substrate-specific chemical reactions to generate/cleave covalent bonds in physiological conditions (Table 4.2). In this chapter, different enzyme-mediated

Table 4.2 Classification of enzymes considering the catalysed reaction.

Enzyme class	Type of reaction catalyzed	Examples
Oxidoreductases	Transfer of electrons or hydrogen atoms from one substrate to another	**Dehydrogenase** – oxidizes a substrate by reducing an electron acceptor **Oxidase** – catalyzes oxidation–reduction reaction using O_2 as an electron donor
Transferases	Transfer of a functional group from one substrate to another	**Kinase** – transfers a phosphate group **Transaminase** – transfers an amino group
Hydrolases	Break down a chemical bond, usually involve the transfer of functional groups to water	**Lipase** – breaks down lipid molecules **Protease** – breaks down proteins into smaller polypeptide or single amino acids
Lyase	Addition of a group to a double bond or removal of group to form double bond	**Decarboxylase** – adds or cleaves a carboxyl group
Isomerases	Rearrangement of atoms within a molecule	**Phosphohexoisomerase** – catalyzes the isomerization of glucose-6-phosphate to fructose-6-phosphate reversibly
Ligases	Binds two or more substrates together	**DNA polymerase** – synthesis of DNA molecules from deoxyribonucleotides **DNA ligase** – join DNA strands by catalyzing the formation of a phosphodiester bond

approaches for hydrogel formation targeting TE and RM applications will be reviewed.

4.2 Enzymatically Cross-Linked Hydrogels

Enzymatic cross-linking is a mild and eco-efficient synthetic alternative route for hydrogels formation [37–39]. The highly specific enzymatic reactions generate new chemical bonds forming a polymeric network under physiological conditions (Figure 4.2), avoiding side reactions or intrinsic toxicity.

The enzyme activity controls the cross-linking reaction in terms of gelation rate, and thus the hydrogel can be tailored to ensure localized drug delivery, obtain a suitable cell distribution, and properly integrate with the surrounding tissues. The versatility of the enzymatic tools to generate hydrogels with tunable

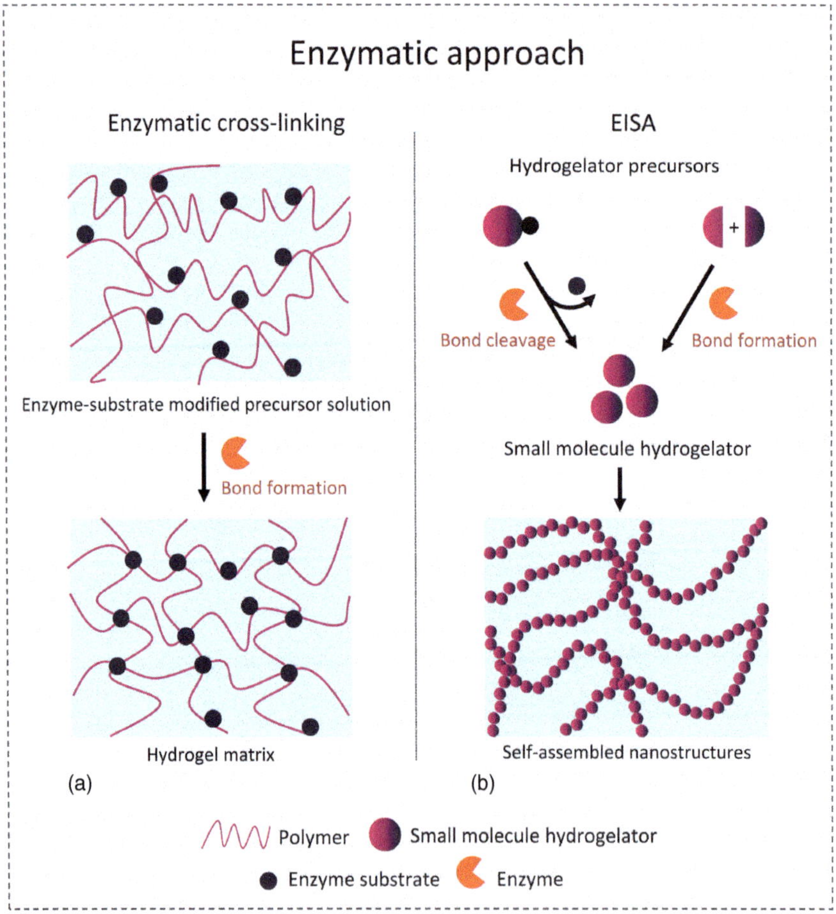

Figure 4.2 Schematic presentation of enzymatic approaches for hydrogel formation by (a) chemical crosslinking and (b) enzyme-assisted supramolecular polymerization.

properties allows the production of injectable materials, adhesives, site-defect matching scaffolds, and 3D cell culture media for TE and RM applications (Table 4.3) [121].

4.2.1 Oxidoreductases

Oxidoreductases catalyze oxidation and reduction reactions by the exchange of electrons or redox equivalents between a donor and an acceptor molecule (Table 4.2) [122]. They have been applied in a wide range of industrial applications, such as lignocellulosic transformation, textile and food application, or detergent formulations [122]. Among the enzymes belonging to this family, horseradish peroxidase (HRP) and tyrosinase are commonly employed to produce hydrogels (Table 4.3). Less exploited enzymes, such as lysyl oxidase (LO) and plasma oxidase (PO), have also been proposed as candidates for hydrogel formation [92].

4.2.1.1 Peroxidases – HRP

Peroxidases are a wide family of oxidoreductases that typically catalyze the reaction ROOR′ + electron donor (2e−) + 2H + → ROH + R′OH (Figure 4.3a) [124]. Although these enzymes generally do not require cofactors, most of them use H_2O_2 as a substrate. HRP is the most used enzyme to synthesize hydrogels with short gelation time and high and controllable mechanical strength suitable for encapsulation of therapeutics (drugs, cells, peptides, or proteins) [125]. The HRP/H_2O_2 complex mainly oxidases phenol and aniline derivatives [126]. The oxidative catalysis of hydroxyphenil groups produces quinones that spontaneously react with nucleophiles (hydroxyl groups, amines, and thiols) through Michael addition and Schiff base allowing the cross-linking of several biomolecules and derivative polymers.

The most exploited strategy to develop hydrogels via HRP-mediated redox system is by grafting phenolic functionality (mainly tyramine and hydroxyphenylpropionic acid (HPA)) on polymers (dextran, chitosan, alginate, collagen, or polyethylene glycol [PEG]) followed by an enzymatic action on the grafted functionalities (Figure 4.3a). This method has been applied for development of many hydrogel systems for TE and RM applications, such as wound healing, tissue adhesiveness, vascularization, and encapsulation (Table 4.3). Jin et al. exploited the combination of different biopolymers such as dextran, hyaluronic acid (HA), and heparin modified with HRP substrates to produce scaffolds that mimic the molecular structure of the extracellular matrix (ECM) for cartilage TE applications [54, 55]. Dextran-tyramine gels containing bovine chondrocytes with good mechanical properties and swelling capacity have been produced by controlled HRP-catalyzed cross-linking. The obtained 3D matrices allowed for nutrients exchange resembling the cartilage tissue performance during chondrogenesis differentiation [54]. In a similar approach, Kim et al. described the synthesis of an injectable HA-tyramine-based hydrogel as a carrier of the anti-inflammatory agent dexamethasone for the treatment of rheumatoid arthritis [47]. Another example of the application of this catalytic system with modified polymers is the synthesis of

Table 4.3 Enzymatically generated hydrogels and potential applications.

Hydrogel matrix material	Enzyme type	Application
Functionalized polyaspartic acid polymers with phenol aromatic motifs	Peroxidases	Drug delivery, wound healing, and TE [40]
Hyaluronic acid-tyramine	HRP	Drug delivery and nonspecific TE [41, 42], injectable [43–45], cartilage repair [46, 47]
PEG–HPA/hyaluronic-tyramine	HRP	Intervertebral disk regeneration [48]
PLG-g-tyramine/PEG	HRP	TE scaffolds [49]
ε-polylysine-PEG/tyramine	HRP	Tissue adhesive [50]
ε-polylysine-HPA	HRP	Bioadhesive and wound infection prevention [51]
Dextran-tyramine	HRP	Drug delivery and nonspecific TE [52], cartilage tissue repair [53]
Dextran-tyramine/hyaluronic acid-tyramine or heparin-tyramine	HRP	Cartilage tissue repair [54, 55]
Carboxymethylcellulose-tyramine	HRP	Biomedical applications [56], multicellular spheroids for TE [57]
Gelatin-tyramine	HRP	Osteoblast delivery vehicle [58]
Gelatin-HPA	HRP	Fibroblast delivery on wound healing [59], tissue adhesiveness [60], cartilage tissue repair [61], brain tissue regeneration [62], diabetic wound healing [63]
Gelatin-HPA	HRP/GalOx	Dermal tissue regeneration [64]
Gelatin/alginate-tyramine	HRP	Microcapsules, fabricated cell sheets, and spherical tissues [65]
Collagen-tyramine	HRP	Vascularized TE [66]
Glycol chitosan-HPA	HRP	Bone regeneration [67]
Thiolated chitosan/EGCG nanospheres	HRP	Chronic wound management [68]
PEG-tyramine/ chitosan-4-hydroxyphenil acid	HRP	Drug delivery and TE [69]
Chitosan-HPA	HRP	Drug delivery and nonspecific TE [70]
Alginatedopamine	HRP	TE scaffold (adhesive) [71]
Tetronic–tyramine conjugates	HRP	Drug delivery and nonspecific TE [72]
Polyvinyl alcohol-tyramine	HRP/GOx	Dressing hydrogel triggered by wound exudate [73]

Table 4.3 (Continued)

Hydrogel matrix material	Enzyme type	Application
PEGmetacrylate	HRP/GOx	Biocatalyst and TE [74]
PEG/gelatin-norbornene	HRP/GOx	Dynamically cross-linked hydrogels [75]
Chitosan/gelatin	Tyrosinase	TE approaches [76], wound dressing [77], film biofabrication [78, 79]
Chitosan/dopamine	Tyrosinase	Tissue glue [80]
Silk fibroin/chitosan	Tyrosinase	Scaffold for TE [81]
Tyrosine containing peptide/chitosan	Tyrosinase	Protein immobilization [82]
Chondroitin sulfate-tyramine	Tyrosinase	Drug release and TE [83]
HA-tyramine/gelatin	tyrosinase	Tissue adhesive and sprayable hydrogel [84]
PEG-peptide	mshTyr/SrtA	*In situ* cell encapsulation and investigation of cell behavior [85]
Chitosan/gelatin/phenolic compound	Laccase	Chronic wound management [86]
Thiolated chitosan/phenolic compound	Laccase	Chronic wound management [87, 88]
Chitosan/phenolic compound	Laccase	Drug release [89]
O-Carboxymethyl chitosan/phenolic compound	Laccase	Wound management [90]
PVA/ferulic acid	Laccase	Ophthalmic applications [91]
Nanofibrous lysine-rich peptide hydrogels	LO/PO	No application described [92]
Fibrin gel	FXIIIa	Neurite extension [93], angiogenesis [94], cartilage repair [95, 96]
	TG	Cardiovascular TE [97]
PEG-peptide	tTG	Gelation model [98, 99], surgical tissue adhesive [100], cartilage tissue repair [101]
	FXIIIa	Smart implants for TE [102], drug delivery systems [103], vascularization [104], *in situ* cell manipulation [105]
Hyaluronic acid-PEG	FXIIIa	Injectable matrix for RM [106]
Gelatin	mTG	Scaffold for TE [107, 108], sustained drug delivery [109], dermal healing [110], microfluidic biosensor [111], 3D TE [112]
Gelatin/chitosan	tTG	*In situ* applications [77]

(continued)

Table 4.3 (Continued)

Hydrogel matrix material	Enzyme type	Application
Elastin-like polypeptide gels	tTG	Cartilage tissue repair [113]
Lysine and glutamine hydrogel	tTG	TE applications [114]
Casein	mTG	Sustained drug delivery [115]
Hyaluronic acid-peptide motifs	FXIIIa	3D neuronal cultures [116]
Collagen	mTG	Injectable hydrogel for skin TE [117], TE and cancer therapy [118]
Chitosan/cellulose/collagen	tTG	Composite membrane for postsurgical peritoneal adhesion prevention [119]
CoA-functionalized PEG	Phosphopantetheinyl transferase	Cell biology and TE [120]

Abbreviations: CoA: coenzyme A, EGCG: epigallocatechin gallate, FXIIIa: transglutaminase isoenzyme factor XIIIa, GalOx: galactose oxidase, GOx: glucose oxidase, HPA: hydroxyphenylpropionic acid, HRP: horseradish peroxidase, LO: lysyl oxidase, mshTyr: mushroom tyrosinase, mTG: microbial transglutaminase, PEG: polyethyleneglycol, PLG: poly(L-glutamic acid), PO: plasma amine oxidase, PVA: polyvinyl alcohol, SrtA: bacterial transpeptidase sortase A, RM: regenerative medicine, TE: tissue engineering, tTG: tissue transglutaminase.

an injectable gelatin-HPA hydrogel to encapsulate adult neural stem cells. This tunable biocompatible hydrogel showed superior resistance to oxidative stress and matched the storage modulus of neural tissue in adult brain. Moreover, the embedded cells displayed higher gene expression for the neuronal lineage markers [62]. Yoon et al. synthesized a chemokine-containing gelatin-hydroxyphenyl hydrogel that enhanced the re-epithelialization, neovascularization, and collagen deposition in type I diabetic-induced mice reducing the diabetic wound area [63]. The authors hypothesized that the encapsulated chemokines (IL-8 and MIP-3α) were able to recruit endogenous cells promoting tissue healing. Wang et al. oxidized ε-poly-L-lysine conjugated with HPA and demonstrated the antibacterial efficacy of this hydrogel after subcutaneous injection into a mice model [51]. Our group has also reported the HRP/H_2O_2 enzymatic-assisted cross-linking of thiolated chitosan to *in situ* incorporate epigallocathechin gallate nanospheres for chronic wound management. The scaffolds exhibited intrinsic antioxidant and antibacterial properties and ability to inhibit deleterious wound enzymes [68].

Other authors have described the combination and dual action of HRP and glucose oxidase (GOx) [73–75] or galactose oxidase (GalOx) [64] to *in situ* generate H_2O_2. Sakai et al. showed *in situ* dual-enzymatic polymerization of polyvinyl alcohol–phenolic conjugates (PVA–Ph) to generate dressings for wound management [73]. Hydrogel formation was initiated immediately after the contact of a PVA–Ph aqueous solution containing GOx and HRP with the wound exudate. Encapsulated GOx oxidized glucose from the exudate generating H_2O_2

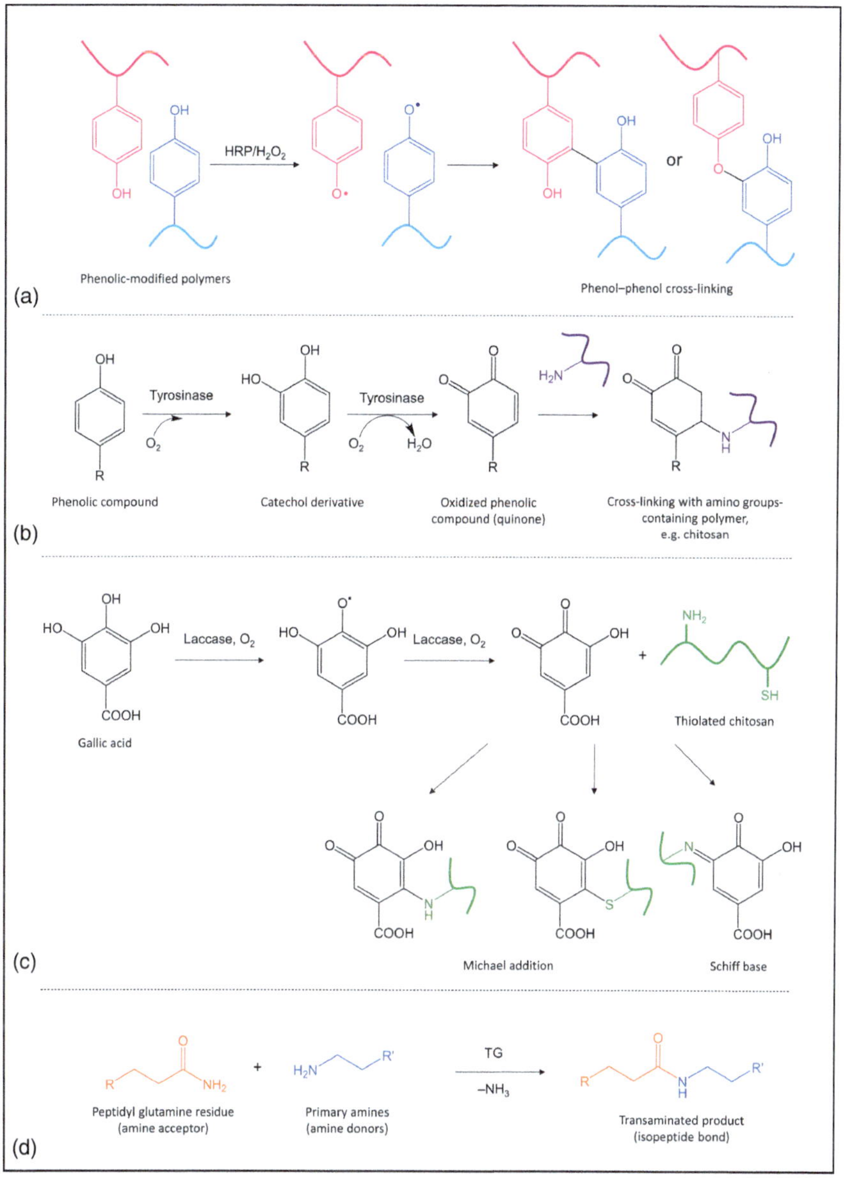

Figure 4.3 Enzymatic cross-linking via HRP (a), tyrosinase (b), laccase (Source: Based on Hoang Thi et al. [123].) (c), and transglutaminase (d).

that was used by the embedded HRP to cross-link PVA–Ph within 20 seconds at physiological glucose concentrations. The developed wound dressing material displayed faster closure of full-thickness wounds in rats than commercially available hydrogel dressings [73]. The same GOx/HRP catalytic system was employed to achieve chemical cross-linking polymerization of previously self-assembled 3D printable acrylic-modified hydrogelators. The 3D polymeric constructs combined the properties of supramolecular hydrogels with the advantages of enzymatic cross-linking, providing superior mechanical strength and higher density [74]. Another promising scaffold for tissue regeneration was synthesized via HRP/GalOx dual-enzymatic cross-linking of HPA-gelatin polymer for encapsulation of bone mesenchymal stem cells [64]. The injectable hydrogel exhibited rapid gelation rates and excellent biocompatibility and promoted the wound healing process.

4.2.1.2 Tyrosinase

Tyrosinase is a copper-containing enzyme that catalyzes the hydroxylation of monophenols to *o*-diphenols and the oxidation of *o*-diphenols to *o*-quinones by using oxygen (O_2) as an electron acceptor [127]. Tyrosinase-catalyzed cross-linking mainly proceeds by phenol oxidation of tyrosines from proteins or other phenolic moieties (e.g. dopamine or tyramine) into quinones. These highly reactive species will further react with nucleophile groups as hydroxyl, amino, or thiol groups via Michael-type addition and Schiff base reaction (Figure 4.3b).

Jin et al. developed a biocompatible enzymatically cross-linked tyramine-chondroitin scaffold for encapsulation of fibroblasts cells and control drug release [128]. Modified tyramine-HA oxidized by tyrosinase reacted with gelatin, thus forming injectable and sprayable gels for drugs and cells localized delivery system, or surgical glue applications [84]. Tyrosinase has been also explored to cross-link tyrosine residues from silk or fibroin to obtain protein–polysaccharides conjugates [81, 129, 130].

Arkenberg et al. reported a dual-enzymatic procedure to tune PEG-derived hydrogels properties. First, bacterial transpeptidase sortase A (SrtA) was employed to conjugate two PEG-peptide macromers into a 3D matrix. Then, mushroom tyrosinase was used oxidize the tyrosine residues from the peptides into di-tyrosine and thus to tune the stiffness of this hydrogel. This post-gelation reaction played a crucial role in inhibiting cell spreading and controlling cell morphology by mimicking the ECM dynamic stiffening process [85]. These studies indicated that tyrosine-catalyzed reactions have the potential for the development of wound dressings [77], film-forming materials [78, 79], adhesives [80], or other applications involving protein immobilization (Table 4.3) [82].

4.2.1.3 Laccase

Laccase is a copper-depending enzyme that catalyzes the monoelectronic oxidation of a substrate to form the corresponding reactive radical using O_2 as the final electron donor and producing H_2O as a byproduct (Figure 4.3c). The main substrates of these enzymes are phenols and amines [131]. Our group exploited laccase-assisted cross-linking reaction between natural biopolymers, as a bulk material, and polyphenolic compounds, as cross-linkers, for the generation of multifunctional and bioactive chronic wound dressing materials [86–88]. Rocasalbas et al. prepared chitosan/gelatin-based hydrogels coupled with proanthocyanidins extracted from the plant *Hamamelis virginiana* through quinone/amino reaction via Michael addition mechanism [86]. The phenolic compounds loaded in the hydrogels have a double role (i) as a structural component that increases hydrogel stability and

(ii) as a bioactive element to inhibit deleterious wound enzymes and bacterial growth stimulating the wound healing process [86]. Multifunctional thiolated chitosan hydrogels were also synthesized utilizing natural phenolic compounds, gallic acid and chicoric acid as cross-linkers. Quinones reacted with nucleophilic groups (–SH and –NH_2) from the thiolated chitosan through Schiff base and 1–4 Michael-type addition to form the gel matrix. The developed hydrogel dressing showed high antioxidant activity and efficacy to eradicate medically relevant bacterial pathogens. Moreover, the scaffold was validated *ex vivo* as a dressing material for wound management using chronic wound exudates [87, 88]. The versatility of chitosan-based hydrogels properties was further explored using different phenolic compounds to control the mechanical properties and drug release [89, 90]. In another example, Bersanetti et al. reported the formation of tunable hydrogels after laccase-mediated cross-linking of PVA and ferulic acid as a prospective candidate for biomedical applications [91].

4.2.2 Transferases: Transglutaminase

Transferases catalyze the transfer of a functional group (amine, carboxyl, carbonyl, phosphoryl, methyl, acyl, and glycosyl) from a donor substrate to an acceptor molecule [132]. Transglutaminase (TG) is the most widely used transferase enzyme for the enzymatically generation of hydrogels; however, other transferases, such as phosphopantetheinyl transferase, have also been employed for TE applications (Table 4.3).

TGs catalyze the isopeptide bond formation in proteins, covalent conjugation of polyamines, lipid esterification, or deamination of glutamine residues. Amide linkage between a protein γ-carboxamide group and free primary amines are formed in the TG-catalyzed reaction (Figure 4.3d) [98]. TGs are responsible for some biochemical reactions such as fibrin clots and cornified epidermis formation stimulating wound healing [133]. Different TGs have been exploited to prepare hydrogels based on fibrin [93–97], polypeptide [113], PEG [98–101], and natural polymers, such as gelatin [107–112]. The TG-promoted reaction provides (i) resistance to proteolytic degradation bonds, (ii) effective cross-linking of small substrates without addition of cofactors, and (iii) fast gelation rates [106].

Many authors have exploited the role of factor XIII, a TG isozyme involved in fibrin clot stabilization [106], to prepare fibrin-based matrices with improved mechanical properties for nerve repair [93], angiogenesis [94], cartilage TE [95, 96], and cardiovascular TE [97]. Early studies showed the ability of fibrin-based scaffolds to covalently incorporate morphoregulatory proteins-derived oligopeptides via factor XIII catalysis to promote cell differentiation [93, 94]. More recently, Williams et al. developed an injectable cardiac ECM-fibrin-based scaffold with tunable biochemical composition and stiffness that mimicked myocardium tissue and promoted the expression of endothelial and smooth muscle cell genes [97].

TG has also been employed to functionalize injectable PEG-derived hydrogels with growth factors and cell-derived proteins [98–106]. PEG is commonly modified with glutamine, poly-L-lysine, or other peptides as TG substrates [98–105]. An elegant strategy has been applied by Ehbar et al. to produce dual-enzymatic-responsive hydrogels using peptide-conjugated PEG. The hydrogel building block precursors were functionalized to be cross-linked via FXIIIa and susceptible to degradation by matrix metalloproteinases (MMPs) under physiological conditions [102]. Site-specific cell adhesion ligands were simultaneously cross-linked with multiarm PEG macromers conjugated to FXIIIa substrate, enabling extensive cell spreading, proliferation, and migration, as well as tunable proteolytic matrix degradation by cell-secreted MMPs. Sala et al. also employed an enzymatic tethering approach for site-specific and properly oriented immobilization of biologically active molecules on FXIII-catalyzed PEG-glutamine hydrogels [103]. The exposure of morphogenes or adhesive sites, such as RDG-fibronectin motifs, to cells induced cellular proliferation and differentiation [103]. More recently, the coculture of mesenchymal and endothelial cells (hBM-MSCS and HUVEC) in biologically inert TG-cross-linked PEG scaffolds has been reported [104]. The embedment of bone morphogenic protein-2 (BMP-2) or fibroblasts growth factors promoted the osteogenic differentiation of both cells. More advanced systems have been proposed for biomolecules tethering and *in situ* cell manipulation through enzymatic hydrogel photopatterning. Mosiewicz et al. presented a PEG-based hydrogel with photocontrollable physicochemical properties. In this approach, an FXIIIa substrate protected with a photolabile cage was covalently incorporated in a PEG 3D network. Local photoactivation led to the exposure of the FXIII substrate enabling enzymatic cross-linking and the adhesion of proteins and growth factors into the PEG hydrogels [105].

Biopolymers, such as collagen, gelatin, HA, or chitosan have been also applied as polymer precursors of enzymatically TG-generated hydrogels. Cai et al. produced composite membranes combining carboxymethyl chitosan, carboxymethyl cellulose, and collagen to prevent postsurgical peritoneal adhesion [119]. These membranes were applied between the injured site and the adjacent tissue in a mice model. The biocompatible antiadhesion films decreased the deposition of ECM components, responsible for peritoneum adhesion, and the inflammatory response. Zhao et al. also used TG to prepare injectable collagen-based hydrogels [117]. This scaffold was tested for skin tissue regeneration demonstrating cell survival, growth, and proliferation within the hydrogel matrix. Li et al. synthesized another collagen-based hydrogel in the presence of a biocompatible ionic liquid via microbial transglutaminase (mTG)-mediated cross-linking [118]. The generated 3D structure governed the cellular fate of cancer and fibroblast cell lines. Scaffolds inhibited cancer cells development but promoted the adhesion and proliferation of normal-shaped fibroblast cells. The use of the ionic liquid also imbued the hydrogels with degradation resistance and anti-inflammatory properties after subcutaneous injection into mice. Gelatin hydrogels have also been prepared via TGs for cell encapsulation. Chen et al. were able to fabricate large, perfusable, macroporous, HUVEC cells-laden hydrogels able to maintain sufficient oxygen delivery and mass transfer and promote microvasculature network formation [112].

HA derivatives are excellent candidates to cross-link with TG. HA-peptide-modified polymers have been reported to form FXIIIa-cross-linked hydrogels for 3D neural cell cultures [116]. This scaffold featured injectability, tuneable gelling speed, and covalent attachment to ECM fibrin ensuring good tissue adhesiveness. HA have also been proposed as novel building blocks to prepare hybrid PEG-based artificial ECMs for RM applications. Ranga et al. described the preparation of hybrid HA–PEG hydrogels via TG cross-linking of PEG–peptide and HA–glutamine conjugates [106]. The injectable and biocompatible hydrogels regulated the cellular phenotype of human mammary cancer epithelial cells.

4.3 Supramolecular Enzyme-Driven Hydrogelation

Supramolecular hydrogels are formed by the self-assembly of molecular building blocks called hydrogelators. Unlike chemically cross-linked hydrogels, the network formation in supramolecular hydrogels is entirely via noncovalent interactions of small molecules and polymeric hydrogelators. These hydrogelators self-assemble into an organized supramolecular structure through noncovalent interactions, such as hydrogen bonding, electrostatic, van der Waals, hydrophobic–hydrophilic, and/or π–π interactions. Different physical or chemical perturbation (e.g. change of pH, temperature, or ionic strength) can be used to trigger supramolecular hydrogelation. Enzymes catalysis boosts the supramolecular gelation by regulating the hydrophobicity/hydrophilicity balance of the precursors via chemical bond cleavage or formation (Figure 4.2). Enzyme-instructed self-assembly (EISA) of small-molecule building blocks provides a route to design a wide range of molecular hydrogelators with controllable gelation in response to biological environments (Table 4.4).

4.3.1 Hydrolases

Hydrolases catalyze the cleavage of chemical bonds using water. Phosphatases, thermolysin, and β-lactamase can change the amphiphilicity of small molecules triggering self-assembly that ultimately may lead to supramolecular hydrogel formation.

4.3.1.1 Phosphatases

Phosphatases represent a large family of enzymes able to catalyze the cleavage of hydrophilic phosphate groups (dephosphorylation) from a variety of substrates. These enzymes have been used to control the hydrophilicity/hydrophobicity balance, converting a precursor to a hydrogelator and trigger gel formation. In early works, Yang et al. demonstrated the enzyme-directed supramolecular hydrogelation of small molecules, such as Fmoc-tyrosine, utilizing alkaline phosphatase [134]. Dephosphorylation reaction via alkaline phosphatase increased the hydrophobicity of the simple amino acid derivative Fmoc-tyrosine phosphate, simultaneously forming self-assembled nanofibers and inducing hydrogelation [135].

EISA has been exploited to assist the formation of supramolecular hydrogels from highly hydrophobic compounds [137, 138]. Conversion of the precursor to hydrogelator upon enzymatic action is crucial for hydrogelation, since other methods assayed as mixing, heating–cooling cycles, pH adjustment, or sonication of both

Table 4.4 EISA-generated hydrogels and potential application.

Hydrogel matrix material	Enzyme	Application
Fmoc-peptide derivative hydrogels	Phosphatase	Assay platform for enzyme inhibitors [134, 135], Scaffolds to assist biomineralization [136], nonspecific application [137]
Taxol-peptide derivate	Phosphatase	Delivery system for hydrophobic drugs [138, 139]
Nap-peptide derivatives	Phosphatase	Nonspecific application [140]
β-Aminoacid derivatives	Phosphatase	*In vivo* hydrogelation, long-term biostability [141, 142]
Nap-peptide derivatives	Phosphatase	Intracellular hydrogelation to inhibit bacterial growth [143, 144]
Carbohydrate derivative hydrogelator	Phosphatase	Cancer cell therapy [145]
Mithocrondrial targeting-ligand (TTP) phosphorylated precursor	Phosphatase	Cancer cell therapy [146]
Phenylalanine dipeptide conjugated with TTP	Phosphatase	Cancer cell therapy [147]
Pentapeptidic hydrogelator (Nap-FFGEY)	Kinase/phosphatase	Nonspecific TE applications [148]
Nap-peptide derivatives	Esterase	Intracellular hydrogelation [149]
Precursor sensitive to MMP-7 (palmytoil-GGGHGPLGLARK-$CONH_2$)	MMP-7	Cancer cell therapy [150]
Precursor sensitive to MMP-9 (FFFFCGLDD)	MMP-9	Cancer cell therapy [151]
Precursor sensitive to MMP-7 (Palmitoyl-GGGH)	MMP-7	Diagnostic sensor, cancer cell therapy [152]
Precursor sensitive to MMP-9 (GPKG–LKGA)	MMP-9	Diagnosis of cancer and other diseases [153]
Precursor sensitive to MMP-9 (GFFLGLDD)	MMP-9	Drug delivery systems for cancer therapy [154]
Fmoc-peptide-ester hydrogels	Thermolysin	Biosensing, wound healing management [155]
Ionic peptides	Thermolysin	Enzyme detection and TE [156]
Precursor containing β-lactamase responsive cephem unit	β-Lactamase	Screen inhibitors [157]
Y-shaped DNA sequence	DNA polymerase	Nonspecific application [158]
DNA sequence	DNA polymerase	Bioelectronic interface, drug release, cell therapy [159]
DNA sequence	DNA polymerase	Nonspecified application [160]

Abbreviations: Fmoc: fluorenylmethyloxycarbonyl, Nap: naphthalene, TTP: triphenyl phosphinium, F: phenylalanine, G: glycine, E: glutamic acid, Y: tyrosine, H: histidine. P: proline, L: leucine, R: arginine, K: lysine, D: aspartic acid.

components are not cytocompatable and often lead to components precipitation failing to form supramolecular hydrogels [137]. Gao et al. produced a hydrogel precursor with therapeutic properties by conjugating a highly hydrophobic anti-neoplastic drug as taxol to a self-assembling motif and a phosphatase substrate (Figure 4.4a) [138]. Other research groups also engineered hydrophilic supramolecular hydrogels from highly hydrophobic small-molecule derivative therapeutics [139, 140, 161]. Hydrogels made of hydrophobic peptides are promising drug delivery systems due to their excellent stability in aqueous environments both *in vitro* and *in vivo* [140].

Phosphatase-instructed self-assembly of Fmoc-tyrosine derivatives, have been explored to screen inhibitors as a therapeutic tools to attenuate the abnormal activity or overexpression of some enzymes involved in specific diseases and disorders (Figure 4.4a) [135]. Since the presence of a certain inhibitor concentration will prevent the gelation process, hydrogelation can be used as a visual readout assay to identify prospective enzyme inhibitors [135]. Schnepp et al. fabricated supramolecular Fmoc-tyrosine 3D structures containing calcified nanofilaments. Upon phosphatase cleavage of Fmoc-tyrosine phosphate, the released phosphate ions remain in the self-assembled gel matrix. Further addition of calcium resulted in the deposition of inorganic mineral (calcium phosphate) on the hydrogel nanofibers [136]. This biomineralization process significantly modified the hybrid composite matrix morphology improving stiffness, critical strain, thermal stability, and dynamic storage and loss moduli. Inspired by this, Rauner et al. used alkaline phosphatase to catalyze the formation of amorphous calcium phosphate nanostructures in previously photopolymerized hydrogels containing acrylate and acrylamide derivatives. The developed biocompatible 3D matrices exhibited higher scaffold stiffness due to the calcium phosphate deposition [162]. This *in situ* mineralization within the gels might be further exploited for the generation of implant materials with tunable mechanical properties, stiff scaffolds for RM, and cell growth or drug delivery carriers [162].

EISA also offers a unique opportunity to explore *in vivo* extracellular and intracellular hydrogelation in response to specific enzymatic biological processes. Yang et al. built a precursor from two β-amino acid derivatives (β^3-homo-phenylglycine), to confer proteolytic resistance in biological environments, and a tyrosine phosphate residue as an enzyme substrate. Phosphatase also triggered the supramolecular hydrogel formation in complex biological fluids such as blood, and after injection in the extracellular subcutaneous tissue of a mouse [141, 142]. Controlled *in vivo* hydrogelation with such excellent stability in biological environments renders β-peptide derivatives as a potential candidates for long-term and enzyme-responsive biomedical applications. Xu laboratory has reported examples of enzyme-responsive materials where the supramolecular hydrogelation occurs intracellularly in both bacterial and mammalian cells, leading to inhibition of growth or the induction of apoptosis, respectively. A requirement to form an intracellular hydrogel is to design a soluble precursor modified with a substrate group of an intracellular enzyme. The endogenous biocatalyst should convert the soluble precursor into a hydrogelator that self-assembles into nanofibers or some other higher ordered structures. Yang

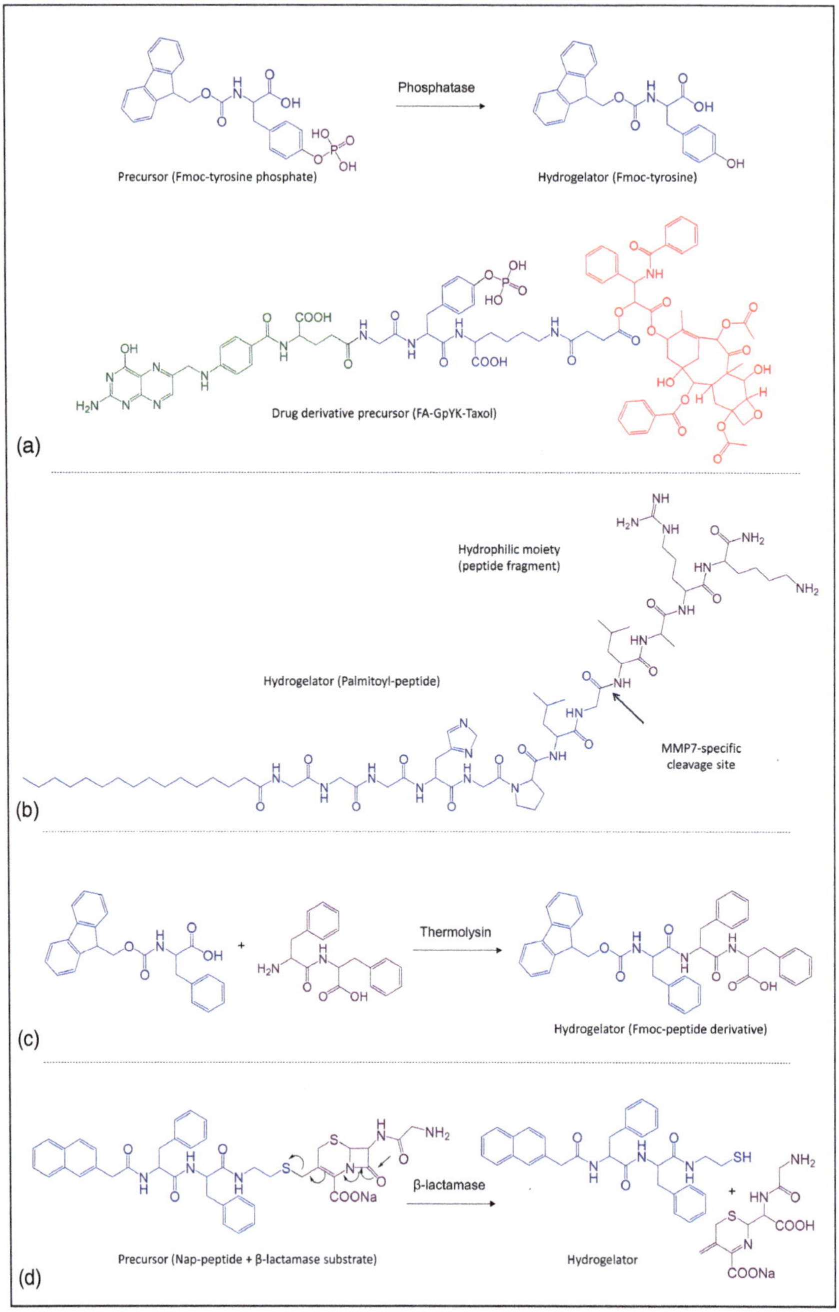

Figure 4.4 Enzymatic-assisted hydrogelation via (a) phosphatases (Source: Based on Yang et al. [134] and Wang et al. [139].), (b) MMPs (Source: Based on Tanaka et al.[150].), (c) thermolysin (Source: Based on Das et al. [155].), and (d) β-lactamase (Source: Based on Hoang Thi et al. [123].).

et al. synthesized an esterase substrate-conjugated hydrogelator able to penetrate the cell membrane. The endogenous esterase catalyzed the hydrogelator release and triggered the supramolecular hydrogel formation. As a result, the viscosity changes in the cytoplasm induced cell death [149]. Interestingly, intracellular enzymatic hydrogelation depends on the levels of enzyme expression (e.g. esterases) in different cell lines offering a new way to specifically cause cell death. Authors further demonstrated the intracellular hydrogelation in *Escherichia coli*. Upon precursor diffusion into the bacterial cells, endogenous phosphatase reaction triggered the intracellular assembly of nanostructures inhibiting bacterial growth [143]. This approach can be exploited with any small substrate precursor molecule susceptible to bacterial enzymes to design potential antimicrobial agents.

Other studies took advantage of phosphatase overexpression in cancer cells as a powerful tool for diagnostic and cancer therapy (details of this approach can be found in Chapter 8). Cells overexpressing phosphatase were able to generate fluorescent nanofibers from a fluorophore-conjugated peptide [144]. In another work, Pires et al. used an aromatic amphiphile carbohydrate derivative that self-assembled into nanofibers around osteosarcoma cancer cells (Saos2 cells), inducing selective cell death without affecting the surrounding healthy cells viability. Targeting organelles from cancer cells by EISA is another promising approach to selectively kill cancer cells and minimize drug resistance [145]. Recently, Xu laboratory built a mitochondrial-targeting ligand conjugated to a phosphorylated peptide precursor able to self-assemble in the pericellular space of Saos2 cancer cells by phosphatase reaction. The generated nanoscale assemblies were incorporated by the cells through endocytosis, ultimately accumulating in the mitochondria. The subcellular accumulation of nanofibers via EISA promoted cell death without inducing drug resistance [146]. Jeena et al. also used controlled molecular self-assembly associated with enzyme overexpression inside organelle cells to inhibit cancer cell growth. They designed a phenylalanine dipeptide conjugated with the mitochondrial targeting signal triphenylphosphonium (TPP) which self-assembled and accumulate in mitochondria [147].

Most of the studies report enzymatic-driven hydrogelation triggered by the action of one enzyme. However, in biological systems, multiple enzymes work antagonistically. The phosphatase/kinase catalyzing system is involved in the regulation of cell signal transduction where kinase forms and phosphatase cleaves phosphate–protein bonds. Yang et al. designed the pentapeptidic compound Nap-FFGEY to regulate supramolecular hydrogel formation *in vitro* and *in vivo*. Controlled dissociation/formation of the self-assembled nanostructures occurs by either adding or removing the hydrophilic phosphate group via tyrosine kinase or tyrosine phosphatase. Furthermore, the combination of both enzymes tuned the gelation process *in vivo* after subcutaneous injection [148]. Enzymatic cyclical reversibility of sol–gel–sol phase transition of small molecular precursors/hydrogelators offers desirable response to some diseases associated with abnormal enzyme expression level or activity, e.g. cancer, diabetes, or multiple sclerosis.

4.3.1.2 Metalloproteinases

Other extracellular enzymes overexpressed and secreted by cancer cells are the MMPs. Like phosphatases, MMPs have been explored to induce cancer cells death and to assist delivery of drugs. Tanaka et al. developed a peptide lipid precursor sensitive to high levels of MMP7 (Figure 4.4b) [150]. The incubation of several cell lines with the generated precursor showed a selective extracellular hydrolysis only around cancer cell lines overexpressing MMP7. After enzymatic cleaving of the hydrophilic moiety from the precursor, the resulting hydrogelator is released, further internalized and self-assembled inside cancer cells causing cellular death. This strategy based on a synthesized precursor composed of a supramolecular gelator region conjugated to a hydrophilic fragment was also exploited by other authors as enzyme substrates for MMPs in cancer cell therapy [151, 152], as method to detect protease activity via hydrogelation [153] and to nanoencapsulate and release a chemotherapy drug (Table 4.4) [154].

4.3.1.3 Thermolysin

Thermolysin, a bacterial thermostable extracellular protease, catalyzes the formation of covalent bonds between two substrates (e.g. peptides) by reverse hydrolysis in aqueous solution. Proteases normally hydrolyze peptide bonds in aqueous medium; however, the formation of a thermodynamically more stable and higher ordered structure, as supramolecular hydrogel, shifts the reaction equilibrium favoring peptide ligation (Figure 4.4c) [163]. Toledano et al. described this conceptually novel approach by using thermolysin to produce *in situ* amphiphilic Fmoc-tripeptides hydrogelators. Nongelling Fmoc–amino acids conjugates were linked to dipeptides and further self-assembled into 3D fibril supramolecular network for cell culture applications [164]. This elegant strategy of EISA has been further explored to synthesize Fmoc-peptide-esters fibrous hydrogels via amide bond formation for potential applications in TE or enzyme detection [155] and gelation of ionic peptides [156].

4.3.1.4 β-Lactamases

β-Lactamases are bacterial enzymes able to catalyze the disruption of β-lactam antibiotics such as penicillin or cephalosporin, deactivating the antibacterial properties and causing widespread antimicrobial drug resistance. A hydrogelator bound to a β-lactamase responsive cephem unit was synthesized (Figure 4.4d). Upon β-lactamase treatment, the hydrogelator is released and self-assembled to yield supramolecular hydrogels [157]. These authors demonstrated that EISA is a powerful alternative tool for the detection of β-lactamases-producing bacteria and screening for new β-lactamases inhibitors.

4.3.2 DNA Polymerases

DNA is a strong hydrophilic polyelectrolyte consisting of a small set of complementary nucleotide monomers. Highly specific interactions between monomers (adenine–thymine and guanine–cytosine) facilitate the design of synthetic self-assembled 2D and 3D structures in solution. DNA is an excellent candidate for the construction of supramolecular hydrogels due to their relatively easy modification by specific enzymes, such as polymerases, ligases, endonucleases, and exonucleases. The generated hydrogels have adjustable mechanical properties, controlled biodegradability, and self-healing and stimuli-responsive properties [165]. Accessibility to larger DNA quantities owed to the significant advances in the chemical synthesis and biotechnological production prompted the incorporation of this biomolecule as a bulk material in hydrogels. The embedment of nanoparticles [166] or proteins [167–169] allowed for DNA scaffolds upgrading.

DNA building blocks are assembled through enzymatic ligation or hybridization of DNA ends and/or intercalated motifs [165]. Luo laboratory covalently cross-linked 3D-branched DNA molecules via ligase leading to a biodegradable and easily molded gel matrix [166]. The adjustment of DNA concentrations and sequence result in the formation of tunable hydrogels for applications such as 3D cell culture, cell transplant therapy, or controlled drug delivery, TE, among others [165]. DNA hydrogels have also been generated *in situ* through polymerase chain reaction (PCR). Thermally stabilized branched Y-shaped DNA sequences served as a PCR primers, instead of standard linear primers. When linked together, they form a 3D network. The PCR process also enabled the coupling of multiple sequences of modified monomers, such as nucleotides conjugated to fluorescent dyes, onto a single PCR product [158]. DNA polymerization can result in gels with metamaterial behavior, acting as solid in aqueous solution, liquid-like upon water removal and presenting shape-memory properties when re-hydrated. These meta-hydrogels were explored as a bioelectronic interface to create an electric circuit that uses water as a switch. Upon water removal, the hydrogel became "liquid-like" conforming a channel shape that linked two electrodes, turning on the circuit. In presence of water, the meta-hydrogel presented "solid-like" properties receding from the electrodes and shutting off the current. These metaproperties can also be exploited in biomedical applications for controlled drug release or cell therapy [159]. In another approach, Chen and Romesberg functionalized nucleotidic monomers with an azide group. Upon DNA polymerization, each modified monomer incorporated a 5′-alkyne-modified single-stranded molecule via click chemistry. Then, these single-strain polynucleotides were converted to a double-stranded DNA by DNA polymerase creating an original bottlebrush DNA architecture that able to generate hydrogels [160].

4.4 Conclusions

As outlined, enzyme-mediated hydrogel formation has become an interesting synthetic route to prepare soft materials for various biomedical applications, especially in the TE and RM field. Hydrogel matrix formation is triggered by specific enzyme-catalyzed chemical reactions that enable the physical or chemical cross-linking of different precursors, e.g. covalently cross-linked macromolecular polymers or by self-assembling of small molecules into supramolecular structures. Regardless the different enzymatic approaches used to generate hydrogels, these strategies share the following common characteristics: (i) control over the gelation kinetics, (ii) mild reaction conditions that allow for the encapsulation of bioactive molecules and cells without compromising their bioactivity, and (iii) tunable mechanical and swelling properties suitable for controlled drug delivery.

Enzymatically cross-linked hydrogels are mainly used as injectable scaffolds, drug and bioactive delivery vehicles, wound dressings, muco/bioadhesive, or cell encapsulation systems. HRP, TG, and tyrosinase can be highlighted as the most studied enzyme systems due to (i) their commercial availability (extraction, purification, and stability), (ii) well-known activity (reaction conditions, enzyme substrates, and mechanisms of action), (iii) compatible with a wide range of precursors (e.g. polymers, biopolymers, proteins, or other macromolecules), and (iv) the simple synthetic routes to design and modify precursors with enzyme substrates. However, there are still many unexplored enzymes that would expand the existing toolbox for enzymatically cross-linked scaffolds formation. Despite the major advances and advantages of this strategy, there are still challenges to overcome such as (i) the stability and availability of the enzymes, (ii) limited mechanical properties of some hydrogels, and (iii) the scarcer amount of *in vivo* studies. Moreover, there are some crucial questions that need to be addressed, such as: what happens when the enzyme is embedded in the gel matrix during the hydrogel formation? Some examples clearly demonstrated that enzymes are still active after encapsulation, but it is not clear how these enzymes can affect the biological/biomedical application.

On the other hand, one prominent area of research is enzymatic hydrogelation of small molecules to produce supramolecular hydrogels. Enzyme-triggered formation of hydrogelators: (i) allows minimal invasive delivery of the 3D matrices in form of liquid precursors, (ii) offers a superior opportunity to generate/degrade hydrogels in response to a biological stimulus, (iii) prepare hydrophilic hydrogels from hydrophobic drug derivative compounds or macromolecules, and (iv) since small molecules can also enter the cell, the enzymatic reaction can occur in intra or extracellular environments. Phosphatase, thermolysin, β-lactamase, MMPs, and DNA polymerase are the most representative enzymes to produce supramolecular hydrogels by noncovalent interactions; however, any endogenous enzyme susceptible to be overexpressed/downregulated due to a medical condition, such as cancer, cardiovascular disease, osteoarthritis, or Alzheimer, is also a good candidate. However, the lack of information related to the enzymes activity, mechanism of action, or participation in a specific biological event limits the application of this enzymatic approach. Supramolecular hydrogels versatility makes them good candidates also for (i) diseases treatment and diagnosis, (ii) enzyme inhibitors screening in visual readout assays, (iii) biomineralization in skeletal TE, and (iv) the development of bioelectronic interfaces devices. Despite these advantages, there are still many challenges such as control over the diffusion of the precursors, improvement of the stability of the precursors, and monitoring the kinetics *in vivo*.

References

1 Hoffman, A.S. (2012). Hydrogels for biomedical applications. *Adv. Drug Delivery Rev.* 64 (suppl): 18–23. https://doi.org/10.1016/j.addr.2012.09.010.

2 Nguyen, M.K. and Lee, D.S. (2010). Injectable biodegradable hydrogels. *Macromol. Biosci.* 10 (6): 563–579. https://doi.org/10.1002/mabi.200900402.

3 Nguyen, Q.V., Huynh, D.P., Park, J.H., and Lee, D.S. (2015). Injectable polymeric hydrogels for the delivery of therapeutic agents: a review. *Eur. Polym. J.* 72: 602–619. https://doi.org/10.1016/j.eurpolymj.2015.03.016.

4 Nguyen, M. and khan; Eben Alsberg. (2014). Bioactive factor delivery strategies from engineered polymer hydrogels for therapeutic medicine. *Prog. Polym. Sci.* 39 (7): 1236–1265. https://doi.org/10.1016/j.progpolymsci.2013.12.001.Bioactive.

5 Balakrishnan, B., Joshi, N., Jayakrishnan, A., and Banerjee, R. (2014). Self-crosslinked oxidized alginate/gelatin hydrogel as injectable, adhesive biomimetic scaffolds for cartilage regeneration. *Acta Biomater.* 10 (8): 3650–3663. https://doi.org/10.1016/j.actbio.2014.04.031.

6 Jeznach, O. and Sajkiewicz, P. (2018). Review article injectable hydrogels and nanocomposite hydrogels for cartilage regeneration. *J. Biomed. Mater. Res. Part A* https://doi.org/10.1002/jbm.a.36449.

7 Van Tomme, S.R., Storm, G., and Hennink, W.E. (2008). In situ gelling hydrogels for pharmaceutical and biomedical applications. *Int. J. Pharm.* 355 (1, 2): 1–18. https://doi.org/10.1016/j.ijpharm.2008.01.057.

8 Nezhad-Mokhtari, P., Ghorbani, M., Roshangar, L., and Soleimani Rad, J. (2019). Chemical gelling of hydrogels-based biological macromolecules for tissue engineering: photo- and enzymatic-crosslinking methods. *Int. J. Biol. Macromol.* 139: 760–772. https://doi.org/10.1016/j.ijbiomac.2019.08.047.

9 Liu, G., Ding, Z., Yuan, Q. et al. (2018). Multi-layered hydrogels for biomedical applications. *Front. Chem.* 6: 1–10. https://doi.org/10.3389/fchem.2018.00439.

10 Xu, X., Sun, H., Wang, Y. et al. (2020). Fabrication of a multifunctional hydrogel with a robust interface bioinspired by the structure of the dentogingival junction. *Chem. Commun.* 56 (25): 3633–3636. https://doi.org/10.1039/d0cc00907e.

11 Wei, K., Chen, X., Zhao, P. et al. (2019). Stretchable and bioadhesive supramolecular hydrogels activated by a one-stone-two-bird postgelation functionalization method. *ACS Appl. Mater. Interfaces* 11 (18): 16328–16335. https://doi.org/10.1021/acsami.9b03029.

12 Kumar, K., Dhawan, N., Sharma, H. et al. (2014). Bioadhesive polymers: novel tool for drug delivery. *Artif. Cells Nanomed. Biotechnol.* 42 (4): 274–283. https://doi.org/10.3109/21691401.2013.815194.

13 Tan, H. and Marra, K.G. (2010). Injectable, biodegradable hydrogels for tissue engineering applications. *Materials* 3 (3): 1746–1767. https://doi.org/10.3390/ma3031746.

14 Jiang, Y., Chen, J., Deng, C. et al. (2014). Click hydrogels, microgels and nanogels: emerging platforms for drug delivery and tissue engineering. *Biomaterials* 35 (18): 4969–4985. https://doi.org/10.1016/j.biomaterials.2014.03.001.

15 Bruggeman, K.F., Williams, R.J., and Nisbet, D.R. (2018). Dynamic and responsive growth factor delivery from electrospun and hydrogel tissue engineering materials. *Adv. Healthc. Mater.* 7 (1): 1–14. https://doi.org/10.1002/adhm.201700836.

16 Scigalkova, I., Bystronova, J., Kovarova, L. et al. (2019). Formulations within soft hydrogels on encapsulated monocytes and incoming immune cells. *RSC Adv.* 9: 21396–21404. https://doi.org/10.1039/c9ra02878a.

17 Eslahi, N., Abdorahim, M., and Simchi, A. (2016). Smart polymeric hydrogels for cartilage tissue engineering: a review on the chemistry and biological functions. *Biomacromolecules* 17 (11): 3441–3463. https://doi.org/10.1021/acs.biomac.6b01235.

18 Maitra, J. and Shukla, V.K. (2014). Cross-linking in hydrogels – a review. *Am. J. Polym. Sci.* 4 (2): 25–31. https://doi.org/10.5923/j.ajps.20140402.01.

19 Hennink, W.E. and van Nostrum, C.F. (2012). Novel crosslinking methods to design hydrogels. *Adv. Drug Delivery Rev.* 64 (Suppl): 223–236. https://doi.org/10.1016/j.addr.2012.09.009.

20 Buwalda, S.J., Boere, K.W.M., Dijkstra, P.J. et al. (2014). Hydrogels in a historical perspective: from simple networks to smart materials. *J. Controlled Release* 190: 254–273. https://doi.org/10.1016/j.jconrel.2014.03.052.

21 Fadeev, M., Davidson-Rozenfeld, G., Biniuri, Y. et al. (2018). Redox-triggered hydrogels revealing switchable stiffness properties and shape-memory functions. *Polym. Chem.* 9 (21): 2905–2912. https://doi.org/10.1039/c8py00515j.

22 Ma, S., Rong, M., Lin, P. et al. (2018). Fabrication of 3D tubular hydrogel materials through on-site surface free radical polymerization. *Chem. Mater.* 30 (19): 6756–6768. https://doi.org/10.1021/acs.chemmater.8b02532.

23 Rodgers, Z.L., Hughes, R.M., Doherty, L.M. et al. (2015). B12-mediated, long wavelength photopolymerization of hydrogels. *J. Am. Chem. Soc.* 139 (9): 3372–3378. https://doi.org/10.1097/CCM.0b013e31823da96d.Hydrogen.

24 Hu, W., Wang, Z., Xiao, Y. et al. (2019). Advances in crosslinking strategies of biomedical hydrogels. *Biomater. Sci.* 7 (3): 843–855. https://doi.org/10.1039/c8bm01246f.

25 Zhang, Z., Loebus, A., De Vicente, G. et al. (2014). Synthesis of poly(ethylene glycol)-based hydrogels via amine-Michael type addition with tunable stiffness and postgelation chemical functionality. *Chem. Mater.* 26 (12): 3624–3630. https://doi.org/10.1021/cm500203j.

26 Li, Y., Liu, C., Tan, Y. et al. (2014). In situ hydrogel constructed by starch-based nanoparticles via a Schiff base reaction. *Carbohydr. Polym.* 110: 87–94. https://doi.org/10.1016/j.carbpol.2014.03.058.

27 Xu, J., Liu, Y., and Hsu, S. (2019). Hydrogels based on Schiff base linkages for biomedical applications. *Molecules* 24 (3005): 1–21.

28 Ding, H., Liang, X., Zhang, X.N. et al. (2019). Tough supramolecular hydrogels with excellent self-recovery behavior mediated by metal-coordination interaction. *Polymer* 171 (February): 201–210. https://doi.org/10.1016/j.polymer.2019.03.061.

29 Ahn, J., Park, S., Lee, J.H. et al. (2013). Fluorescent hydrogels formed by CH–π and π–π interactions as the main driving forces: an approach toward understanding the relationship between fluorescence and structure. *Chem. Commun.* 49 (21): 2109–2111. https://doi.org/10.1039/c2cc37249e.

30 Zhang, J., Wang, N., Liu, W. et al. (2013). Intermolecular hydrogen bonding strategy to fabricate mechanically strong hydrogels with high elasticity and fatigue resistance. *Soft Matter* 9 (27): 6331–6337. https://doi.org/10.1039/c3sm50866h.

31 Xiao, T., Xu, L., Zhou, L. et al. (2019). Dynamic hydrogels mediated by macrocyclic host–guest interactions. *J. Mater. Chem. B* 7 (10): 1526–1540. https://doi.org/10.1039/c8tb02339e.

32 Zhao, X., Huebsch, N., Mooney, D.J., and Suo, Z. (2010). Stress-relaxation behavior in gels with ionic and covalent crosslinks. *J. Appl. Phys.* 107 (6): 1–5. https://doi.org/10.1063/1.3343265.

33 Miyamae, K., Nakahata, M., Takashima, Y., and Harada, A. (2015). Self-healing, expansion–contraction, and shape-memory properties of a preorganized supramolecular hydrogel through host–guest interactions. *Angew. Chem. Int. Ed.* 54 (31): 8984–8987. https://doi.org/10.1002/anie.201502957.

34 Lin, P., Ma, S., Wang, X., and Zhou, F. (2015). Molecularly engineered dual-crosslinked hydrogel with ultrahigh mechanical strength, toughness, and good self-recovery. *Adv. Mater.* 27 (12): 2054–2059. https://doi.org/10.1002/adma.201405022.

35 Wang, B., Xiao, X., Zhang, Y., and Liao, L. (2019). High strength dual-crosslinked hydrogels with photo-switchable color changing behavior. *Eur. Polym. J.* 116: 545–553. https://doi.org/10.1016/j.eurpolymj.2019.04.035.

36 Yang, Y., Wang, X., Yang, F. et al. (2018). Highly elastic and ultratough hybrid ionic–covalent hydrogels with tunable structures and mechanics. *Adv. Mater.* 30 (18): 1–9. https://doi.org/10.1002/adma.201707071.

37 Ren, K., He, C., Xiao, C. et al. (2015). Injectable glycopolypeptide hydrogels as biomimetic scaffolds for cartilage tissue engineering. *Biomaterials* 51: 238–249. https://doi.org/10.1016/j.biomaterials.2015.02.026.

38 He, J., Chen, R., Lu, Y. et al. (2016). Fabrication of circular micro fluidic network in enzymatically-crosslinked gelatin hydrogel. *Mater. Sci. Eng. C* 59: 53–60. https://doi.org/10.1016/j.msec.2015.09.104.

39 Nguyen, D.H., Tran, N.Q., and Nguyen, C.K. (2013). Tetronic-grafted chitosan hydrogel as an injectable and biocompatible scaffold for biomedical applications. *J. Biomater. Sci., Polym. Ed.* 24 (14): 1636–1648. https://doi.org/10.1080/09205063.2013.789356.

40 Sofia, S.J., Singh, A., and Kaplan, D.L. (2002). Peroxidase-catalyzed crosslinking of functionalized polyaspartic acid polymers. *J. Macromol. Sci. Part A Pure Appl. Chem.* 10 (9): 1151–1181. https://doi.org/10.1081/MA-120014843.

41 Darr, A. and Calabro, A. (2009). Synthesis and characterization of tyramine-based hyaluronan hydrogels. *J. Mater. Sci. Mater. Med.* 20 (1): 33–44. https://doi.org/10.1007/s10856-008-3540-0.

42 Lee, F., Chung, J.E., and Kurisawa, M. (2009). An injectable hyaluronic acid-tyramine hydrogel system for protein delivery. *J. Controlled Release* 134 (3): 186–193. https://doi.org/10.1016/j.jconrel.2008.11.028.

43 Kurisawa, M., Chung, J.E., Yang, Y.Y. et al. (2005). Injectable biodegradable hydrogels composed of hyaluronic acid-tyramine conjugates for drug delivery and tissue engineering. *Chem. Commun.* 34: 4312–4314. https://doi.org/10.1039/b506989k.

44 Kurisawa, M., Lee, F., Wang, L.S., and Chung, J.E. (2010). Injectable enzymatically crosslinked hydrogel system with independent tuning of mechanical strength and gelation rate for drug delivery and tissue engineering. *J. Mater. Chem.* 20 (26): 5371–5375. https://doi.org/10.1039/b926456f.

45 Lee, F., Chung, J.E., and Kurisawa, M. (2008). An injectable enzymatically crosslinked hyaluronic acid-tyramine hydrogel system with independent tuning of mechanical strength and gelation rate. *Soft Matter* 4 (4): 880–887. https://doi.org/10.1039/b719557e.

46 Toh, W.S., Lim, T.C., Kurisawa, M., and Spector, M. (2012). Modulation of mesenchymal stem cell chondrogenesis in a tunable hyaluronic acid hydrogel microenvironment. *Biomaterials* 33 (15): 3835–3845. https://doi.org/10.1016/j.biomaterials.2012.01.065.

47 Kim, K.S., Park, S.J., Yang, J.A. et al. (2011). Injectable hyaluronic acid-tyramine hydrogels for the treatment of rheumatoid arthritis. *Acta Biomater.* 7 (2): 666–674. https://doi.org/10.1016/j.actbio.2010.09.030.

48 Frith, J.E., Cameron, A.R., Menzies, D.J. et al. (2013). An injectable hydrogel incorporating mesenchymal precursor cells and pentosan polysulphate for intervertebral disc regeneration. *Biomaterials* 34 (37): 9430–9440. https://doi.org/10.1016/j.biomaterials.2013.08.072.

49 Ren, K., He, C., Cheng, Y. et al. (2014). Injectable enzymatically crosslinked hydrogels based on a poly(L-glutamic acid) graft copolymer. *Polym. Chem.* 5 (17): 5069–5076. https://doi.org/10.1039/c4py00420e.

50 Wang, R., Zhou, B., Liu, W. et al. (2014). Fast in situ generated polylysine-poly(ethylene glycol) hydrogels as tissue adhesives and hemostatic materials using an enzyme-catalyzed method. *J. Biomater. Appl.* 29 (8): 1167–1179. https://doi.org/10.1177/0885328214553960.

51 Wang, R., Xu, D., Liang, L. et al. (2016). Enzymatically crosslinked epsilon-poly-L-lysine hydrogels with inherent antibacterial properties for wound infection prevention. *RSC Adv.* 6: 8620–8627. https://doi.org/10.1039/C5RA15616E.

52 Jin, R., Hiemstra, C., Zhong, Z., and Feijen, J. (2007). Enzyme-mediated fast in situ formation of hydrogels from dextran – tyramine conjugates. *Biomaterials* 28: 2791–2800. https://doi.org/10.1016/j.biomaterials.2007.02.032.

53 Jin, R. (2010). Hydrogels as injectable scaffolds. *Tissue Eng. Part A* 16: 8. https://doi.org/10.1089/ten.tea.2009.0764.

54 Jin, R., Moreira Teixeira, L.S., Dijkstra, P.J. et al. (2010). Enzymatically-crosslinked injectable hydrogels based on biomimetic dextran-hyaluronic acid conjugates for cartilage tissue engineering. *Biomaterials* 31 (11): 3103–3113. https://doi.org/10.1016/j.biomaterials.2010.01.013.

55 Jin, R., Moreira Teixeira, L.S., Dijkstra, P.J. et al. (2011). Chondrogenesis in injectable enzymatically crosslinked heparin/dextran hydrogels. *J. Controlled Release* 152 (1): 186–195. https://doi.org/10.1016/j.jconrel.2011.01.031.

56 Ogushi, Y., Sakai, S., and Kawakami, K. (2007). Synthesis of enzymatically-gellable carboxymethylcellulose for biomedical applications. *J. Biosci. Bioeng.* 104 (1): 30–33. https://doi.org/10.1263/jbb.104.30.

57 Sakai, S., Ito, S., Ogushi, Y. et al. (2009). Enzymatically fabricated and degradable microcapsules for production of multicellular spheroids with well-defined diameters of less than 150 mm. *Biomaterials* 30 (30): 5937–5942. https://doi.org/10.1016/j.biomaterials.2009.07.031.

58 Amini, A.A. and Nair, L.S. (2012). Enzymatically cross-linked injectable gelatin gel as osteoblast delivery vehicle. *J. Bioact. Compat. Polym.* 27 (4): 342–355. https://doi.org/10.1177/0883911512444713.

59 Lee, Y., Bae, W., Lee, W., and Dong, K. (2014). Enzyme-catalyzed in situ forming gelatin hydrogels as bioactive wound dressings: effects of fibroblast delivery on wound healing efficacy. *J. Mater. Chem. B* 7712–7718. https://doi.org/10.1039/C4TB01111B.

60 Lee, Y. (2013). In situ forming gelatin-based tissue adhesives and their phenolic content-driven properties. *J. Mater. Chem. B* 2407–2414. https://doi.org/10.1039/c3tb00578j.

61 Wang, L.S., Du, C., Toh, W.S. et al. (2014). Modulation of chondrocyte functions and stiffness-dependent cartilage repair using an injectable enzymatically crosslinked hydrogel with tunable mechanical properties. *Biomaterials* 35 (7): 2207–2217. https://doi.org/10.1016/j.biomaterials.2013.11.070.

62 Lim, T.C., Toh, W.S., Wang, L.S. et al. (2012). The effect of injectable gelatin-hydroxyphenylpropionic acid hydrogel matrices on the proliferation, migration, differentiation and oxidative stress resistance of adult neural stem cells. *Biomaterials* 33 (12): 3446–3455. https://doi.org/10.1016/j.biomaterials.2012.01.037.

63 Yoon, D.S., Lee, Y., Ryu, H.A. et al. (2016). Cell recruiting chemokine-loaded sprayable gelatin hydrogel dressings for diabetic wound healing. *Acta Biomater.* 38: 59–68. https://doi.org/10.1016/j.actbio.2016.04.030.

64 Yao, M., Zhang, J., Gao, F. et al. (2019). New BMSC-laden gelatin hydrogel formed in situ by dual-enzymatic cross-linking accelerates dermal wound healing. *ACS Omega* 4 (5): 8334–8340. https://doi.org/10.1021/acsomega.9b00878.

65 Liu, Y., Sakai, S., and Taya, M. (2013). Impact of the composition of alginate and gelatin derivatives in bioconjugated hydrogels on the fabrication of cell sheets and spherical tissues with living cell sheaths. *Acta Biomater.* 9 (5): 6616–6623. https://doi.org/10.1016/j.actbio.2013.01.037.

66 Kuo, K., Lin, R., Tien, H. et al. (2015). Bioengineering vascularized tissue constructs using an injectable cell-laden enzymatically crosslinked collagen hydrogel derived from dermal extracellular matrix. *Acta Biomater.* https://doi.org/10.1016/j.actbio.2015.09.002.

67 Gohil, S.V., Brittain, S.B., Kan, H.M. et al. (2015). Evaluation of enzymatically crosslinked injectable glycol chitosan hydrogel. *J. Mater. Chem. B* 3 (27): 5511–5522. https://doi.org/10.1039/c5tb00663e.

68 Petkova, P., Francesko, A., and Tzanov, T. (2015). Enzyme-assisted formation of hybrid biopolymer hydrogels incorporating active phenolic nanospheres. *Eng. Life Sci.* 15 (4): 416–424. https://doi.org/10.1002/elsc.201400143.

69 Tran, N.Q., Joung, Y.K., Lih, E. et al. (2010). Supramolecular hydrogels exhibiting fast in situ gel forming and adjustable degradation properties. *Biomacromolecules* 11 (3): 617–625. https://doi.org/10.1021/bm100047y.

70 Sakai, S., Yamada, Y., Zenke, T., and Kawakami, K. (2009). Novel chitosan derivative soluble at neutral pH and in-situ gellable via peroxidase-catalyzed enzymatic reaction. *J. Mater. Chem.* 19 (2): 230–235. https://doi.org/10.1039/b812086b.

71 Hou, J., Li, C., Guan, Y. et al. (2015). Polymer chemistry improved adhesion properties. *Polym. Chem.* 6: 2204–2213. https://doi.org/10.1039/c4py01757a.

72 Park, K.M., Shin, Y.M., Joung, Y.K. et al. (2010). In situ forming hydrogels based on tyramine conjugated 4-arm-PPO-PEO via enzymatic oxidative reaction. *Biomacromolecules* 11 (3): 706–712. https://doi.org/10.1021/bm9012875.

73 Sakai, S. (2013). Polyvinyl alcohol-based hydrogel dressing gellable on-wound via a co-enzymatic reaction triggered by glucose in the wound exudate. *J. Mater. Chem. B* 5067–5075. https://doi.org/10.1039/c3tb20780c.

74 Wei, Q., Xu, M., Liao, C. et al. (2016). Printable hybrid hydrogel by dual enzymatic polymerization with superactivity. *Chem. Sci.* 7 (4): 2748–2752. https://doi.org/10.1039/c5sc02234g.

75 Nguyen, H.D., Liu, H., Hudson, B.N., and Lin, C. (2019). Enzymatic cross-linking of dynamic thiol-norbornene click hydrogels. *ACS Biomater. Sci. Eng.* 5: 1247–1256. https://doi.org/10.1021/acsbiomaterials.8b01607.

76 Choi, Y.R., Kim, E.H., Lim, S., and Choi, Y.S. (2018). Efficient preparation of a permanent chitosan/gelatin hydrogel using an acid-tolerant tyrosinase. *Biochem. Eng. J.* 129: 50–56. https://doi.org/10.1016/j.bej.2017.10.016.

77 Chen, T., Embree, H.D., Brown, E.M. et al. (2003). Enzyme-catalyzed gel formation of gelatin and chitosan: potential for in situ applications. *Biomaterials* 24 (17): 2831–2841. https://doi.org/10.1016/S0142-9612(03)00096-6.

78 Chen, T., Embree, H.D., Wu, L., and Payne, G.F. (2002). Protein – polysaccharide conjugation: tyrosinase-catalyzed conjugation of gelatin and chitosan. *Biopolym. Orig. Res. Biomol.* 64: 292–302. https://doi.org/10.1002/bip.10196.

79 Wu, L.Q., Bentley, W.E., and Payne, G.F. (2011). Biofabrication with biopolymers and enzymes: potential for constructing scaffolds from soft matter. *Int. J. Artif. Organs* 34 (2): 215–224. https://doi.org/10.5301/IJAO.2011.6406.

80 Yamada, K., Chen, T., Kumar, G. et al. (2000). Chitosan based water-resistant adhesive. Analogy to mussel glue. *Biomacromolecules* 1 (2): 252–258. https://doi.org/10.1021/bm0003009.

81 Gyung, D.K., Ki, H.L., Chang, S.K. et al. (2004). Silk fibroin/chitosan conjugate crosslinked by tyrosinase. *Macromol. Res.* 12 (5): 534–539.

82 Demolliens, A., Boucher, C., Durocher, Y. et al. (2008). Tyrosinase-catalyzed synthesis of a universal coil-chitosan bioconjugate for protein immobilization. *Bioconjugate Chem.* 19 (9): 1849–1854. https://doi.org/10.1021/bc800066b.

83 Jin, R. and Lin, C. (2013). Tyrosinase-mediated in situ forming hydrogels from biodegradable chondroitin sulfate–tyramine conjugates. *J. Am. Chem. Soc.* 2011: 353–361. https://doi.org/10.1002/pi.4306.

84 Kim, S., Lee, S., Lee, J. et al. (2018). Tissue adhesive, rapid forming, and sprayable ECM hydrogel via recombinant tyrosinase crosslinking. *Biomaterials* 178: 401–412. https://doi.org/10.1016/j.biomaterials.2018.04.057.

85 Arkenberg, M.R. and Lin, C.C. (2017). Orthogonal enzymatic reactions for rapid crosslinking and dynamic tuning of PEG-peptide hydrogels. *Biomater. Sci.* 5 (11): 2231–2240. https://doi.org/10.1039/c7bm00691h.

86 Rocasalbas, G., Francesko, A., Touriño, S. et al. (2013). Laccase-assisted formation of bioactive chitosan/gelatin hydrogel stabilized with plant polyphenols. *Carbohydr. Polym.* 92 (2): 989–996. https://doi.org/10.1016/j.carbpol.2012.10.045.

87 Stefanov, I., Hinojosa-Caballero, D., Maspoch, S. et al. (2018). Enzymatic synthesis of a thiolated chitosan-based wound dressing crosslinked with chicoric acid. *J. Mater. Chem. B* 6 (47): 7943–7953. https://doi.org/10.1039/c8tb02483a.

88 Stefanov, I., Pérez-Rafael, S., Hoyo, J. et al. (2017). Multifunctional enzymatically generated hydrogels for chronic wound application. *Biomacromolecules* 18 (5): 1544–1555. https://doi.org/10.1021/acs.biomac.7b00111.

89 Huber, D., Tegl, G., Baumann, M. et al. (2017). Chitosan hydrogel formation using laccase activated phenolics as cross-linkers. *Carbohydr. Polym.* 157: 814–822. https://doi.org/10.1016/j.carbpol.2016.10.012.

90 Huber, D., Grzelak, A., Baumann, M. et al. (2018). Anti-inflammatory and anti-oxidant properties of laccase-synthesized phenolic-*O*-carboxymethyl chitosan hydrogels. *New Biotechnol.* 40: 236–244. https://doi.org/10.1016/j.nbt.2017.09.004.

91 Bersanetti, P.A., Escobar, V.H., Nogueira, R.F. et al. (2019). Enzymatically obtaining hydrogels of PVA crosslinked with ferulic acid in the presence of laccase for biomedical applications. *Eur. Polym. J.* 112: 610–618. https://doi.org/10.1016/j.eurpolymj.2018.10.024.

92 Bakota, E.L., Aulisa, L., Galler, K.M., and Hartgerink, J.D. (2011). Enzymatic cross-linking of a nanofibrous peptide hydrogel. *Biomacromolecules* 12 (1): 82–87. https://doi.org/10.1021/bm1010195.

93 Schense, J.C., Bloch, J., Aebischer, P., and Hubbell, J.A. (2000). Enzymatic incorporation of bioactive peptides into fibrin matrices enhances neurite extension. *Nat. Biotechnol.* 18 (4): 415–419. https://doi.org/10.1038/74473.

94 Hall, H., Baechi, T., and Hubbell, J.A. (2001). Molecular properties of fibrin-based matrices for promotion of angiogenesis in vitro. *Microvasc. Res.* 62 (3): 315–326. https://doi.org/10.1006/mvre.2001.2348.

95 Peretti, G.M., Xu, J.W., Bonassar, L.J. et al. (2006). Review of injectable cartilage engineering using fibrin gel in mice and swine models. *Tissue Eng.* 12 (5): 1151–1168. https://doi.org/10.1089/ten.2006.12.1151.

96 Eyrich, D., Brandl, F., Appel, B. et al. (2007). Long-term stable fibrin gels for cartilage engineering. *Biomaterials* 28 (1): 55–65. https://doi.org/10.1016/j.biomaterials.2006.08.027.

97 Williams, C., Budina, E., Stoppel, W.L. et al. (2015). Cardiac extracellular matrix – fibrin hybrid scaffolds with tunable properties for cardiovascular tissue engineering. *Acta Biomater.* 14: 84–95. https://doi.org/10.1016/j.actbio.2014.11.035.

98 Sperinde, J.J. and Griffith, L.G. (1997). Synthesis and characterization of enzymatically-cross-linked poly(ethylene glycol) hydrogels. *Macromolecules* 9297 (97): 5255–5264. https://doi.org/10.1021/ma970345a.

99 Sperinde, J.J. and Griffith, L.G. (2000). Control and prediction of gelation kinetics in enzymatically cross-linked poly(ethylene glycol) hydrogels. *Macromolecules* 5476–5480.

100 Hu, B. and Messersmith, P. (2005). Enzymatically cross-linked hydrogels and their adhesive strength to biosurfaces. *Orthod. Craniofac. Res.* 8: 145–149.

101 Jones, M.R. (2008). Facile coupling of synthetic peptides and peptide-polymer conjugates to cartilage via transglutaminase enzyme. *Biomaterials* 28 (35): 5215–5224.

102 Ehrbar, M., Rizzi, S.C., Schoenmakers, R.G. et al. (2007). Biomolecular hydrogels formed and degraded via site-specific enzymatic reactions. *Biomacromolecules* 8 (10): 3000–3007. https://doi.org/10.1021/bm070228f.

103 Sala, A., Ehrbar, M., Trentin, D. et al. (2010). Enzyme mediated site-specific surface modification. *Langmuir* 26 (13): 11127–11134. https://doi.org/10.1021/la1008895.

104 Blache, U., Metzger, S., Vallmajo-Martin, Q. et al. (2016). Dual role of mesenchymal stem cells allows for microvascularized bone tissue-like environments in PEG hydrogels. *Adv. Healthc. Mater.* 5 (4): 489–498. https://doi.org/10.1002/adhm.201500795.

105 Mosiewicz, K.A., Kolb, L., Van Der Vlies, A.J. et al. (2013). In situ cell manipulation through enzymatic hydrogel photopatterning. *Nat. Mater.* 12 (11): 1072–1078. https://doi.org/10.1038/nmat3766.

106 Ranga, A., Lutolf, M.P., Hilborn, J., and Ossipov, D.A. (2016). Hyaluronic acid hydrogels formed in situ by transglutaminase-catalyzed reaction. *Biomacromolecules* 17 (5): 1553–1560. https://doi.org/10.1021/acs.biomac.5b01587.

107 Crescenzi, V., Francescangeli, A., and Taglienti, A. (2002). New gelatin-based hydrogels via enzymatic networking. *Biomacromolecules* 21: 1384–1391. https://doi.org/10.1021/bm025657m.

108 Yung, C.W., Wu, L.Q., Tullman, J.A. et al. (2007). Transglutaminase crosslinked gelatin as a tissue engineering scaffold. *J. Biomed. Mater. Res. Part A* 83 (4): 1039–1046. https://doi.org/10.1002/jbm.a.

109 Yung, C.W., Bentley, W.E., and Barbari, T.A. (2010). Diffusion of interleukin-2 from cells overlaid with cytocompatible enzyme-crosslinked gelatin hydrogels. *J. Biomed. Mater. Res. Part A* 95 (1): 25–32. https://doi.org/10.1002/jbm.a.32740.

110 Broderick, E.P., Halloran, D.M.O., Rochev, Y.A. et al. (2004). Enzymatic stabilization of gelatin-based scaffolds. *J. Biomed. Mater. Res. Part B* 37–42. https://doi.org/10.1002/jbm.b.30119.

111 Chen, T., Small, D.A., McDermott, M.K. et al. (2003). Enzymatic methods for in situ cell entrapment and cell release. *Biomacromolecules* 4 (6): 1558–1563. https://doi.org/10.1021/bm034145k.

112 Chen, P., Yang, K., Wu, C. et al. (2014). Fabrication of large perfusable macroporous cell-laden hydrogel scaffolds using microbial transglutaminase. *Acta Biomater.* 10 (2): 912–920. https://doi.org/10.1016/j.actbio.2013.11.009.

113 Hale, M.K.M.C., Setton, L., and Chilkoti, A. (2005). Synthesis and in vitro evaluation of enzymatically cross-linked elastin-like polypeptide gels for cartilaginous tissue repair. *Tissue Eng. Part A* 11 (11): 1768–1779.

114 Davis, N.E., Ding, S., Forster, R.E. et al. (2012). Modular enzymatically crosslinked protein polymer hydrogels for in situ gelation. *Biomaterials* 31 (28): 7288–7297. https://doi.org/10.1016/j.biomaterials.2010.06.003.Modular.

115 Song, F., Zhang, L., Shi, J., and Li, N. (2010). Novel casein hydrogels: formation, structure and controlled drug release. *Colloids Surf. B* 79 (1): 142–148. https://doi.org/10.1016/j.colsurfb.2010.03.045.

116 Broguiere, N., Isenmann, L., and Zenobi-Wong, M. (2016). Novel enzymatically cross-linked hyaluronan hydrogels support the formation of 3D neuronal networks. *Biomaterials* 99: 47–55. https://doi.org/10.1016/j.biomaterials.2016.04.036.

117 Zhao, L., Li, X., Zhao, J. et al. (2016). A novel smart injectable hydrogel prepared by microbial transglutaminase and human-like collagen: its characterization and biocompatibility. *Mater. Sci. Eng. C* 68: 317–326. https://doi.org/10.1016/j.msec.2016.05.108.

118 Li, X. and Fan, D. (2019). Smart collagen hydrogels based on 1-ethyl-3-methylimidazolium acetate and microbial transglutaminase for potential applications in tissue engineering and cancer therapy. *ACS Biomater. Sci. Eng.* 5 (7): 3523–3536. https://doi.org/10.1021/acsbiomaterials.9b00393.

119 Cai, X., Hu, S., Yu, B. et al. (2018). Transglutaminase-catalyzed preparation of crosslinked carboxymethyl chitosan/carboxymethyl cellulose/collagen composite membrane for postsurgical peritoneal adhesion prevention. *Carbohydr. Polym.* 201 (2): 201–210. https://doi.org/10.1016/j.carbpol.2018.08.065.

120 Mosiewicz, K.A., Johnsson, K., and Lutolf, M.P. (2010). Phosphopantetheinyl transferase-catalyzed formation of bioactive hydrogels for tissue engineering. *J. Am. Chem. Soc.* 5972–5974.

121 El-Sherbiny, I.M. and Yacoub, M.H. (2013). Hydrogel scaffolds for tissue engineering: progress and challenges. *Global Cardiol. Sci. Pract.* 3: 316–342. https://doi.org/10.5339/gcsp.2013.38.

122 Xu, F. (2000). Applications of oxidoreductases: recent progress. *Ind. Biotechnol.* 1: 38–50.

123 Hoang Thi, T.T., Lee, Y., Le Thi, P., and Park, K.D. (2019). Engineered horseradish peroxidase-catalyzed hydrogels with high tissue adhesiveness for biomedical applications. *J. Ind. Eng. Chem.* 78: 34–52. https://doi.org/10.1016/j.jiec.2019.05.026.

124 Ryan, B.J., Carolan, N., and Ó'Fágáin, C. (2006). Horseradish and soybean peroxidases: comparable tools for alternative niches? *Trends Biotechnol.* 24 (8): https://doi.org/10.1016/j.tibtech.2006.06.007.

125 Hollmann, F. and Arends, I.W.C.E. (2012). Enzyme initiated radical polymerizations. *Polymers* 759–793. https://doi.org/10.3390/polym4010759.

126 Kobayashi, S., Uyama, H., and Kimura, S. (2001). Enzymatic polymerization. *Chem. Rev.* 101 (12): 3793–3818. https://doi.org/10.1021/cr990121l.

127 Sugumaran, M. (2016). Reactivities of quinone methides versus *o*-quinones in catecholamine metabolism and eumelanin biosynthesis. *Int. J. Mol. Sci.* 1–23. https://doi.org/10.3390/ijms17091576.

128 Jin, R., Lou, B., and Lin, C. (2013). Tyrosinase-mediated in situ forming hydrogels from biodegradable chondroitin sulfate-tyramine conjugates. *Polym. Int.* 62 (3): 353–361. https://doi.org/10.1002/pi.4306.

129 Freddi, G., Anghileri, A., Sampaio, S. et al. (2006). Tyrosinase-catalyzed modification of *Bombyx mori* silk fibroin: grafting of chitosan under heterogeneous reaction conditions. *J. Biotechnol.* 125 (2): 281–294. https://doi.org/10.1016/j.jbiotec.2006.03.003.

130 Anghileri, A., Lantto, R., Kruus, K. et al. (2007). Tyrosinase-catalyzed grafting of sericin peptides onto chitosan and production of protein-polysaccharide bioconjugates. *J. Biotechnol.* 127 (3): 508–519. https://doi.org/10.1016/j.jbiotec.2006.07.021.

131 Riva, S., Molecolare, R., and Bianco, V.M. (2006). Laccases: blue enzymes for green chemistry. *Trends Biotechnol.* 24 (5): https://doi.org/10.1016/j.tibtech.2006.03.006.

132 Blanco, A. and Blanco, G. (2017). Enzymes. In: *Medical Biochemistry* (ed. A. Blanco and G. Blanco), 153–175. Cambridge, Massachusetts, United States: Academic press, Elsevier Inc. https://doi.org/10.1016/B978-0-12-803550-4/00008-2.

133 Griffin, M., Casadio, R., and Bergamini, C.M. (2002). Transglutaminases: nature's biological glues. *Biochem. J.* 396: 377–396.

134 Yang, Z., Gu, H., Fu, D. et al. (2004). Enzymatic formation of supramolecular hydrogels. *Adv. Mater.* 16 (16): 1440–1444. https://doi.org/10.1002/adma.200400340.

135 Yang, Z. and Xu, B. (2004). A simple visual assay based on small molecule hydrogels for detecting inhibitors of enzymes. *Chem. Commun.* 10 (21): 2424–2425. https://doi.org/10.1039/b408897b.

136 Schnepp, Z.A.C., Gonzalez-McQuire, R., and Mann, S. (2006). Hybrid biocomposites based on calcium phosphate mineralization of self-assembled supramolecular hydrogels. *Adv. Mater.* 18 (14): 1869–1872. https://doi.org/10.1002/adma.200502545.

137 Gao, J., Wang, H., Wang, L. et al. (2009). Enzyme promotes the hydrogelation from a hydrophobic small molecule. *J. Am. Chem. Soc.* 131 (32): 11286–11287. https://doi.org/10.1021/ja9042142.

138 Gao, Y., Kuang, Y., Guo, Z.F. et al. (2009). Enzyme-instructed molecular self-assembly confers nanofibers and a supramolecular hydrogel of taxol derivative. *J. Am. Chem. Soc.* 131 (38): 13576–13577. https://doi.org/10.1021/ja904411z.

139 Wang, H., Yang, C., Wang, L. et al. (2011). Self-assembled nanospheres as a novel delivery system for taxol: a molecular hydrogel with nanosphere morphology. *Chem. Commun.* 47 (15): 4439–4441. https://doi.org/10.1039/c1cc10506j.

140 Wang, H., Yang, C., Tan, M. et al. (2011). A structure-gelation ability study in a short peptide-based "super hydrogelator" system. *Soft Matter* 7 (8): 3897–3905. https://doi.org/10.1039/c0sm01405b.

141 Yang, Z., Liang, G., and Xu, B. (2006). Supramolecular hydrogels based on β-amino acid derivatives. *Chem. Commun.* 7: 738–740. https://doi.org/10.1039/b516133a.

142 Yang, Z., Liang, G., Ma, M. et al. (2007). In vitro and in vivo enzymatic formation of supramolecular hydrogels based on self-assembled nanofibers of a β-amino acid derivative. *Small* 3 (4): 558–562. https://doi.org/10.1002/smll.200700015.

143 Yang, Z., Liang, G., Guo, Z. et al. (2007). Intracellular hydrogelation of small molecules inhibits bacterial growth. *Angew. Chem. Int. Ed.* 46 (43): 8216–8219. https://doi.org/10.1002/anie.200701697.

144 Gao, Y., Shi, J., Yuan, D., and Xu, B. (2012). Imaging enzyme-triggered self-assembly of small molecules inside live cells. *Nat. Commun.* 3: https://doi.org/10.1038/ncomms2040.

145 Pires, R.A., Abul-Haija, Y.M., Costa, D.S. et al. (2015). Controlling cancer cell fate using localized biocatalytic self-assembly of an aromatic carbohydrate amphiphile. *J. Am. Chem. Soc.* 137 (2): 576–579. https://doi.org/10.1021/ja5111893.

146 Wang, H., Feng, Z., Wang, Y. et al. (2016). Integrating enzymatic self-assembly and mitochondria targeting for selectively killing cancer cells without acquired drug resistance. *J. Am. Chem. Soc.* 138 (49): 16046–16055. https://doi.org/10.1021/jacs.6b09783.

147 Jeena, M.T., Palanikumar, L., Go, E.M. et al. (2017). Mitochondria localization induced self-assembly of peptide amphiphiles for cellular dysfunction. *Nat. Commun.* 8 (1): 1–9. https://doi.org/10.1038/s41467-017-00047-z.

148 Yang, Z., Liang, G., Wang, L., and Xu, B. (2006). Using a kinase/phosphatase switch to regulate a supramolecular hydrogel and forming the supramolecular hydrogel in vivo. *J. Am. Chem. Soc.* 128 (9): 3038–3043. https://doi.org/10.1021/ja057412y.

149 Yang, Z., Xu, K., Guo, Z. et al. (2007). Intracellular enzymatic formation of nanofibers results in hydrogelation and regulated cell death. *Adv. Mater.* 19 (20): 3152–3156. https://doi.org/10.1002/adma.200701971.

150 Tanaka, A., Fukuoka, Y., Morimoto, Y. et al. (2015). Cancer cell death induced by the intracellular self-assembly of an enzyme-responsive supramolecular gelator. *J. Am. Chem. Soc.* 137 (2): 770–775. https://doi.org/10.1021/ja510156v.

151 Yang, Z., Ma, M., and Xu, B. (2009). Using matrix metalloprotease-9 (MMP-9) to trigger supramolecular hydrogelation. *Soft Matter* 5 (13): 2546–2548. https://doi.org/10.1039/b908206a.

152 Koda, D., Maruyama, T., Minakuchi, N. et al. (2010). Proteinase-mediated drastic morphological change of peptide-amphiphile to induce supramolecular hydrogelation. *Chem. Commun.* 46 (6): 979–981. https://doi.org/10.1039/b920359a.

153 Bremmer, S.C., McNeil, A.J., and Soellner, M.B. (2014). Enzyme-triggered gelation: targeting proteases with internal cleavage sites. *Chem. Commun.* 50 (14): 1691–1693. https://doi.org/10.1039/c3cc48132h.

154 Kalafatovic, D., Nobis, M., Son, J. et al. (2016). MMP-9 triggered self-assembly of doxorubicin nanofiber depots halts tumor growth. *Biomaterials* 98: 192–202. https://doi.org/10.1016/j.biomaterials.2016.04.039.

155 Das, A.K., Collins, R., and Ulijn, R.V. (2008). Exploiting enzymatic (reversed) hydrolysis in directed self-assembly of peptide nanostructures. *Small* 4 (2): 279–287. https://doi.org/10.1002/smll.200700889.

156 Guilbaud, J.B., Vey, E., Boothroyd, S. et al. (2010). Enzymatic catalyzed synthesis and triggered gelation of ionic peptides. *Langmuir* 26 (13): 11297–11303. https://doi.org/10.1021/la100623y.

157 Yang, Z., Ho, P., Liang, G. et al. (2007). Using lactamase to trigger supramolecular hydrogelation. *J. Am. Chem. Soc.* 266–267. https://doi.org/10.1021/ja0675604.

158 Hartman, M.R., Yang, D., Tran, T.N.N. et al. (2013). Thermostable branched DNA nanostructures as modular primers for polymerase chain reaction. *Angew. Chem. Int. Ed.* 52 (33): 8699–8702. https://doi.org/10.1002/anie.201302175.

159 Lee, J.B., Peng, S., Yang, D. et al. (2012). A mechanical metamaterial made from a DNA hydrogel. *Nat. Nanotechnol.* 7 (12): 816–820. https://doi.org/10.1038/nnano.2012.211.

160 Chen, T. and Romesberg, F.E. (2017). Enzymatic synthesis, amplification, and application of DNA with a functionalized backbone. *Angew. Chem. Int. Ed.* 56 (45): 14046–14051. https://doi.org/10.1002/anie.201707367.

161 Li, X., Wang, Y., Yang, C. et al. (2014). Supramolecular nanofibers of triamcinolone acetonide for uveitis therapy. *Nanoscale* 6 (23): 14488–14494. https://doi.org/10.1039/c4nr04761c.

162 Rauner, N., Meuris, M., Zoric, M., and Tiller, J.C. (2017). Enzymatic mineralization generates ultrastiff and tough hydrogels with tunable mechanics. *Nature* 1–6. https://doi.org/10.1038/nature21392.

163 Williams, R.J., Smith, A.M., Collins, R. et al. (2009). Enzyme-assisted self-assembly under thermodynamic control. *Nat. Nanotechnol.* 4 (1): 19–24. https://doi.org/10.1038/nnano.2008.378.

164 Toledano, S., Williams, R.J., Jayawarna, V., and Ulijn, R.V. (2006). Enzyme-triggered self-assembly of peptide hydrogels via reversed hydrolysis. *J. Am. Chem. Soc.* 128 (4): 1070–1071. https://doi.org/10.1021/ja056549l.

165 Gačanin, J., Synatschke, C.V., and Weil, T. (2020). Biomedical applications of DNA-based hydrogels. *Adv. Funct. Mater.* 30 (4): https://doi.org/10.1002/adfm.201906253.

166 Um, S.H., Lee, J.B., Park, N. et al. (2006). Enzyme-catalysed assembly of DNA hydrogel. *Nat. Mater.* 5 (10): 797–801. https://doi.org/10.1038/nmat1741.

167 Meng, H.M., Liu, H., Kuai, H. et al. (2016). Aptamer-integrated DNA nanostructures for biosensing, bioimaging and cancer therapy. *Chem. Soc. Rev.* 45 (9): 2583–2602. https://doi.org/10.1039/c5cs00645g.

168 Nimjee, S.M., White, R.R., Becker, R.C., and Sullenger, B.A. (2017). Aptamers as therapeutics. *Annu. Rev. Pharmacol. Toxicol.* 57: 61–79. https://doi.org/10.1146/annurevpharmtox-010716-104558.

169 Lai, J., Li, S., Shi, X. et al. (2017). Displacement and hybridization reactions in aptamer-functionalized hydrogels for biomimetic protein release and signal transduction. *Chem. Sci.* 8 (11): 7306–7311. https://doi.org/10.1039/c7sc03023a.

5

Hierarchical Peptide- and Protein-Based Biomaterials: From Molecular Structure to Directed Self-assembly and Applications

Yinchen Yuan, Yejiao Shi, and Helena S. Azevedo

Queen Mary University of London, Institute of Bioengineering, School of Engineering and Materials Science, Mile End road, London E1 4NS, UK

5.1 Introduction

Hierarchical materials, with dimensions of features ranging from the nano- to the macroscale, are extremely common in nature to provide properties of interest. For example, macromolecules such as collagen and cellulose are nanoscale building blocks of human tissues and higher plants, which play critical roles in their organization, properties, and function.

The extracellular matrix (ECM) of tissues is a dynamic and hierarchically organized nanocomposite that regulates essential cell functions such as adhesion, migration, proliferation, and differentiation. Engineering complex tissues requires biomaterial scaffolds that recapitulate the structure and composition of the ECM to provide cells with physical and biochemical signals that are important for tissue development and organization. Much of the functionality in cells and tissues are maintained and/or result from self-assembly of their individual constituents [1]. In fact, self-assembly has been exploited to fabricate biomaterials as they are typically formed of a network of interwoven nanofibers reminiscent of the filamentous structures found in the ECM. However, 3D scaffolds, in which cells are randomly distributed, offer limited control over spatial cell organization and tissue architecture. Nano/microscale control over biomaterial composition and architecture may enable improved regulation of cell–material interactions and cell–cell contacts.

Alignment of nanostructures provides a strategy to control materials properties and macroscale cell behavior. Different strategies have been investigated to create hierarchical organization in self-assembling biomaterials, including the use of concentration gradients, controlled diffusion/mobility of molecules [2, 3], and supramolecular aggregates that can be generated under specific environmental conditions (e.g. temperature, mechanical agitation, electrical fields, space confinement). In the following sections, we attempt to identify rules that govern self-assembly across different length scales.

Multifunctional Hydrogels for Biomedical Applications, First Edition.
Edited by Ricardo A. Pires, Iva Pashkuleva, and Rui L. Reis.

5.2 Molecular Design/Selection of Building Blocks for Hierarchical Self-assembly

Self-assembly, a widely existing process in nature, is a facile and versatile method for the bottom–up fabrication of functional biomaterials [4]. Among different building blocks used in molecular self-assembly, peptides have drawn great attention and been extensively utilized for diverse applications in biomedicine because of their good biocompatibility and biodegradability, structural and functional programmability, as well as their synthetic simplicity and affordability [5]. Through rational design, a variety of peptide nanostructures, such as fibers, tubes, tapes, micelles, could be generated by self-assembly through the subtle balance of noncovalent forces, including electrostatic, hydrophobic, hydrogen bonding, van der Waals interactions, and aromatic stacking [6].

Synthetic peptides are built up by natural or nonnatural amino acids. In nature, there are 20 different amino acids which have the same basic structure, with an amine group, a carboxyl group, a hydrogen atom, and a side chain covalently attached to a central carbon atom. Their unique characteristics derive from their variable side chains, which can be divided into three different categories (Figure 5.1) [7]. Hydrophobic amino acids, with aliphatic side chains (A, V, L, I, and M), can provide hydrophobic interactions, while the ones with aromatic side chains (F, Y, and W) can be engaged in π–π stacking in addition. Hydrophilic amino acids with uncharged side chains can create hydrogen bonds through either hydroxyl (S and T) or amide (N and Q) groups, while the ones with either positively charged (K, R, and H) or negatively charged (E and D) can also be involved in electrostatic interactions. On the other hand, glycine, with no side chain, and proline with its side chain being covalently linked to the amine terminus can be utilized to balance the structure rigidity of the peptide molecules due to its flexible and locked conformation, respectively. All these interactions and conformations imposed by the different amino acids can govern the self-assembly of peptides and influence the hierarchical order of peptide-based materials. Therefore, the realization of hierarchical self-assembly of peptides hinges upon rational molecular design of the peptide sequences and selection of specific building blocks, which can control the different noncovalent interactions promoting the multiscale hierarchical assembly for the formation of anisotropic materials.

In this section, we summarize and discuss various peptide designs based on the selection of different categories of amino acids, which have been explored to influence the self-assembly of peptides from the supramolecular level to micro length scale and lead to the generation of highly ordered architectures (Table 5.1). We aim to provide a toolbox for building anisotropy in peptide materials based on a directed self-assembly process.

5.2.1 Hydrophobic Aromatic Amino Acids

Owing to the high diamagnetic susceptibility of aromatic rings, peptides containing aromatic amino acids have been frequently utilized as building blocks for magnetic

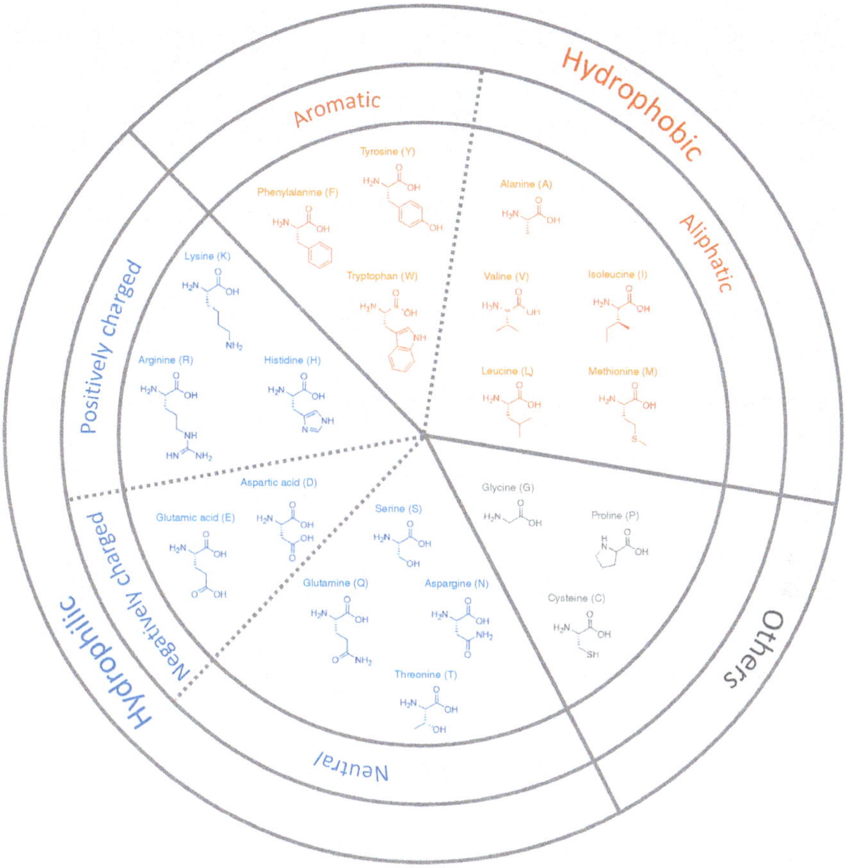

Figure 5.1 The 20 natural amino acids grouped into three main categories: their common names, one letter abbreviations, and chemical structures are given. Source: Based on Fleming and Ulijn [7].

alignment of peptide assemblies as the magnetic susceptibility is amplified when in the assembled state. For example, Tendler and collaborators reported the alignment of self-assembled aromatic dipeptide (FF) nanotubes under a magnetic field ($B > 7$ T) with their long axis parallel to the magnetic field direction [16]. Alignment of self-assembled naphthalene diphenylalanine (Nap-FF) worm-like micelles under magnetic field was also described by Adams and coworkers, and the aligned structures could be further retained upon transformation to anisotropic hydrogel with the addition of $CaCl_2$ or reduction of pH [17].

In addition to magnetic field, Yan's group demonstrated that the aromatic dipeptide Fmoc-FF could also respond to ultrasonic waves and undergo solid–solid phase transition. Ultrasound was suggested to cause high temperature and pressure locally, produced by cavitation effects, disrupt the hydrophobic and π–π stacking intermolecular interactions involved in one phase state of the dipeptide and then rearrange the molecular packing to form another well-ordered crystalline structure [26].

Table 5.1 Rational molecular design of peptides responsive to different environmental manipulations for their hierarchical assembly.

Environmental manipulation	Peptide sequence/ assembly units	Assembly pathway	Final organization	References
Temperature	$C_{15}H_{31}$CONH-AAAAAKK-$CONH_2$	Thermal annealing induced enhanced nanofiber alignment	Aligned nanofibers	[8]
	NH_2-FF-COOH	Thermal annealing induced hexagonal microtubes	Hexagonally packed nanotubes	[9]
Temperature + shear force	$C_{15}H_{31}$CONH-VVVAAAEEE-COOH	Heating charged PA solutions at 80 °C and gradual cooling down to RT formed a liquid crystal. Injecting this liquid crystal into a $CaCl_2$ solution promoted self-assembly and gelification. Shear force generated during injection led to macroscopic alignment of nanofibers parallel to the direction of the applied shear force	Noodle-shaped hydrogels with oriented nanofibers	[10]
	HOOC-EAA-OT4-AAE-COOH (OT4: α-quaterthiophene)	Same as above	Same as above	[11]
Temperature + circumferential shear force + template	$C_{15}H_{31}$CONH-VVVAAAEEE-COOH	Same as above. Using the heated PA solutions, circumferential anisotropic tubes were fabricated in a shear flow chamber with rotating inner rod	Tubular hydrogels with circumferentially aligned nanofibers	[12]
pH	$C_{11}H_{23}$CONH-GAGAGAGY-COOH	pH-induced assembly and alignment of PA due to the different acid dissociation constant of the carboxylic acid at the C-terminus and phenolic hydroxyl groups on tyrosine residue	Well-dispersed cylindrical nanofibers at pH 11; bundles of parallel nanoribbons at pH 8; self-supporting gel ($pH < 8$)	[13]

Table 5.1 (Continued)

Environmental manipulation	Peptide sequence/ assembly units	Assembly pathway	Final organization	References
	$C_{15}H_{31}$CONH-AAAAKKKKG (RADA)$_n$-NH_2 ($n = 1, 2$, and 3); $C_{15}H_{31}$CONH-AAAAKKKKGRGDS-NH_2	Lateral assembly of nanofibers due to electrostatic interactions between complementary sequences designed on the surface region of the PA molecules	Laterally assembled nanofibers	[14]
Enzyme catalysis	Nap-FFF-K-pY-COOH (high birefringence); Nap-FF-K-pY-COOH (little birefringence) p = $PO(OH)_2$	An anisotropic hydrogel spontaneously formed after the treatment with alkaline phosphatase because of enhanced interfiber aromatic–aromatic interactions	Anisotropic hydrogel of aligned nanofibers	[15]
Magnetic field	NH_2-FF-COOH	Aligned nanotubes under magnetic field ($7\,T < B < 12\,T$) with their long axis parallel to the field direction due to the large diamagnetic anisotropy of phenylalanine	Aligned nanotubes	[16]
Magnetic field + pH (or addition of counter ions)	Nap-FF-COOH	When self-assembling into worm-like micelles, the presence of aromatic rings enabled the peptide alignment under magnetic field (9.4 T). The anisotropy was retained upon transformation into hydrogel by addition of $CaCl_2$ or reduction of pH	Aligned supra-molecular hydrogels	[17]

(Continued)

Table 5.1 (Continued)

Environmental manipulation	Peptide sequence/ assembly units	Assembly pathway	Final organization	References
Magnetic field + temperature + UV light	$C_{12}H_{25}$-(diacetylene)-C_8H_{17}CONH-GANPNAAG-COOH	Thermal treatment (90 °C) was conducted to disassemble PA nanofibers followed by cooling in the magnetic field (20 T) and resulting in significant nanofiber alignment. UV irradiation was applied to enable intermolecular cross-linking between PA alkyl tails within the aligned nanofibers	Nanofibers aligned along the magnetic field direction	[18]
Magnetic field (with liquid crystal template) + temperature + UV light	$C_{12}H_{25}$-(diacetylene)-C_8H_{17}CONH-GAGAK-COOH + disodium cromoglycate (LC)	Alignment of PA nanofibers induced by a combination of magnetic field (2 T) and liquid crystal template after thermal treatment (80 °C). The presence of LC template allowed alignment in lower fields. Photopoly-merization of aligned PA bundles was achieved by UV irradiation	Aligned PA nanofibers on centimeter scale and oriented parallel to the LC template (perpendicu-lar to the magnetic field direction) and with improved mechanical stability	[19]
Electric field	$C_{15}H_{31}$CONH-VVVAAAKKK-$CONH_2$ (+) + $(C_{14}H_{22}NO_{11})_n$ (HA, −)	Co-assembly of building blocks with different molecular sizes and opposite charge was directed under the electric field. The strengths and directions of electric field affected nanofiber growth	Membranes with different nanofiber orientation and physical properties (thickness, mechanical properties).	[20]

Table 5.1 (Continued)

Environmental manipulation	Peptide sequence/ assembly units	Assembly pathway	Final organization	References
Electric field + shear force (electro-spinning)	$C_{15}H_{31}$CONH-EEVVV-COOH $C_{15}H_{31}$CONH-VVVAAAEEE-COOH	Electric field applied to PA nanofibers with high surface charge density (electrospinning) induces orientation of PA nanofibers along the spinning direction through shear forces generated at the cone-jet	Electrospun PA fibers made of aligned nanofiber bundles	[21]
X-ray	$C_{15}H_{31}$CONH-AAAAAAEEE-COOH	Crystallization of PA filaments mediated by enhanced electrostatic repulsions induced by X-ray irradiation	Crystallized PA filaments	[22]
Shear force	KK(SLXL)$_3$KK; X = serine (no benzyl ring but a hydroxyl group), or phenylalanine (a benzyl ring but no hydroxylation), or tyrosine (one benzyl ring and one hydroxyl group), or DOPA (one benzyl ring and two hydroxyl groups)	When X = DOPA, shear force assisted in forming anisotropic hydrogel string; DOPA can also be oxidized to initiate covalent cross-linking which enhanced the gel birefringence and structure integrity	X = serine or DOPA, similar nanofibers; X = phenylalanine, shorter and more Rigid nanofibers; X = tyrosine, longer and more flexible nanofibers	[23]
	HOOC-VEVAG-OPV3-GAVEV-COOH (OPV3: 1,4-distyryl-benzene)	Non-heated peptide-chromophore solution dispensed into HCl solution	Noodle-like hydrogel with oriented nanofibers	

(Continued)

Table 5.1 (Continued)

Environmental manipulation	Peptide sequence/ assembly units	Assembly pathway	Final organization	References
Ultrasound	$C_{15}H_{31}$CONH-AAAAGGGpSRGD-COOH (more hydrophilic, less β-sheet and shorter persistence length); $C_{15}H_{31}$ CONH-AAAA GGGEIKVAV-COOH (more hydrophobic, more β-sheet; and longer persistence length)	Ultrasonic agitation enhanced the alignment of stiffer PA nanofibers (with higher hydrophobicity, more β-sheet character, and longer persistence length) on PDMS pattern	Patterned and aligned nanofibers	[24]
	NH_2-^{D}FFD-COOH (organogel in methanol); NH_2-^{D}FFI-COOH (hydrogel in water)	One-directional ultrasound assisted anisotropic arrangement of supramolecular interactions (highly related to the peptide sequence and solvent environment)	Aligned fibrous structures	[25]
	Fmoc-FF-COOH	Ultrasound directed solid–solid transformation of dipeptide to crystalline nanobelt structures	Crystalline dipeptide nanobelts	[26]
Substrate patterned by soft lithography	Ac-KKQLQLQ-LQLQLQLKK-$CONH_2$ (+) + HA (−)	The co-assembly of building blocks with opposite charge was performed by casting on PDMS molds with different topographical patterns	Membranes with nanofibrous structure and defined topographical micropatterns	[27]

Table 5.1 (Continued)

Environmental manipulation	Peptide sequence/ assembly units	Assembly pathway	Final organization	References
Substrate patterned by soft lithography + UV light	KKLLA(K)-(COC_8H_{16})-diacetylene-($C_{12}H_{25}$); RGDSKKLA(K)-(COC_8H_{16})-diacetylene-($C_{12}H_{25}$)	Patterns were created using PDMS mold during PA self-assembly and gelation with NH_4OH. UV-triggered polymerization of diacetylene groups enhanced the mechanical properties of gels	Micropatterned self-assembling nanofibrous PA gels over large areas	[28]
Substrate patterned by soft lithography + temperature	NH_2-FF-COOH	Amorphous thin peptide film on Si substrate converted into crystalline peptide nanowires through high-temperature aniline vapor aging under anhydrous conditions. Surface-mediated nucleation and vertical growth driven by high temperature and aniline vapor. The use of micro-patterned PDMS allowed the growth of aligned nanowires on patterned areas	Vertically aligned peptide nanowires on Si substrate	[29]

Crystallization of the aromatic dipeptide has also been reported to be induced during the thermal annealing process. Robust hexagonal hollow microtubes were observed to form as a result of the confined organization of the FF nanotubes self-assembled in a hexagonal packing pattern with thermal treatment. These crystalline peptide microtubes with hexagonal dimensions have been shown with active optical waveguiding capacity, allowing their potential utility in photonic and electronic devices [9]. When aged in a high-temperature aniline vapor, the aromatic dipeptide FF was found to grow vertically into well-aligned peptide nanowires with a high aspect ratio (at least 100) and a long persistence length (more than 10 μm) [29].

Shao's work reported changes in peptide amphiphile (PA, $C_{11}H_{23}$CONH-GAGAGAGY-COOH) assemblies from well-dispersed cylindrical nanofibers at pH 11 to nanoribbons aggregated in parallel bundles at pH 8, due to the neutralization of phenolic hydroxyl groups on tyrosine residues. Neutralization of the carboxyl group on terminal carboxyl groups also occurred with further pH decrease, resulting in a hierarchically structured robust and plastic PA hydrogel [13]. Moreover, the self-assembly behavior of peptide molecules can also be influenced by the number of hydroxyl groups in the phenolic ring of amino acid side chain. Hartgerink's group designed and characterized a series of multidomain peptides (MDPs) with the general sequence of $K_2(SLXL)_3K_2$, where X = serine, phenylalanine, tyrosine, or 3,4-dihydroxylphenylalanine (DOPA). When X = phenylalanine, with a benzyl ring but no hydroxyl group, shorter and more rigid nanofibers were observed to form, while when X = tyrosine, with a benzyl ring and one hydroxyl group, longer and more flexible nanofibers were obtained. However, when these MDP solutions were injected into HBSS buffer, strings were formed but not strong enough to be lifted from solution and also did not show birefringence. When X = DOPA, with a benzyl ring and two hydroxyl groups, similar long nanofibers were observed to form as when X = serine, with no benzyl ring but one hydroxyl group. Contrary to serine containing MDP, when the DOPA containing MDP solution was sheared into HBSS buffer, anisotropic hydrogel strings composed of parallel aligned nanofibers were generated. This result indicates that the DOPA aromatic side chain is key for the nanofiber alignment. Upon DOPA oxidation, covalent cross-linking within and between these aligned nanofibers could also be initiated, allowing enhanced birefringence and structural integrity of the anisotropic hydrogel strings [23].

Favoring π–π interactions can also induce alignment of peptide assemblies. Xu's group demonstrated that the hydrogelator bearing three phenylalanine residues (Nap-FFF-K-pY-COOH) displayed stronger intermolecular aromatic–aromatic interactions compared to the hydrogelator bearing two phenylalanine residues. These enhanced interactions were believed to be responsible for the alignment of the nanofibers formed during enzymatic hydrogelation (Table 5.1) and thus the generation of anisotropic supramolecular hydrogel [15].

5.2.2 Hydrophobic Aliphatic Amino Acids

Ulijn's and Bai's groups demonstrated that one-directional ultrasonic waves could induce the alignment of the tripeptide (^{D}FFD) assemblies and form highly ordered microfibrous in methanol. However, similar behavior was not observed for ^{D}FFD in water due to the hydrophilic charged aspartic acid in the peptide sequence. By changing the hydrophilic aspartic acid to more hydrophobic isoleucine, the ultrasonic alignment and gelation process could be observed again in water, indicating that the anisotropic arrangement of supramolecular interactions is highly dependent on the peptide sequence and solvent environment [25].

The Stupp's group has demonstrated that PAs can be simultaneously aligned and patterned within microchannels during their self-assembly based on a novel technique called sonication-assisted solution embossing. The process was believed to be driven by a synergistic interaction between the liquid crystal transition and spatial confinement [30]. The group has further reported that more hydrophobic and β-sheet containing PAs interact strongly with the polydimethylsiloxane (PDMS) surface of the stamp, hindering the ability of the PA nanofibers to reorient at a higher degree of confinement with sonication-assisted solution embossing. The more hydrophilic and less β-sheet containing PA nanofibers were easier to cleave, rotate, and align on the PDMS pattern even without the aid of ultrasonication [24].

5.2.3 Hydrophilic Charged Amino Acids

The amine groups at the side chains of lysine, arginine, and histidine residues, as well as the carboxyl groups in glutamic acid and aspartic acid residues, are not only donors or acceptors for intermolecular hydrogen bonds but can also be involved in electrostatic interactions. The protonation and deprotonation state of these amino acids can be selectively altered as the pH is raised above or below their pK_a values, allowing the screening of their charges and the regulation of their interactions. As a consequence, the hierarchical self-assembly of peptides containing these amino acids can be directed through subtle pH changes. Based on this rationale, a series of pH-sensitive PAs, with alternating arginine and aspartic acid in the surface region of the molecule, were designed, $C_{15}H_{31}$CONH-AAAAKKKKG(RADA)$_n$-CONH$_2$ (n = 1, 2, and 3). When the environmental pH was adjusted to 11, the lateral assembly of PA nanofibers into higher order structures was observed due to the attractive electrostatic interactions between the complementary sequences designed in the surface region [14].

Apart from environmental pH manipulation, X-ray irradiation has also been reported to deprotonate the carboxyl group in glutamic acid containing PAs ($C_{15}H_{31}$CONH-AAAAAAEEE-COOH). Upon X-ray irradiation, the electrostatic repulsive forces among the high aspect ratio filaments were enhanced, leading to the compressive rearrangement of the PA filaments into aligned bundles that trapped within a 3D network, leading to the observed crystallization [22]. Additionally, the electrostricted water molecules around charged amino acid residues on the surface of supramolecular assemblies can be dehydrated at elevated temperature, leading to their close aggregation. Stupp's group discovered a thermal pathway that can convert isotropic PA ($C_{15}H_{31}$CONH-VVVAAAEEE-COOH) solutions first into 2D plaques with filamentous texture, when the temperature is increased to 80 °C, then spontaneously align into long-range bundled nanofibers upon cooling to 25 °C [10]. Lysine-containing PA ($C_{15}H_{31}$CONH-AAAAAKK-CONH$_2$) nanofibers were also shown to align when subjected to heat treatment [8]. Combination of heat treatment with shear flow has also been applied on charged peptide–π–peptide conjugates (HOOC-EAA-OT4-AAE-COOH, Table 5.1) to prepare macroscopic noodle hydrogels composed of aligned nanofibers [11].

Charged PAs ($C_{15}H_{31}$CONH-VVVAAAKKK-CONH$_2$) were found to be key in the formation of highly ordered architectures, such as sacs and membranes, during their co-assembly with polyelectrolytes bearing opposite charge, such as hyaluronic acid (HA) [2]. The hierarchical self-assembly was driven by a dynamic synergy between the static self-assembly and excess osmotic pressure of counterions.

5.2.4 Others

The peptide bond has been used to promote alignment of PA nanofibers under strong magnetic field (Table 5.1) [18]. Restuccia et al. synthesized glycosylated self-assembling peptide ("Q11") to generate peptide nanofibers displaying *N*-acetylglucosamine (GlcNAc) on their surface through linkage to asparagine. In crowded conditions (presence of macromolecules), the glycosylated nanofibers laterally pack and align without external intervention, while in dilute conditions, they remain disperse. The GlcNAc moiety interacts strongly with water forming a hydration layer that reduces nanofiber nonspecific association under dilute conditions. Crowded environments produce excluded volume effects and promote the formation of nanofiber bundles and short-range interfiber interactions that facilitate long-range alignment [31].

5.3 Hierarchical Assembly Through Environmental Manipulation

5.3.1 Temperature

Anisotropy in self-assembling systems can be obtained by controlling the temperature, which may be related to the internal solvent evaporation. Stupp's group found a thermal pathway to obtain a long-range aligned PA hydrogel (Table 5.1) [10]. By heating PA solutions to 80 °C and then cooling down to room temperature, aligned nanofiber bundles were observed and an anisotropic hydrogel was formed by injecting treated PA solutions into electrolyte solutions ($CaCl_2$). It was assumed that the thermal treatment caused internal dehydration of PA assemblies, which allows close interaction between fibers leading to the formation of liquid crystalline-like structures. Similar thermal treatment was also applied to a positively charged PA ($C_{15}H_{31}$CONH-AAAAAKK-$CONH_2$), and enhanced nanofiber alignment was observed upon the temperature increase [8]. Yan et al. reported a hexagonal FF microtube with hierarchical structure after thermal treatment [9]. A collagen vitrigel membrane with homogeneous morphology was developed by Guo et al. produced via gelation, vitrification, and rehydration. After gelation was completed, the collagen membrane was dried under controlled vitrification conditions (temperature, relative humidity, and time) before rehydration. The evaporation of trapped moisture in the membrane influenced the self-assembly, enabling reorganization of the collagen fibrils leading to the increasing density and the formation of parallel fibril arrays [32].

5.3.2 Magnetic Field

It is well known that molecules exhibit anisotropic diamagnetism, indicating that they could potentially align under a high magnetic field [33]. The capacity of molecules to align in magnetic fields depends on the energy differences between two orthogonal molecular axes, as molecules prefer the orientation with the smallest energy. Energy differences, ΔE, are determined by Equation (5.1).

$$\Delta E = -\Delta\chi B^2 \tag{5.1}$$

where $\Delta\chi$ is the difference of molecular diamagnetic susceptibility between two orthogonal axes ($\Delta\chi = \chi\| - \chi\perp$) and B is the magnetic induction. However, the energy differences for a single molecule are much smaller compared to the thermal energy. Magnetic orientation is likely to be achieved by the following three approaches: large molecules, like molecular assemblies and macromolecules; pre-assembled molecules such as liquid crystals; molecules containing high magnetic susceptibility units [18, 34]. Magnetic anisotropy in biomolecules such as collagen, silk, and muscle fiber has been reported since 1930s. More recently, it was found that some peptide assemblies were also able to orient in the magnetic field. Magnetic anisotropy in proteins and peptides has been attributed to the diamagnetic anisotropy of the planar peptide bonds. Both β-sheet and α-helix produce anisotropy, though the latter has larger anisotropy because the planar peptide bonds are oriented parallel to the helix axis [35].

Amyloid fibrils can align parallel to the magnetic field due to the β-sheet structure [36]. A 2 T magnetic field was used to pre-align β-amyloid (Aβ) peptides to obtain oriented fibrils for X-ray diffraction, which was introduced by Inouye et al. in 1993 when studying the structure of Aβ amyloid fibril [37]. However, magnetic orientation is more difficult for longer and more physiological peptides. It was found that the ability of Aβ(1–40) and Aβ(11–25) fibers to orient in the magnetic field was enhanced by aging the peptide solutions before the magnetic field was applied, as the long-term storage would promote the formation of liquid crystalline domains [38].

As benzene has a large $\Delta\chi$ of 60×10^{-6} cm^3/mol (about 10 times higher than a peptide bond), magnetic alignment of aromatic peptides has attracted attention [34]. Tendler and coworkers reported the ability of assembled diphenylalanine (FF) tubes to align under magnetic field, with their long axis parallel to the magnetic field direction when $B > 7$ T. The alignment largely owes to the diamagnetic anisotropy of the aromatic rings, since no alignment was observed in peptides with low aromatic content [16]. Magnetic field was also used by Adams and collaborators to align a supramolecular hydrogel by gelling Nap-FF solutions in the magnetic field. At high pH, the formation of long worm-like micelles allowed the naphthalene-functionalized dipeptide to display an anisotropic structure, which was considered as the prerequisite to enable the magnetically alignment [17].

PA nanoribbons with crystal-like molecular order (without aromatic groups) were shown to adopt a high level of alignment in a strong magnetic field of 20 T. The PA, with a GANPNAAG sequence and an N-terminal conjugated hydrophobic alkyl chain containing polymerizable diacetylene moiety, was able to disassemble when heated to 90 °C. The disassembled PA developed an anisotropic structure in the magnetic field during the cooling process since there is no motion restriction caused by fiber entanglement. Since UV light triggers the polymerization of the diacetylene in the PA alkyl tails, this anisotropic would transfer to the polymer backbone [18]. However, as the diamagnetic susceptibility of PA is still very small

($\Delta\chi \approx -611 \times 10^{-12}$ cm^3/mol), a lyotropic chromonic liquid crystal (disodium cromoglycate, $\Delta\chi \approx 1226 \times 10^{-12}$ cm^3/mol) was introduced as template to direct the magnetic alignment of PA assemblies. PA nanofibers were able to align in lower magnetic field (2 T), which was 10 times lower than the previous one [19].

5.3.3 Electric Field

Electric field is also regarded as a powerful method to control the self-assembly process and create ordered assemblies. It is assumed that the electrostatic interactions between charged nanofibers and electric field create the alignment [39]. Type-I collagen was able to assemble into highly oriented and densely packed elongated bundles when electric field was applied, where the electrochemical process induced the differential charging of collagen thereby controlling the self-assembly [40]. An anisotropic hydrogel produced by negatively charged silk nanofiber under the effect of electric field has also been reported [39]. Stupp's group employed electrospinning technique to fabricate microfibers composed of highly aligned bundles of individual PA nanofibers that showed birefringence in polarizing optical microscopy. In this work, negatively charged PAs were used which possess high conductivity and adequate viscosity for electrospinning [21].

Electric field was also found to modify the kinetics of PA–HA membrane assembly since this system involved molecular co-assembly and diffusion of charged species. An increase of aligned fibers was observed when an electric field with certain orientation and strength was applied [41].

Strong electric fields are required to align peptide nanofibers because of their low susceptibility to the field, which may cause, however, detrimental effects such as heating and electrochemical degradation of the peptide, limiting the usage of electric field in orienting peptide nanofibers [20]. The use of liquid crystal template can overcome these drawbacks, guiding the macroscopic alignment of PA bundles formed in the electric field [20].

5.3.4 Patterned Substrates

Soft lithography is a patterning technique that uses a flexible elastomeric master to transfer the pattern to the substrate. The most commonly used elastomeric material is PDMS. There are many patterning techniques, such as dip-pen nanolithography and electron-beam lithography, which have been successfully used to fabricate hierarchical peptide and protein biomaterials [42–44]. Soft lithography has the advantage of producing self-assemblies with flexible orientations and complex organizations, and it is also a low-cost and easily-applied technique [45]. For example, using a PDMS stamp with parallel channels, self-assembling nanofibers were forced to align along the channels within stamps by steric repulsion in confined spaces [24]. The technique is more effective when the width of the confining channel is smaller than the persistence length of nanofiber [24, 30].

Stupp's group combined soft lithography with sonication to guide PA nanofiber alignment and achieve different 2D patterns (e.g. turn-like pattern), in which PA's self-assembly was influenced by both steric confinement and liquid crystal transition within the microchannel of the stamp [30]. The group further used the technology to orient a photosensitive polymerizable PA followed by photo-crosslinking with UV light, creating highly ordered 3D PA structures with various topographies [28]. The PA topographical features were shown to affect stem cell morphology, alignment, and differentiation. More recently, Mata and collaborators fabricated patterned membranes by co-assembling HA and MDPs on PDMS substrates patterned by soft lithography (Table 5.1). Stem cells cultured on the patterned membranes adapted their morphology depending on the topographical patterns they were cultured on [27]. Ryu et al. prepared micropatterned peptide (FF) thin films on silicon (Si) substrate and subjected to high temperature (150 °C) under aniline vapor. Peptide nanowires were found to grow only on the patterned areas (Table 5.1) [29].

5.3.5 Shear Forces

External shearing forces, which can be generated using various approaches, including extruding, drawing, microfluid, and electrospinning, offer the possibility to create long-range aligned nanofibers. Once the shear force is applied, assemblies are forced to align along the direction of the shear. For example, electrospinning was combined with self-assembly to induce alignment of PA nanofibers in the micrometer-scale. The large shear force produced at the cone-jet aligns the PA nanofibers in the direction of the electrospinning jet [21]. However, the extremely high shear forces and voltage required in this technique make it unsuitable for direct encapsulation of cells during the alignment process [12]. Here, we mainly focus on low-speed mechanical approaches, easily accessible in the laboratory, which have successfully been used to fabricate ordered collagen scaffolds but are now being applied to peptide nanofibers [46].

Hartgerink's group reported macroscopic anisotropy in MDPs assisted by shearing forces through syringe delivery. MDPs were also found to form parallel bundles and exhibit shear-thinning and shear recovery properties, which is believed to be related to the shear-induced alignment [23]. Furthermore, the low strain forces produced when dragging a solution of thermally treated liquid crystalline PA from a pipette tip also contributed to the macroscopic alignment and formation of anisotropic self-assembled hydrogel [10]. The similar procedure could also be used to produce tubular PA gels with circumferentially aligned nanofibers in custom-made shear flow chamber [11] and create the macroscopic alignment of peptide motifs bearing π-conjugated functionality [12]. However, the shear-induced long-range alignment was still largely related to the peptide sequence and is more likely to be effective when peptide assemblies have already exhibited some level of anisotropy.

5.3.6 pH

pH changes can affect the self-assembly of charged peptides since amino acid side chains with charged groups can be in either a protonated or deprotonated state, depending on the pH, so that the surface charge of the individual amino acids can be selectively altered as the pH is raised above or below their pK_a value [14, 47]. Therefore, by rationally designing peptides with charged groups, the electrostatic interactions between neighboring peptides can be controlled, which makes it possible to induce the hierarchical self-assembly at certain pHs. Chen et al. designed a series of PAs with the charged region having four consecutive lysine residues and the surface region consisted of RADA segments. It was found that the PA nanofiber was aggregated in a parallel fashion into a network of bundles when the pH was adjusted to 11. At such pH, the charge of lysine residues was screened, which encouraged the nanofiber formation, while the arginine residues remained protonated. The alternating positive and negative charge of RADA sequence at the surface region promoted their lateral assembly [14]. Guo et al. developed $C_{11}H_{23}$CONH-GAGAGAGY-COOH PA and also observed a similar parallel aggregation at pH 11 because of hydrogen bonding formed between surface phenolic hydroxyl groups and carboxyl groups [13].

5.3.7 Ultrasound

In a biomaterial laboratory, the application of ultrasound is not limited to the material dissolution. It can also be used to manipulate the self-assembly process as the high-frequency waves would overcome energy barriers and break intermolecular interactions [25]. Ultrasonic cavitation could also generate local temperatures of up to 5000 K and pressures of several hundred atmospheres in the sample, and the extreme condition may induce changes in the self-assembly behavior [48, 49]. Stupp's group found that PAs were able to align in microchannel patterns, with the aid of sonication, in which the ultrasound broke and reorganized the PA assemblies [24]. Song et al. reported the utility of sonication to direct solid–solid transition of Fmoc-FF organization, in which the isotropic nanosheets would transfer into anisotropic nanobelt with 10-minute ultrasonic irradiation [26]. Pappas et al. utilized one-direction ultrasonic approach to achieve highly ordered tripeptide structures, and apart from peptide sequence, the solvent environment was also believed to influence the anisotropic arrangement [25].

5.3.8 Other Methods

Stupp's group reported the packing of PA filaments into aligned bundles triggered by X-ray because X-ray exposure caused high charge density on the surface of the filaments (Table 5.1), which led to increased electrostatic repulsive force among filaments enabling the crystallization. Addition of ions that screened the charges on the filaments suppressed the formation of crystalline structures [22]. Xu's group developed an enzymatic pathway to fabricate anisotropic hydrogels using rationally designed aromatic peptide containing a tyrosine phosphate moiety. The nanofiber spontaneously aligns during the gelation upon the addition of the enzyme alkaline phosphatase. It was assumed that the anisotropy is the result of both aromatic–aromatic interaction triggered by enzyme catalysis [15].

5.4 Techniques for the Characterization of Hierarchically Organized Biomaterials

5.4.1 Polarized Light Microscopy

Polarized light is especially effective to analyze anisotropic samples such as biological macromolecular assemblies as they are structurally birefringent. These anisotropic samples are capable of separating the incident light into two rays with orthogonal vibration directions and different refractive indices, named ordinary ray and extraordinary ray. The anisotropy of the bulk sample could be observed by directly placing the sample between cross polarizers, which has the advantage of revealing the anisotropy of the whole sample instead of focusing on a small local area [15].

Polarized light microscopy is equipped with a polarizer (positioned in the light path somewhere before the specimen) and an analyzer (in the optical pathway between the objective rear aperture and the observation tubes or camera port) which are at right angle to each other (Figure 5.2a) [15]. The polarizer produces the polarized light entering into the sample, while the analyzer recombines the two out-of-phase rays emerged from the anisotropic sample into a single ray. Polarizing microscopy can be used with either reflected or transmitted mode, which makes it suitable for both transparent and opaque materials. The technique is also very cost-effective and easy to learn. However, like other optical microscopes, it only offers a limited resolution.

Polarizing microscopy has been used to study the structure of highly ordered tissues such as cornea (Figure 5.2c) [50], cartilage [52], and muscle fiber [53], as well as artificial anisotropic biomaterials. For example, different shapes of anisotropic PA hydrogels produced by thermal annealing display bright colors when observed under polarizing microscopy (Figure 5.2b), while isotropic counterparts were invisible [10]. The polarizing color generated from the anisotropic area depends on the relative retardation of the slow ray relative to the fast ray, which increases with the rise of sample thickness and birefringence [51].

Quantitative image analysis enables studying the birefringence and molecular orientation based on the polarizing color. For example, the orientation of collagen fibers in the marginal rib of the dogfish egg could be determined (Figure 5.2e) [51]. Moreover, the birefringence magnitude of anisotropic samples can be determined by quantitative analysis and retardation calculations. Polarized images of supramolecular peptide hydrogel could illustrate the retardation of every resolved point with an OpenPolScope method (Figure 5.2d) [15]. By studying the maximum retardations of magnetic field-induced alignment in different magnetic fields, the effect of magnetic field strengths on the alignment can be known [18]. With the polarized luminescence property, birefringent self-assembling peptides have a further application in *in vivo* bioimaging. Biocompatible peptide Fmoc-FF nanobelts mixed with living cells showed a clear cell image under polarized microscope without the usage of fluorescent dyes [26].

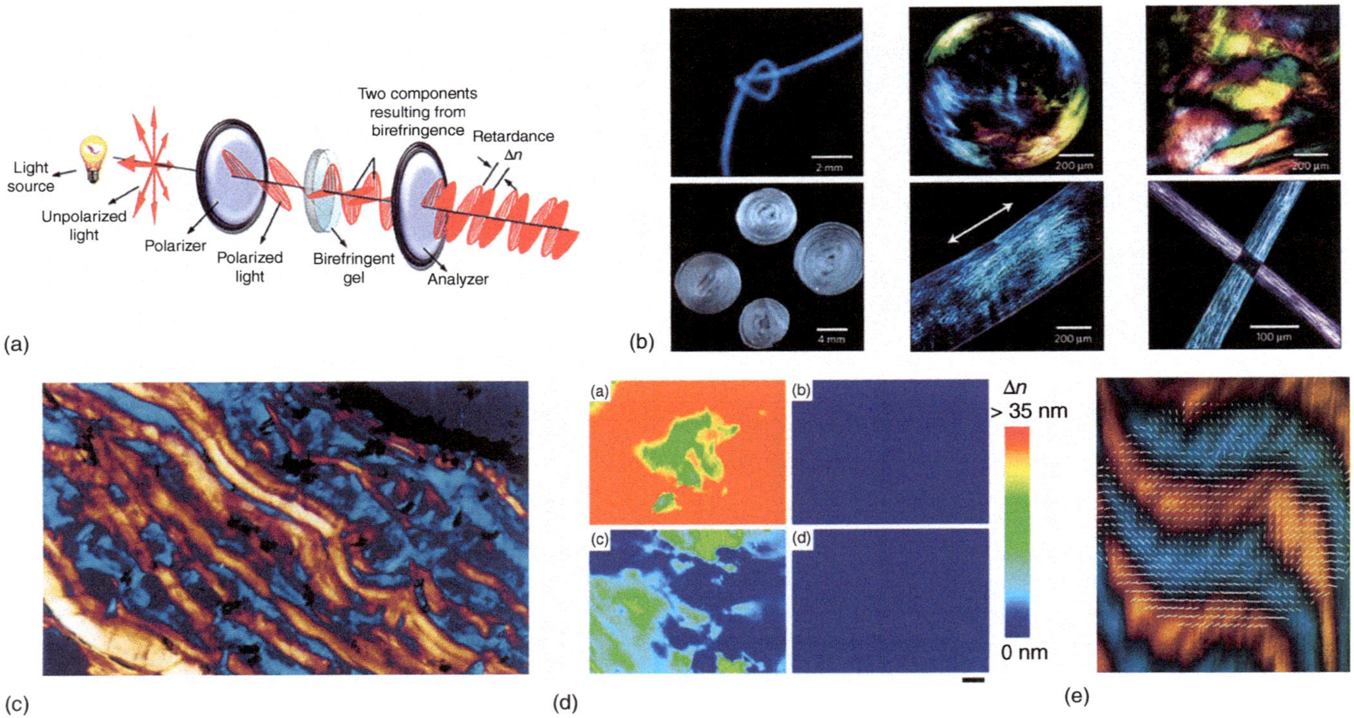

Figure 5.2 (a) The configuration of polarized light microscope. Source: Zhou et al. [15]. (b) Birefringence of anisotropic PA hydrogels of different shapes formed from heated PA solutions and observed between cross polarizers. Source: Zhang et al. [10] / with permission of Springer Nature. (c) Color contrast polarized light microscopy of cross section of bovine sclera showing the collagen orientation. Collagen in the blue regions was at right angles to the collagen in the yellow regions. Source: Meek et al. [50] / with permission of Elsevier. (d) Polarized optical microscopy retardance (Δn) images of four peptide hydrogels (scale bar = 100 μm) used to quantify their birefringence (hydrogel in day 1 had larger birefringence than day 4, while hydrogels in day 2, and day 4 were nonbirefringent) [15]. (e) Vectors on the polarized image of marginal rib of the dogfish egg were obtained from the polarizing color, which illustrated the orientation of collagen fibrils. Source: Ross et al. [51] / with permission of Royal Microscopical Society.

5.4.2 High-Resolution Microscopy (AFM, TEM, and SEM)

Atomic force microscopy (AFM), transmission electron microscopy (TEM), and scanning electron microscopy (SEM) are the most common microscopy methods for direct imaging of nanostructured materials. Compared to optical microscopy, high-resolution microscopy can provide structure information at much smaller length scales, but it also has a few drawbacks. Since most biomimetic constructs are water-content, dehydration is required for electron microscopies so artifacts are often unavoidable (though cryo-SEM and -TEM allow wet samples to be frozen at low temperature) [6]. To study the nanostructure of self-assembling peptides, AFM has mainly been used to image assemblies from solutions dried onto planar solid substrates, such as mica, while the investigation of peptide solutions is also accessible [54]. Conventional TEM enables visualization of dried films on holey grids, with samples usually stained with heavy-metal-containing compounds to enhance contrast [54]. SEM is more intensively used to examine larger assemblies such as films and hydrogels. Because SEM is performed under vacuum, specimens need to be in the dry state. Dehydration followed by critical point drying is often conducted to prevent collapse of the specimens, followed by coating with a few nanometers of electrically conducting metals. High-resolution microscopy is typically focused on local structures at nanoscale, so analyzing the anisotropy of inhomogeneous samples solely based on images provided by AFM, TEM, and SEM can sometimes be misleading [55]. Nonetheless, the hierarchical structure of self-assembled PA–HA membranes was elucidated by TEM and SEM [2].

5.4.3 Small-Angle X-ray Scattering (SAXS)

Small-angle X-ray scattering (SAXS) uses X-rays with the wavelength of 0.07–0.2 nm to study the structure of protein and peptide assemblies [56]. When X-rays travel through the specimen, the intensity and pattern of the scattered X-ray can be recorded. The nanostructure of the sample can be quantified by plotting the curve $I(q)$ against q (I is the scattering intensity and q is the scattering vector determined by $2\sin\,\theta/\lambda$, where λ and θ represent X-ray wavelength and scattering angle, respectively), as $I(q)$ is highly related to the geometric parameters [57]. Anisotropy of biological samples typically shows an ellipsoid-like behavior of $I(q)$ at low q conferred by $I(q) \sim q^{-4}$ [58]. For example, Stupp and coworkers used SAXS to investigate the orientation and order in monodomain gels of aligned nanofibers [10]. The slope of $I(q)$ curve (in double-logarithmic scale) at low q range was −4 at 25 °C (before and after heating) and also at 80 °C (for two minutes), indicating the presence of large and stable aggregates. On the other hand, the q value where a broad scattering was found in the intermediate q range revealed the size of single nanofibers. SAXS experiments on X-ray triggering peptide crystallization studies, showed a series of Bragg peaks with characteristic position of a highly ordered 2D hexagonal lattice after successive irradiation [22]. Techniques utilized to examine the hierarchical structures are summarized in Table 5.2.

Table 5.2 Comparison of different techniques used for the characterization of hierarchical self-assembled peptide- and protein-based biomaterials

	SAXS	AFM	TEM	SEM	Polarized microscopy	References
Resolution	1–100 nm	0.2 nm (XY) 0.05 nm (Z)	0.2 nm	2 nm	0.2–0.5 μm	[54, 55]
Physical principle	Scattering of X-rays	Physical interaction with sample	Scattering of electrons	Emission of electrons	Transmission or reflection of polarized light	[54, 55]
Sample type	Any form of solid, hydrogel, foam, powder, or liquid	Dried or wet sample attached to the substrate	Heavy-metal stained dried film with thickness ideally 30–60 nm	Dried sample. For nonconductive samples, electrically conducting metal coating is required	Any forms	[55]
Representative data	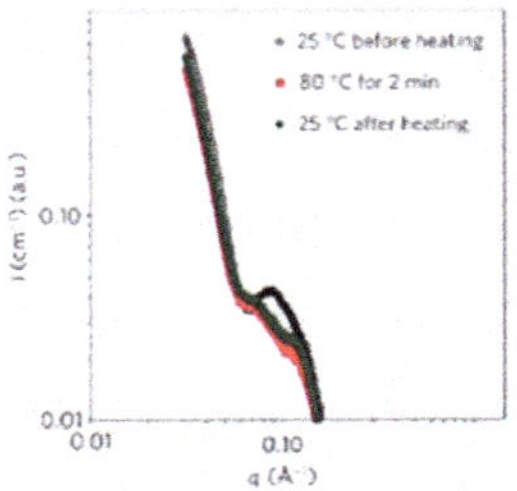	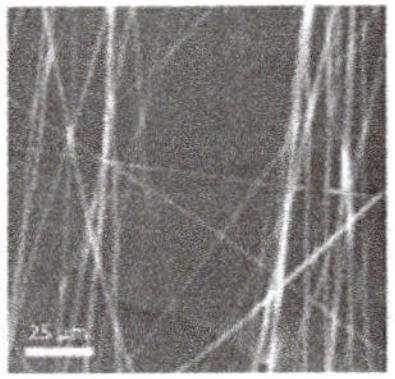	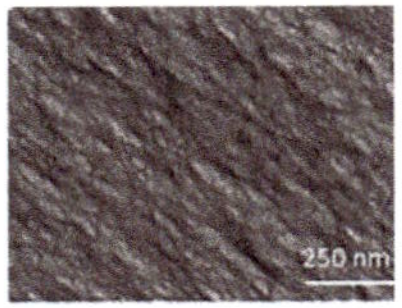	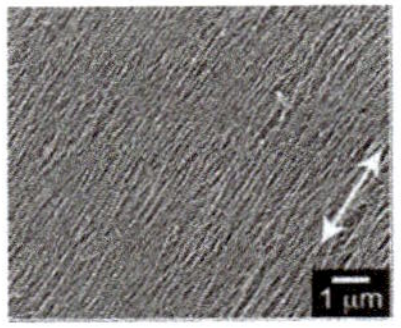	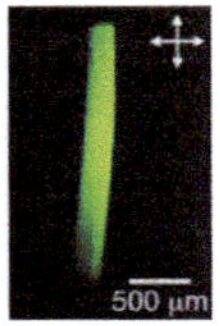	[10, 11, 15, 16]

5.5 Application of Hierarchical Self-assembling Peptide- and Protein-Based Biomaterials in Tissue Regeneration

Hierarchical organization is a common feature of many human tissues (bone, tendons, annulus fibrosus, cornea, muscle, blood vessels). Mimicking the structural organization of tissues via biomaterials approach is believed to foster their regeneration. In this section, we describe the application of hierarchical biomaterials, based on self-assembling peptides and proteins, in the regeneration of tissues for which their use has been reported.

5.5.1 Cornea

The cornea primarily consists of three layers separated by the Bowman's and Descemet's membrane: an outer layer containing an epithelium, a middle stromal layer consisting of a collagen-rich ECM interspersed with keratocytes, and an inner layer of endothelial cells (ECs) [59]. The stroma, which comprises about 90% of the cornea thickness, consists of about 200 sheets of lamellae formed by highly aligned collagen fibrils (predominantly type I, with smaller amounts of types V, VI, XII, XIII, XIV, and XXIV) with uniform spacing, and each lamellae is orientated in a direction orthogonal to the adjacent one [60, 61]. Currently, stromal replacements rely on cornea transplantation, but the limited number of donors cannot meet the large demand. The problem of donor shortage could be solved through the development of artificial or engineered corneas.

The unique structure of the stroma is important for corneal function, as the intricate collagen network endows cornea with strength, resilience, and transparency, with the cell alignment regulating cell phenotype and ECM organization [62]. However, it is extremely challenging to develop such a complex construct in the laboratory. Organized collagen-based constructs appear to be the most popular options in corneal regeneration studies. Guo et al. fabricated cell seeded collagen vitrigels with organized microstructures and high density of collagen fibers. In their *in vitro* study, it was found that human corneal fibroblasts (hCFs) tended to have a morphology resembling native stromal cells when they were in the vitrigels which shared more similarities with the natural stroma [32]. The breakthrough work came from Griffith et al. using synthetic cross-linked recombinant human collagen type III (RHC-III) hydrogel, which showed high transparency to the visible light as the native cornea. Though the clinical study showed its ability to successfully guide the regeneration of corneal tissue, after four-year implantation in humans, the collagen fibrils in the RHC-III hydrogel exhibited preferred alignment in one direction, which differs significantly from the biaxial alignment structure in human corneal stroma [61, 63]. The structure difference is arguably one of the factors leading to the lower mechanical strength of RHC-III hydrogel, compromising its potential utility as a permanent implant [61].

Stacking of artificial anisotropic 2D lamellae into multilayer architecture has been investigated to recreate the highly organized 3D corneal structure. For example, Torbet et al. reported a stroma-like scaffold consisting of a stack of orthogonally disposed sheets of magnetically aligned collagen fibrils. *In vitro* studies showed alignment of hCFs in the direction of fibrils and primary epithelium differentiated on top. However, *in vivo* implantation was only successful in one out of five rabbits, while the other four lost the implant shortly after the surgery [64, 65]. Kaplan and colleagues produced patterned silk film with aligned hCFs and stacked the films together to create a 3D corneal construct. Cell attachment, differentiation, and alignment could be enhanced by modifying the silk construct with RGD peptide motif [66–68].

Self-assembling collagen-like peptides (CLPs) proposed by Hartgerink were also considered as a promising building block to fabricate corneal substitutes [69]. Islam et al. conjugated CLPs to an eight-armed polyethylene glycol to create hydrogel by self-assembly. However, the presence of nanofibers and their microscopic alignment was not shown [70]. The application of PAs has also attracted attention in corneal tissue engineering. It is found that PA with bioactive sequences (e.g. fibronectin and laminin-derived bioactive sequence) could play an important role in enhancing hCFs' adhesion and proliferation and ECM deposition [71]. PAs with MMP-1 cleavable and cell adhesive (RGDS) motifs were also used to coat surfaces [72] and create different anisotropies (oriented stripes) [73]. These surfaces were shown to regulate the phenotype of corneal stromal cells and promote the production of self-releasing tissues with organization similar to the corneal stroma. Recently, curved PA-coated surfaces were used to replicate the natural curvature of the cornea. The curvature was shown to be an important factor for inducing alignment of human corneal stromal cells, which produced highly oriented ECM [62]. Furthermore, when mixed with collagen, a PA was shown to inhibit the contraction of collagen gels and modulate their shape and stiffness through defined PA localization within composite gels. These differences in local stiffness were able to control the differentiation of human limbal epithelial stem cells [74].

5.5.2 Blood Vessels

Increasing research has been conducted to develop artificial vascular scaffolds as the demand of vascular transplantation is raising. Though large artificial blood vessels made of polyethylene terephthalate (PET) and expandable polytetrafluoroethylene (ePTFE) have been clinically approved, the fabrication of small-diameter vessels still remains a challenge [75]. Notably, the development of artificial scaffolds with similar structure to native vessels has been extensively studied. Artery is a major type of blood vessel, and it is typically composed of three concentric layers named the tunica intima, media, and adventitia [76]. Tunica intima is the luminal layer containing a single layer of ECs on the internal elastic lamina. The media is in the middle layer formed by a single or multiple layers of medial lamellar unit, and the quantities vary in number according to the size of the vessel. In each medial layer, all three primary constituents (elastin, smooth muscle cells [SMCs], collagen) are preferential orientated in the circumferential direction [77]. Therefore, it is important to design hierarchical vascular scaffolds to guide cellular organization as well as the formation of cell-mediated *de novo* matrix [78].

The 2D microfabrication technique has been applied to create patterned collagen or polymer substrate to align SMCs. However, the anisotropic monolayer model could not mimic the 3D tissue architecture [79–82]. Thus, a layer-by-layer process has been introduced to build 3D vascular construct. Feng et al. first aligned SMCs on the patterned scaffold and then created multilayer structure with alternative SMC layers and cell-free collagen layers, where the collagen layer acted as a new substrate for SMC seeding. After incubation, each layer of the 3D construct contained aligned elongated SMCs, indicating successful mimicking of the vascular medial layer [83]. However, the multilayer structure was formed on a planar surface so that cannot regenerate the circumferential anisotropic of blood vessel. More recently, bi-layered tubular vascular scaffolds were developed by Nakayama et al. using a bi-layered construct with the luminal layer consisted of longitudinal-aligned collagen nanofibrils and ECs and the outer layer made from circumferentially oriented collagen nanofibrils with SMCs [84]. While both layers' alignment was induced by shear-based extruding, the bi-layer structure was formed by wrapping the outer layer in the circumferential direction. Nguyen et al. further incorporated the insoluble elastin into the bi-layered scaffold to better resemble the composition of native vessels, in which the inner layer was composed of dense collagen lumen and the electrochemical aligned collagen-elastin fiber was wound outside in circumferential or longitudinal direction [78]. It was found that circumferential orientation significantly improved the mechanical properties and anisotropic structure favoring SMC growth as well as ECM deposition.

Since certain bioactive peptide sequences are known to improve biocompatibility and EC adhesion, they are frequently used to modify the surface of artificial vascular grafts [85]. These peptides include REDV, RGD, and GRGDSP from fibronectin, IKLLI, IKVAV, PDSGR, and YIGSR from laminin, and collagen I derived sequence DGEA [85]. A hydrogel formed by a MDP presenting a VEGF-165 peptide mimic was found to be highly angiogenic [86]. However, very few self-assembling peptide vascular scaffolds with ordered structure have been reported. Stupp's group fabricated self-assembling tubular PA hydrogel with circumferentially aligned nanofibers (produced by ionic cross-linking of heated PA solutions under shear in a customized chamber with rotating rod Table 5.1), as potential arterial scaffolds. SMCs encapsulated in the tube wall were observed to align along the PA fibrils in the circumferential direction [12]. Using elastin-like recombinamers and PAs of opposite charge, Mata and coworkers developed self-assembling tubular structures with hierarchical order. These capillary-like structures have shown to support the attachment and proliferation of human umbilical vascular ECs [3].

5.5.3 Skeletal Muscle

Skeletal muscle is a multi-unit hierarchical structure mainly composed of longitudinally aligned myofibrils (1–2 μm), muscle fibers (20–100 μm, also called muscle cell) and fascicles. Though the skeletal muscle possesses a self-repairing mechanism, clinical treatment of large-scale muscle injuries (e.g. volumetric muscle loss) is still relatively unestablished and the development of biomaterials capable of guiding muscle regeneration could be a promising treatment [87]. Due to the highly ordered structure of the muscle fibers, cell alignment is required for obtaining effective regeneration process, which could be achieved by directional guidance by anisotropic scaffolds. Shear-induced fibrin microthreads have a native hierarchical structure, which could longitudinally align cells and be loaded with growth factor to enhance regeneration [88, 89]. Hierarchical 3D nanofibrillar collagen scaffolds aligned by shear-based extrusion and spatial pattern have been successfully fabricated, and long myotubes organized along the direction of the nanofibril orientation [90, 91]. Compared to random-oriented scaffolds, anisotropic scaffolds enhanced regeneration by promoting the density of perfused microvessels [90, 91]. Stupp tested the potential of aligned nanofibrous PA scaffolds produced by annealing (Table 5.1) to mimic the organization and stiffness of myofibers in muscle. These biomimetic scaffolds supported the survival, proliferation alignment, and maturation of myogenic cells *in vitro*, while enhancing engraftment of encapsulated muscle stem cells into endogenous muscle myofibers *in vivo*. The scaffold is injectable, not requiring surgical implantation, biodegradable and growth factor encapsulated in the scaffold could effectively promote the differentiation and maturation of the muscle stem cells [92].

5.6 Conclusions

Engineering long-range order in supramolecular assemblies requires the use of building blocks capable of assembling into discrete structures and responding to external manipulation. Directed self-assembly also involves selection of suitable actuators and their spatio-temporal control. While in many cases molecular design was not considered prior to the application of the external actuation, the remarkable results obtained in some studies described in this chapter provide insights on design rules to direct molecular self-assembly across the length scales. Most studies integrate more than one type of external manipulation which work independently or synergistically to create and maintain long-range order. While the field seems to be based in empirical research, computational studies may shed light on how to predict the behavior of selected building blocks under different types of actuation, or to design assemblies for specific actuators, and contribute for advances in the development of hierarchical biomaterials.

Acknowledgments

We thank the financial support from The Royal Society (Research Grant RSG\R1\180005). Y.Y. acknowledges the China Scholarship Council for her PhD Scholarship (No. 201706630005).

References

1 Azevedo, H.S. (2019). Biomaterials inspired by biology: from molecules to self-assembly. In: *Encyclopedia of Tissue Engineering and Regenerative Medicine* (ed. R.L. Reis), 109–117. Oxford: Academic Press.

2 Capito, R.M., Azevedo, H.S., Velichko, Y.S. et al. (2008). Self-assembly of large and small molecules into hierarchically ordered sacs and membranes. *Science* 319 (5871): 1812–1816.

3 Inostroza-Brito, K.E., Collin, E., Siton-Mendelson, O. et al. (2015). Co-assembly, spatiotemporal control and morphogenesis of a hybrid protein–peptide system. *Nat. Chem.* 7 (11): 897–904.

4 Smith, K.H., Tejeda-Montes, E., Poch, M., and Mata, A. (2011). Integrating top-down and self-assembly in the fabrication of peptide and protein-based biomedical materials. *Chem. Soc. Rev.* 40 (9): 4563–4577.

5 Gazit, E. (2007). Self-assembled peptide nanostructures: the design of molecular building blocks and their technological utilization. *Chem. Soc. Rev.* 36 (8): 1263–1269.

6 Mendes, A.C., Baran, E.T., Reis, R.L., and Azevedo, H.S. (2013). Self-assembly in nature: using the principles of nature to create complex nanobiomaterials. *Wiley Interdiscip. Rev. Nanomed. Nanobiotechnol.* 5 (6): 582–612.

7 Fleming, S. and Ulijn, R.V. (2014). Design of nanostructures based on aromatic peptide amphiphiles. *Chem. Soc. Rev.* 43 (23): 8150–8177.

8 Qin, S.Y., Ding, W.Q., Jiang, Z.W. et al. (2019). Directing an oligopeptide amphiphile into an aligned nanofiber matrix for elucidating molecular structures. *Chem. Commun.* 55 (11): 1659–1662.

9 Yan, X.H., Li, J.B., and Mowald, H. (2011). Self-assembly of hexagonal peptide microtubes and their optical waveguiding. *Adv. Mater.* 23 (25): 2796–2801.

10 Zhang, S., Greenfield, M.A., Mata, A. et al. (2010). A self-assembly pathway to aligned monodomain gels. *Nat. Mater.* 9 (7): 594–601.

11 Wall, B.D., Diegelmann, S.R., Zhang, S.M. et al. (2011). Aligned macroscopic domains of optoelectronic nanostructures prepared via shear-flow assembly of peptide hydrogels. *Adv. Mater.* 23 (43): 5009–5014.

12 McClendon, M.T. and Stupp, S.I. (2012). Tubular hydrogels of circumferentially aligned nanofibers to encapsulate and orient vascular cells. *Biomaterials* 33 (23): 5713–5722.

13 Guo, H., Zhang, J.M., Xu, T. et al. (2013). The robust hydrogel hierarchically assembled from a pH sensitive peptide amphiphile based on silk fibroin. *Biomacromolecules* 14 (8): 2733–2738.

14 Chen, Y.R., Gan, H.X., and Tong, Y.W. (2015). pH-controlled hierarchical self-assembly of peptide amphiphile. *Macromolecules* 48 (8): 2647–2653.

15 Zhou, J., Du, X., Gao, Y. et al. (2014). Aromatic-aromatic interactions enhance interfiber contacts for enzymatic formation of a spontaneously aligned supramolecular hydrogel. *J. Am. Chem. Soc.* 136 (8): 2970–2973.

16 Hill, R.J.A., Sedman, V.L., Allen, S. et al. (2007). Alignment of aromatic peptide tubes in strong magnetic fields. *Adv. Mater.* 19 (24): 4474–4479.

17 Wallace, M., Cardoso, A.Z., Frith, W.J. et al. (2014). Magnetically aligned supramolecular hydrogels. *Chem. Eur. J.* 20 (50): 16484–16487.

18 Lowik, D., Shklyarevskiy, I.O., Ruizendaal, L. et al. (2007). A highly ordered material from magnetically aligned peptide amphiphile nanofiber assemblies. *Adv. Mater.* 19 (9): 1191–1195.

19 van der Asdonk, P., Keshavarz, M., Christianen, P.C.M., and Kouwer, P.H.J. (2016). Directed peptide amphiphile assembly using aqueous liquid crystal templates in magnetic fields. *Soft Matter.* 12 (31): 6518–6525.

20 van der Asdonk, P., Kragt, S., and Kouwer, P.H.J. (2016). Directing soft matter in water using electric fields. *ACS Appl. Mater. Interfaces* 8 (25): 16303–16309.

21 Tayi, A.S., Pashuck, E.T., Newcomb, C.J. et al. (2014). Electrospinning bioactive supramolecular polymers from water. *Biomacromolecules* 15 (4): 1323–1327.

22 Cui, H.G., Pashuck, E.T., Velichko, Y.S. et al. (2010). Spontaneous and X-ray-triggered crystallization at long range in self-assembling filament networks. *Science* 327 (5965): 555–559.

23 Li, I.C. and Hartgerink, J.D. (2017). Covalent capture of aligned self-assembling nanofibers. *J. Am. Chem. Soc.* 139 (23): 8044–8050.

24 Hung, A.M. and Stupp, S.I. (2009). Understanding factors affecting alignment of self-assembling nanofibers patterned by sonication-assisted solution embossing. *Langmuir* 25 (12): 7084–7089.

25 Pappas, C.G., Frederix, P., Mutasa, T. et al. (2015). Alignment of nanostructured tripeptide gels by directional ultrasonication. *Chem. Commun.* 51 (40): 8465–8468.

26 Song, J., Xing, R., Jiao, T. et al. (2018). Crystalline dipeptide nanobelts based on solid–solid phase transformation self-assembly and their polarization imaging of cells. *ACS Appl. Mater. Interfaces* 10 (3): 2368–2376.

27 Mendes, A.C., Smith, K.H., Tejeda-Montes, E. et al. (2013). Co-assembled and microfabricated bioactive membranes. *Adv. Funct. Mater.* 23 (4): 430–438.

28 Mata, A., Hsu, L., Capito, R. et al. (2009). Micropatterning of bioactive self-assembling gels. *Soft Matter.* 5 (6): 1228–1236.

29 Ryu, J. and Park, C.B. (2008). High-temperature self-assembly of peptides into vertically well-aligned nanowires by aniline vapor. *Adv. Mater.* 20 (19): 3754–3758.

30 Hung, A.M. and Stupp, S.I. (2007). Simultaneous self-assembly, orientation, and patterning of peptide–amphiphile nanofibers by soft lithography. *Nano Lett.* 7 (5): 1165–1171.

31 Restuccia, A., Seroski, D.T., Kelley, K.L. et al. (2019). Hierarchical self-assembly and emergent function of densely glycosylated peptide nanofibers. *Commun. Chem.* 2 (1): 53.

32 Guo, Q.Y., Phillip, J.M., Majumdar, S. et al. (2013). Modulation of keratocyte phenotype by collagen fibril nanoarchitecture in membranes for corneal repair. *Biomaterials* 34 (37): 9365–9372.

33 Noor, S. and DWPM, L. (2018). Magnetic fields to align natural and synthetic fibers, chapter 16. In: *Self-Assembling Biomaterials* (ed. H.S. Azevedo and R.M.P. da Silva), 321–340. Woodhead Publishing.

34 Christianen, P.C.M., Shklyarevskiy, I.O., Boamfa, M.I., and Maan, J.C. (2004). Alignment of molecular materials in high magnetic fields. *Physica B* 346: 255–261.

35 Worcester, D.L. (1978). Structural origins of diamagnetic anisotropy in proteins. *Proc. Natl. Acad. Sci. U.S.A.* 75 (11): 5475–5477.

36 Serpell, L.C., Blake, C.C.F., and Fraser, P.E. (2000). Molecular structure of a fibrillar Alzheimer's A beta fragment. *Biochemistry* 39 (43): 13269–13275.

37 Inouye, H., Fraser, P.E., and Kirschner, D.A. (1993). Structure of beta-crystallite assemblies formed by Alzheimer beta-amyloid protein analogues: analysis by X-ray diffraction. *Biophys. J.* 64 (2): 502–519.

38 Malinchik, S.B., Inouye, H., Szumowski, K.E., and Kirschner, D.A. (1998). Structural analysis of Alzheimer's beta(1–40) amyloid: protofilament assembly of tubular fibrils. *Biophys. J.* 74 (1): 537–545.

39 Lu, Q., Bai, S.M., Ding, Z.Z. et al. (2016). Hydrogel assembly with hierarchical alignment by balancing electrostatic forces. *Adv. Mater. Interfaces* 3 (8): 1–6.

40 Cheng, X.G., Gurkan, U.A., Dehen, C.J. et al. (2008). An electrochemical fabrication process for the assembly of anisotropically oriented collagen bundles. *Biomaterials* 29 (22): 3278–3288.

41 Velichko, Y.S., Mantei, J.R., Bitton, R. et al. (2012). Electric field controlled self-assembly of hierarchically ordered membranes. *Adv. Funct. Mater.* 22 (2): 369–377.

42 Denis, F.A., Pallandre, A., Nysten, B. et al. (2005). Alignment and assembly of adsorbed collagen molecules induced by anisotropic chemical nanopatterns. *Small* 1 (10): 984–991.

43 Wilson, D.L., Martin, R., Hong, S. et al. (2001). Surface organization and nanopatterning of collagen by dip-pen nanolithography. *Proc. Natl. Acad. Sci. U.S.A.* 98 (24): 13660–13664.

44 Jiang, H.Z. and Stupp, S.I. (2005). Dip-pen patterning and surface assembly of peptide amphiphiles. *Langmuir* 21 (12): 5242–5246.

45 Xia, Y.N. and Whitesides, G.M. (1998). Soft lithography. *Angew. Chem. Int. Ed. Engl.* 37 (5): 550–575.

46 Yaari, A., Posen, Y., and Shoseyov, O. (2013). Liquid crystalline human recombinant collagen: the challenge and the opportunity. *Tissue Eng. Part A* 19.

47 Aggeli, A., Bell, M., Carrick, L.M. et al. (2003). pH as a trigger of peptide beta-sheet self-assembly and reversible switching between nematic and isotropic phases. *J. Am. Chem. Soc.* 125 (32): 9619–9628.

48 Rae, J., Ashokkumar, M., Eulaerts, O. et al. (2005). Estimation of ultrasound induced cavitation bubble temperatures in aqueous solutions. *Ultrason. Sonochem.* 12 (5): 325–329.

49 Flint, E.B. and Suslick, K.S. (1991). The temperature of cavitation. *Science* 253 (5026): 1397.

50 Meek, K.M. and Fullwood, N.J. (2001). Corneal and scleral collagens – a microscopist's perspective. *Micron* 32 (3): 261–272.

51 Ross, S., Newton, R., Zhou, Y.M. et al. (1997). Quantitative image analysis of birefringent biological material. *J. Microsc.* 187: 62–67.

52 Rieppo, J., Hallikainen, J., Jurvelin, J.S. et al. (2008). Practical considerations in the use of polarized light microscopy in the analysis of the collagen network in articular cartilage. *Microsc. Res. Tech.* 71 (4): 279–287.

53 Swatland, H.J. (1990). Effect of pH on the birefringence of skeletal muscle fibers measured with a polarizing microscope. *Trans. Am. Microsc. Soc.* 109 (4): 361–367.

54 Hamley, I.W. (2007). Peptide fbrillization. *Angew. Chem. Int. Ed.* 46 (43): 8128–8147.

55 Raghuwanshi, V.S. and Garnier, G. (2019). Characterisation of hydrogels: linking the nano to the microscale. *Adv. Colloid Interface Sci.* 274: 102044.

56 Ochbaum, G. and Bitton, R. (2018). Using small-angle X-ray scattering (SAXS) to study the structure of self-assembling biomaterials, chapter 14. In: *Self-Assembling Biomaterials* (ed. H.S. Azevedo and R.M.P. da Silva), 291–304. Woodhead Publishing.

57 Roig-Solvas, B., Brooks, D., and Makowski, L. (2019). A direct approach to estimate the anisotropy of protein structures from small-angle X-ray scattering. *J. Appl. Crystallogr.* 52: 274–283.

58 Kikhney, A.G. and Svergun, D.I. (2015). A practical guide to small angle X-ray scattering (SAXS) of flexible and intrinsically disordered proteins. *FEBS Lett.* 589 (19): 2570–2577.

59 Hassell, J.R. and Birk, D.E. (2010). The molecular basis of corneal transparency. *Exp. Eye Res.* 91 (3): 326–335.

60 Matthyssen, S., Van den Bogerd, B., Ni Dhubhghaill, S. et al. (2018). Corneal regeneration: a review of stromal replacements. *Acta Biomater.* 69: 31–41.

61 Hayes, S., Lewis, P., Islam, M.M. et al. (2015). The structural and optical properties of type III human collagen biosynthetic corneal substitutes. *Acta Biomater.* 25: 121–130.

62 Gouveia, R.M., Koudouna, E., Jester, J. et al. (2017). Template curvature influences cell alignment to create improved human corneal tissue equivalents. *Adv. Biosyst.* 1 (12): 1700135.

63 Fagerholm, P., Lagali, N.S., Ong, J.A. et al. (2014). Stable corneal regeneration four years after implantation of a cell-free recombinant human collagen scaffold. *Biomaterials* 35 (8): 2420–2427.

64 Torbet, J., Malbouyres, M., Builles, N. et al. (2007). Orthogonal scaffold of magnetically aligned collagen lamellae for corneal stroma reconstruction. *Biomaterials* 28 (29): 4268–4276.

65 Builles, N., Janin-Manificat, H., Malbouyres, M. et al. (2010). Use of magnetically oriented orthogonal collagen scaffolds for hemi-corneal reconstruction and regeneration. *Biomaterials* 31 (32): 8313–8322.

66 Lawrence, B.D., Marchant, J.K., Pindrus, M.A. et al. (2009). Silk film biomaterials for cornea tissue engineering. *Biomaterials* 30 (7): 1299–1308.

67 Gil, E.S., Mandal, B.B., Park, S.H. et al. (2010). Helicoidal multi-lamellar features of RGD-functionalized silk biomaterials for corneal tissue engineering. *Biomaterials* 31 (34): 8953–8963.

68 Ghezzi, C.E., Marelli, B., Omenetto, F.G. et al. (2017). 3D functional corneal stromal tissue equivalent based on corneal stromal stem cells and multi-layered silk film architecture. *PLoS One* 12 (1): e0169504.

69 O'Leary, L.E.R., Fallas, J.A., Bakota, E.L. et al. (2011). Multi-hierarchical self-assembly of a collagen mimetic peptide from triple helix to nanofibre and hydrogel. *Nat. Chem.* 3 (10): 821–828.

70 Islam, M.M., Ravichandran, R., Olsen, D. et al. (2016). Self-assembled collagen-like-peptide implants as alternatives to human donor corneal transplantation. *RSC Adv.* 6 (61): 55745–55749.

71 Miotto, M., Gouveia, R.M., and Connon, C.J. (2015). Peptide amphiphiles in corneal tissue engineering. *J. Funct. Biomater.* 6 (3): 687–707.

72 Gouveia, R.M., Castelletto, V., Hamley, I.W., and Connon, C.J. (2015). New self-assembling multifunctional templates for the biofabrication and controlled self-release of cultured tissue. *Tissue Eng. Part A* 21 (11, 12): 1772–1784.

73 Gouveia, R.M., González-Andrades, E., Cardona, J.C. et al. (2017). Controlling the 3D architecture of self-lifting auto-generated tissue equivalents (SLATEs) for optimized corneal graft composition and stability. *Biomaterials* 121: 205–219.

74 Miotto, M., Gouveia, R.M., Ionescu, A.M. et al. (2019). 4D corneal tissue engineering: achieving time-dependent tissue self-curvature through localized control of cell actuators. *Adv. Funct. Mater.* 29 (8): 1807334.

75 Iijima, K., Ichikawa, S., Ishikawa, S. et al. (2019). Preparation of cell-paved and -incorporated polysaccharide hollow fibers using a microfluidic device. *ACS Biomater. Sci. Eng.* 5 (11): 5688–5697.

76 Chan-Park, M.B., Shen, J.Y., Cao, Y. et al. (2009). Biomimetic control of vascular smooth muscle cell morphology and phenotype for functional tissue-engineered small-diameter blood vessels. *J. Biomed. Mater. Res. Part A* 88A (4): 1104–1121.

77 O'Connell, M.K., Murthy, S., Phan, S. et al. (2008). The three-dimensional micro- and nanostructure of the aortic medial lamellar unit measured using 3D confocal and electron microscopy imaging. *Matrix Biol.* 27 (3): 171–181.

78 Nguyen, T.U., Shojaee, M., Bashur, C.A., and Kishore, V. (2019). Electrochemical fabrication of a biomimetic elastin-containing bi-layered scaffold for vascular tissue engineering. *Biofabrication* 11 (1): 015007.

79 Goessl, A., Bowen-Pope, D.F., and Hoffman, A.S. (2001). Control of shape and size of vascular smooth muscle cells in vitro by plasma lithography. *J. Biomed. Mater. Res.* 57 (1): 15–24.

80 Ra, H.J., Picart, C., Feng, H.S. et al. (1999). Muscle cell peeling from micropatterned collagen: direct probing of focal and molecular properties of matrix adhesion. *J. Cell Sci.* 112 (10): 1425–1436.

81 Thakar, R.G., Ho, F., Huang, N.F. et al. (2003). Regulation of vascular smooth muscle cells by micropatterning. *Biochem. Biophys. Res. Commun.* 307 (4): 883–890.

82 Sarkar, S., Dadhania, M., Rourke, P. et al. (2005). Vascular tissue engineering: microtextured scaffold templates to control organization of vascular smooth muscle cells and extracellular matrix. *Acta Biomater.* 1 (1): 93–100.

83 Feng, J., Chan-Park, M.B., Shen, J.Y., and Chan, V. (2007). Quick layer-by-layer assembly of aligned multilayers of vascular smooth muscle cells in deep microchannels. *Tissue Eng.* 13 (5): 1003–1012.

84 Nakayama, K.H., Joshi, P.A., Lai, E.S. et al. (2015). Bilayered vascular graft derived from human induced pluripotent stem cells with biomimetic structure and function. *Regener. Med.* 10 (6): 745–755.

85 Ren, X.K., Feng, Y.K., Guo, J.T. et al. (2015). Surface modification and endothelialization of biomaterials as potential scaffolds for vascular tissue engineering applications. *Chem. Soc. Rev.* 44 (15): 5680–5742.

86 Kumar, V.A., Taylor, N.L., Shi, S.Y. et al. (2015). Highly angiogenic peptide nanofibers. *ACS Nano* 9 (1): 860–868.

87 Haas, G.J., Dunn, A.J., Marcinczyk, M. et al. (2019). Biomimetic sponges for regeneration of skeletal muscle following trauma. *J. Biomed. Mater. Res. Part A* 107 (1): 92–103.

88 Cornwell, K.G. and Pins, G.D. (2007). Discrete crosslinked fibrin microthread scaffolds for tissue regeneration. *J. Biomed. Mater. Res. Part A* 82A (1): 104–112.

89 Cornwell, K.G. and Pins, G.D. (2010). Enhanced proliferation and migration of fibroblasts on the surface of fibroblast growth factor-2-loaded fibrin microthreads. *Tissue Eng. Part A* 16 (12): 3669–3677.

90 Nakayama, K.H., Quarta, M., Paine, P. et al. (2019). Treatment of volumetric muscle loss in mice using nanofibrillar scaffolds enhances vascular organization and integration. *Commun. Biol.* 2 (1): 170.

91 Nakayama, K.H., Alcazar, C., Yang, G. et al. (2018). Rehabilitative exercise and spatially patterned nanofibrillar scaffolds enhance vascularization and innervation following volumetric muscle loss. *npj Regener. Med.* 3 (1): 16.

92 Sleep, E., Cosgrove, B.D., McClendon, M.T. et al. (2017). Injectable biomimetic liquid crystalline scaffolds enhance muscle stem cell transplantation. *Proc. Natl. Acad. Sci. U.S.A.* 114 (38): E7919–E7928.

6

Short Peptide Hydrogels for Biomedical Applications

Priyadarshi Chakraborty[1,2], *Lihi Adler-Abramovich*[2], *and Ehud Gazit*[1,3]

[1] *Tel Aviv University, Shmunis School of Biomedicine and Cancer Research, George S. Wise Faculty of Life Sciences, Tel Aviv 6997801, Israel*
[2] *Tel Aviv University, The Goldschleger School of Dental Medicine, Department of Oral Biology, Sackler Faculty of Medicine, Tel Aviv 6997801, Israel*
[3] *Tel Aviv University, Department of Materials Science and Engineering, Iby and Aladar Fleischman Faculty of Engineering, Tel Aviv 6997801, Israel*

6.1 Introduction

Hydrogels are a unique class of soft material that consist of two different phases: a "liquid-like" phase and a nanoscale "solid-like" fibrous three-dimensional (3D) network encapsulating the liquid and preventing its flow [1]. This network closely resembles the extracellular matrix (ECM), which supports the growth of most cells in our body and provides an intrinsic culture condition that traditional 2D surfaces are unable to reproduce [2]. This resemblance is extremely important as cells recognize the topography of their microenvironment [3, 4], which concurrently impacts their cellular phenotype, differentiation, and gene expression profile [5, 6]. Because of their ECM mimicking properties, hydrogels have been very effective in tissue engineering [7, 8] and other biomedical applications [9–15].

Peptides are fragments of proteins and bear a striking resemblance with these important biomolecules. This chapter deals with hydrogels produced from the self-assembly of peptides with ≤20 amino acid sequences, which are generally defined as short peptides [2]. Self-assembly of short peptides has attracted immense research interest due to their simplistic molecular design, intrinsic biocompatibility, and excellent physical properties [16–20]. Peptide self-assembly yields different nanostructures including nanofibers, nanotapes, nanoparticles, nanotubes, and nanobelts [21], which have been utilized in diverse applications [20, 22–26]. Short peptides are excellent candidates for supramolecular hydrogelation due to their tendency to self-assemble via multiple noncovalent interactions including H-bonding, π-stacking, hydrophobic interactions, and ionic interactions [27–40]. These soft materials often match the mechanical properties of the ECM thus having tremendous prospect as functional biomaterials [41]. The advantages of short peptide-based hydrogels are manifold, e.g. they are biocompatible, biodegradable,

Multifunctional Hydrogels for Biomedical Applications, First Edition.
Edited by Ricardo A. Pires, Iva Pashkuleva, and Rui L. Reis.

and normally non-immunogenic. Moreover, these peptides are synthesized rather easily via solid-phase synthesis with low production cost. The manipulation of the amino acid sequences can also lead to peptides with different properties leading to diverse applications. Compared to conventional cross-linked polymeric hydrogels, short peptide-based supramolecular hydrogels are stimuli-responsive and do not necessitate any chemical cross-linking. These hydrogels are therefore free from cytotoxic components including initiators, enzymes, or catalysts that may be present in cross-linked polymeric hydrogels. These properties allow the short-peptide hydrogels to be applicable in biomedical uses.

Herein, we discuss the biomedical applications of short peptide-based hydrogels. So, the peptides with amino acid residues >20 are beyond the scope of this chapter.

6.2 Short Peptide Hydrogels

Diphenylalanine (FF) is the smallest peptide capable of forming hydrogels. Although FF was identified as the simplest building capable of forming self-assembled nanostructures in 2003 [24], Ulijn and coworkers reported its hydrogelation in 2016 [42]. Fmoc protection of FF at the N-terminal yields nanofibrous hydrogels with excellent potential as functional biomaterials [43, 44]. We first divide short peptide hydrogels into four broad categories and provide a brief introduction on them. Then, we demonstrate their biomedical uses.

6.2.1 Fmoc-Protected Short Peptides

9-Fluorenylmethyloxycarbonyl (Fmoc) is widely used as the amine protecting group during peptide synthesis. The excellent π-stacking ability and hydrophobicity of the fluorenyl ring induce rapid self-assembly and gelation of Fmoc-protected short peptides [45]. Therefore, a plethora of Fmoc-protected short peptide gelators has been reported in the literature. The most studied Fmoc-based short peptide hydrogelator is Fmoc-FF [43, 44]. Several other Fmoc-protected short peptides have been reported to form hydrogels including dipeptide Fmoc-AA [30, 46, 47], Fmoc-GG, Fmoc-AG, and Fmoc-LG [44]; tripeptide Fmoc-RGD [48, 49]; tetrapeptide Fmoc-RGDS and Fmoc-GRDS [50–53], Fmoc-RGDF and Fmoc-FRGD [54]; pentapeptide Fmoc-VTEEI, Fmoc-GVGVP, Fmoc-VPGVG, and Fmoc-VYGGG [55]. More recent studies focus on improving mechanical properties and conferring conductivity to the Fmoc-protected peptide hydrogels by combining them with covalent/conductive polymers [41, 56].

6.2.2 Short Peptide Hydrogels with Alternating Hydrophobic/ Hydrophilic Amino Acid Residues

Some important members of this group are Ac-(AEAEAKAKAEAEAKAK)-NH_2 (EAK16) [57], Ac-(KLDLKLDLKLDL)-NH_2 (KLD12) [58], Ac-(RADARADARADA-RADA)-NH_2 (RAD16-I) [59], and Ac (RARADADARARADADA)-NH_2 (RAD16-II)

[10]. The peptides were designed in such a way that the positive charges are adjacent to the negative ones by placing the hydrophilic and hydrophobic amino acids alternatively. These peptides self-assemble in the presence of salts forming β-sheet hydrogels [60].

6.2.3 β-Hairpin Peptides

These special class of peptides folds into β-hairpins before self-assembly and gelation [61]. The hydrogels produced from these peptides are rich in β-sheets. The archetypal candidate among these class of peptides is MAX1 (VKVKVKVK-V^DPPT-KVKVKVKV-NH_2) [61], the gelation of which could be tuned by external stimuli (temperature, pH, salt). The mechanical rigidity of these gels was tuned by doping with its enantiomer, DMAX1 [62]. To improve the gelation kinetics, the K in position 15 was replaced by E [63]. A three-stranded β-sheet peptide TSS1 (VKVKVKVK-V^DPPT-KVKVKV-K^DPPK-VKVKVKV-NH_2) was also designed extending the similar concept [34] exhibiting temperature and salt-responsive hydrogelation. Another peptide PEP6R, synthesized by the replacement of most lysine residues of MAX1, self-assembled into antibacterial hydrogels [64].

6.2.4 Acetyl-Protected Short Peptides

Hauser and coworkers designed some acetyl-protected short peptides featuring a hydrophobic block comprising amino acid residues organized in a gradient of decreased hydrophobicity, along with a hydrophilic head-group [65, 66]. Primary examples of these peptides are Ac-IVK, Ac-IVD, Ac-LIVAGK-NH_2 (LK_6), Ac-ILVAGK-NH_2 (IK_6), and Ac-LIVAGD (LD_6), which spontaneously formed hydrogels through self-assembly. These hydrogels were further observed to be responsive to metal salts [67]. To increase the mechanical stability of these gels and improve their durability in the presence of cell-culture media, covalent cross-linkings were integrated through cysteine-mediated disulfide bonds [68].

6.3 Biomedical Applications of Short Peptide Hydrogels

Short peptide hydrogels have emerged as excellent candidates for biomedical usage. Herein, we discuss different kinds of biomedical applications of these hydrogels (Scheme 6.1).

6.3.1 2D/3D Cell Scaffolding

Literature reports revealed that the surface stiffness and mechanical rigidity of the scaffolds play an important role in cellular adhesion and morphology [69–72]. Soft hydrogels (rigidity ~1 kPa) exhibit dynamic diffusion and adhesion of cells [73]. Therefore, short peptide-based soft hydrogels are ideal candidates for 2D and 3D cell scaffolding applications [74].

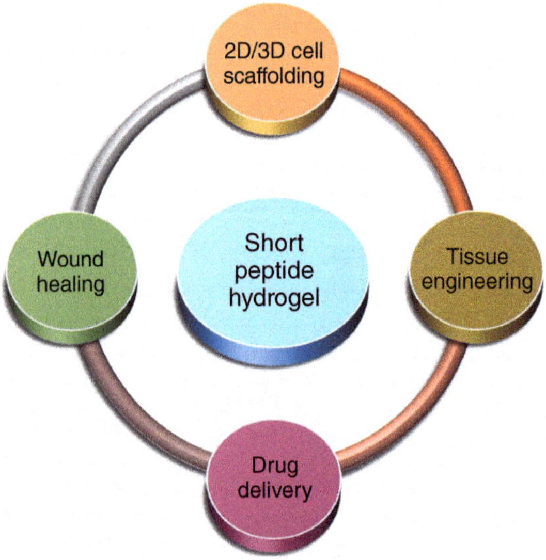

Scheme 6.1 Biomedical applications of short peptide-based supramolecular hydrogels.

Our group reported Fmoc-FF-based hydrogels by solvent switch method, which acted as a 2D scaffold for the growth of CHO cells [43]. Ulijn and coworkers reported 2D and 3D cell culture in Fmoc-FF hydrogels [44]. These hydrogels were prepared by acid–base treatment, and cells were mixed with the hydrogels for the 3D cell culture studies. In another study, Ulijn and coworkers prepared bioactive hydrogels combining Fmoc-FF and Fmoc-RGD building blocks [48]. The hydrogels consisted of fibrous nanostructures with the bioactive RGD ligands exposed on the fiber surface, thus effectively mimicking the ECM. The hydrogel facilitated the 3D spreading and proliferation of dermal fibroblasts through specific RGD-integrin binding.

The self-assembling RAD16-I peptide hydrogels promoted the 3D adhesion and migration of ovarian cancer cells [75]. Chondrocytes maintained their phenotype and produced abundant type II collagen and glycosaminoglycan when cultured in KLD12 hydrogels [58].

MAX1 and MAX8 (VKVKVKVKV^{D}P^{L}PTKVEVKVKV-NH$_2$) peptides could be gelled in the cell culture medium (DMEM) containing C3H10t1/2 mesenchymal stem cells [63, 76–78]. These cells that impregnated gels were mechanically rigid and could be injected to the target sites. The injection procedure did not affect the homogeneous distribution and viability of the cells. Dental pulp stem cells (DPSCs) and growth factors were encapsulated in K(SL)$_3$RG(SL)$_3$KGRGDS peptide-based hydrogel [79]. The cells degraded the hydrogel and exchanged it by a collagenous ECM. Another peptide h9e (FLIVIGSIIGPGGDGPGGD)-based gelator self-assembled into hydrogels in the cell culture medium and Ca^{2+} [80]. To improve the interfiber interactions, the charged Asp residue was further captured [81]. Encapsulation of chondrocytes in a FEFEFKFK octapeptide was reported by Gough and Miller [82]. The cultured cells actively produced collagen type II, along with smaller quantities of collagen type I after 25 days.

3D cell scaffolding in simple nonprotected tripeptide ^{D}LFF was reported by Hartley and coworkers [83]. The hydrogel was prepared by pH tuning technique. Cells cultured on the top of this gel migrated to the bulk with time, allowing 3D culture. This is a simple, convenient, and effective approach to create 3D gel-cell constructs. The migration approach was also adopted by our group, in which, we reported 2D/3D cell scaffolding in a composite hydrogel of Fmoc-RGD and chitosan [56]. In this work, otherwise mechanically weak Fmoc-RGD hydrogels were noncovalently functionalized with chitosan and the resulting composite hydrogels exhibited improved mechanical properties, gelation rate, and cell media durability. Cells (fibroblasts) seeded on the top of these gels migrated into the bulk demonstrating their utility as 3D cell scaffolds.

The integration of conductive inorganic nanomaterials (such as gold nanoparticles and gold nanowires) into otherwise insulating, conventional cardiac tissue engineering scaffolds could offer faster and more synchronized electrical signal propagation in the engineered tissues because of the enhanced electrical coupling between the neighboring cardiac cells [73]. Biocompatible hybrid gels with conductive polymers could act as excellent scaffolds for this application as they offer an all-organic, continuous conducting path compared to the non-continuous, point-to-point connected conducting networks of inorganic nanoparticles. To develop an all-organic, conductive, cytocompatible hydrogel, our research group designed the composite hydrogels of Fmoc-FF and a conductive polymer, polyaniline [41]. The composite hydrogels exhibit self-healing behavior and ohmic conductivity. The elastic nonmetallic nature of this conductive hydrogel allowed its utilization as 2D scaffolds as a conductive interface for electrogenic cardiac cells. The composite hydrogel helped cardiomyocyte organization into a spontaneously contracting system thus demonstrating its potential as a cardiac tissue engineering scaffold (Figure 6.1). Composite hydrogels of Fmoc-FF with Fmoc-R and a hexapeptide were also employed for 2D cell scaffolding [71, 84].

There are some examples of enzyme-triggered hydrogelation of peptides for 3D encapsulation of cells (see Chapter 4) [39, 85–88]. Enzyme-triggered self-assembly can also be utilized to trigger cancer cell death (see Chapter 8). Xu and coworkers demonstrated an enzyme-responsive peptide-based precursor that self-assembled inside living cells by penetrating the cell membrane [89–92]. The promiscuous interactions between nanofibers and cytoskeletal proteins could cause the change of cytoplasm resulting in cell apoptosis [93, 94].

6.3.2 Tissue Engineering

Tissue engineering is one of the most relevant applications of short peptide hydrogels. The remarkable likeness between hydrogel morphology and human tissues inspired scientists to investigate peptide hydrogels as tissue engineering scaffolds. Apart from structural similarity, peptide hydrogels also exhibit striking resemblance in mechanical properties with many tissues. These features along with their intrinsic biocompatibility, cell adhesion, and promoting nutrient transport to cells make peptide hydrogels promising candidates for tissue engineering applications [95–98].

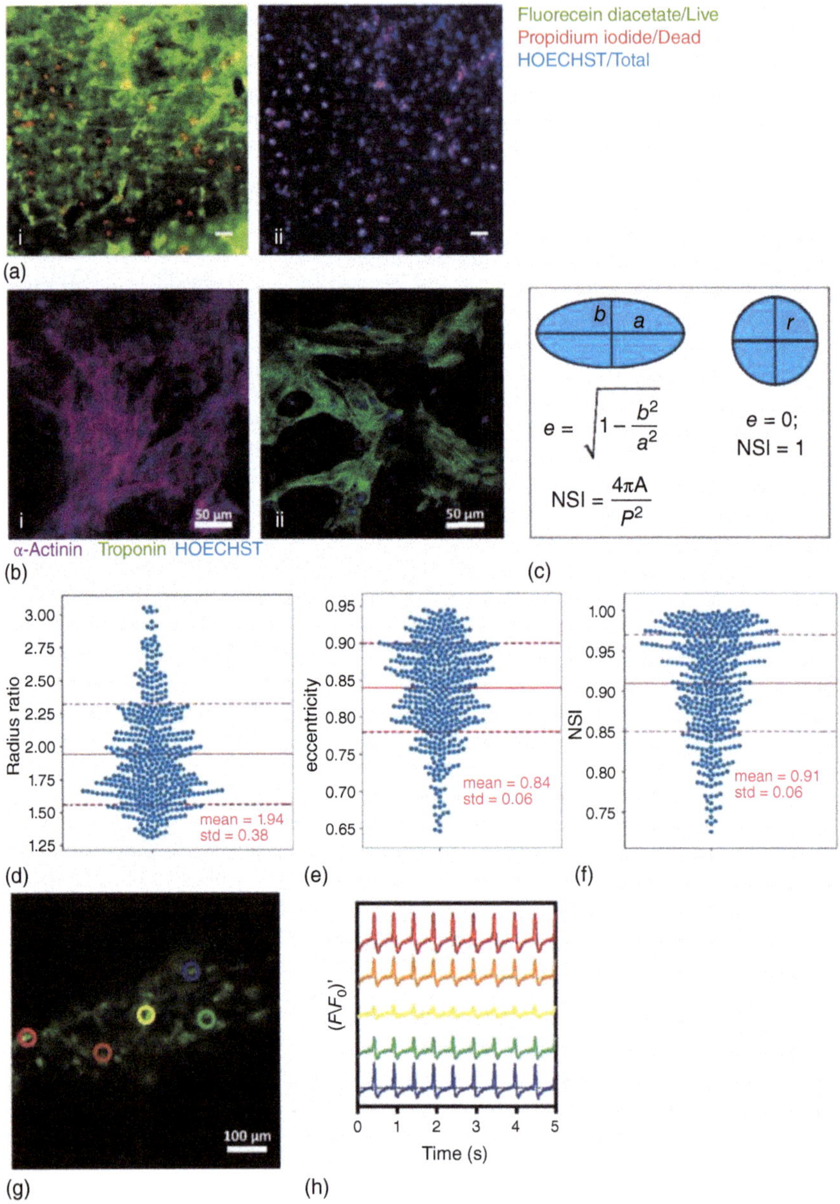
Fluorecein diacetate/Live
Propidium iodide/Dead
HOECHST/Total
i
ii
(a)
i
50 μm
ii
50 μm
α-Actinin Troponin HOECHST
(b)
b
a
r
$e = \sqrt{1 - \frac{b^2}{a^2}}$
$e = 0$;
NSI = 1
$NSI = \frac{4\pi A}{P^2}$
(c)
Radius ratio
mean = 1.94
std = 0.38
(d)
eccentricity
mean = 0.84
std = 0.06
(e)
NSI
mean = 0.91
std = 0.06
(f)
100 μm
(g)
$(F\backslash F_0)'$
Time (s)
(h)

Figure 6.1 Cardiac cell function cultured on the composite gels of Fmoc-FF and polyaniline. (a) Analysis of cardiomyocyte viability by live/dead assay. (i) Live cells stained with fluorecein diacetate (green) and dead cell nuclei stained with PI (red). Source: Gazit, E. et al (2019) / Figure5a(i) / with permission from American Chemical Society. (ii) Hoechst (blue) and PI staining were used for quantifying viability. Scale bar, 50 μm. Source: Gazit, E. et al (2019) / Figure5a(ii) / with permission from American Chemical Society. (b) Cardiac cell staining for alpha actinin (i, purple). Source: Gazit, E. et al (2019) / Figure5b(i) / with permission from American Chemical Society. and troponin-t (ii, green); nuclei are Hoechst-stained (blue). Source: Gazit, E. et al (2019) / Figure5b(ii) / with permission from American Chemical Society. (c) Nuclear stains were used to quantify nuclear morphology. Radius aspect ratio (d), eccentricity (e), and NSI (f) were calculated for nuclei. (g) Calcium transient was assessed at specified points by monitoring calcium dye fluorescence. Source: Gazit, E. et al (2019) / Figure5g / with permission from American Chemical Society. (h) Synchronized calcium signals were observed at all points. F/F_0 refers to measured fluorescence normalized to maximum fluorescence. The colors are correlated with the colored circles in (g). Source: From Chakraborty et al. [41]/with permission of American Chemical Society.

Adler-Abramovich and coworkers reported the application of a composite hydrogel of Fmoc-FF and alginate toward bone tissue regeneration [99]. The MC3T3-E1 preosteoblast cells were observed to be adhered with the hydrogel fibers. Moreover, osteogenic differentiation and calcium mineralization were facilitated by this composite hydrogel thus demonstrating its utilization as a promising scaffold for bone tissue regeneration. Hybrid hydrogel of a peptide (EFK8) and carbon nanotube (SWNT) were utilized by Chen and coworkers for tissue and 3D tumor engineering [100]. The attachment, spreading, proliferation, and movement of NIH-3T3 cells were enhanced by the integration of SWNT with the peptide hydrogel. Moreover, a change in morphology of the A549 lung cancer cells from spheroidal to stretched architectures was also observed because of SWNT integration. Stupp's research group discovered peptide amphiphile (PA)-based hydrogels that were used as scaffolds for muscle stem cell transplantation [101]. The macroscopic degree of cell alignment was determined by the mechanical stiffness of the scaffolds. These scaffolds supported the survival and proliferation of myogenic progenitor cells. Moreover, the optimization of these scaffolds resulted in the differentiation and maturation of cells. The same group utilized a laminin-mimetic IKVAV sequence containing PAs for neural differentiation of human bone marrow mesenchymal stem cells [102].

In an interesting work, silk fibroin (SF) was mixed with a short-peptide gelator NapFF to yield a stable hydrogel at physiological pH [103]. Here, the NapFF peptide was responsible for the supramolecular self-assembly and gelation. Moreover, NapFF caused the conformational transition of SF from random coil to β-sheet. To facilitate the cell adhesion process, a new gelator (NapFFRGD) with the cell attaching RGD sequence was further developed. The composite hydrogel of NapFFRGD and SF (Gel RGD) exhibited excellent cell attachment and spreading. Next, the ability of the Gel RGD to support microvasculature formation was assessed. HUVECs cultured on the surface of the vascular endothelial growth factor (VEGF) encapsulated Gel RGD were observed to form an extensive tubular network within 72 hours. Furthermore, *in vivo* microvasculature formation was also assessed by

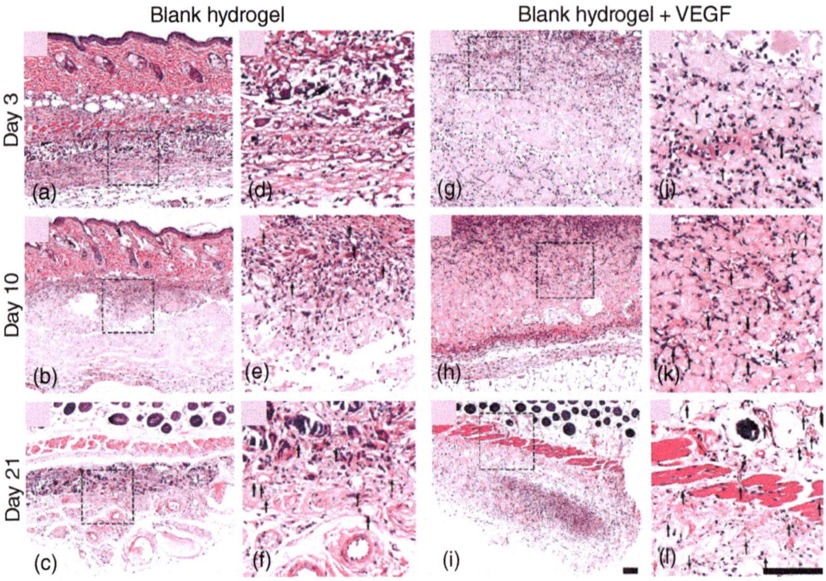

Figure 6.2 Histological images showing blood vessels in implanted hydrogel with/without growth factor loading. (a–c) H&E-stained sections of the implanted Gel RGD hydrogel without growth factor loading on day 3, day 10, and day 21, respectively. (d–f) High-magnification images of the boxed areas shown in parts (a–c). (g–i) H&E-stained sections of the implanted Gel RGD hydrogel loaded with growth factor on day 3, day 10, and day 21, respectively. (j–l) High-magnification images of the boxed areas shown in parts (g–i). Black arrows designate blood vessels. Scale bar = 100 μm. Source: Cheng, B et al (2018) [103] / Figure6 / Reprinted with permission from American Chemical Society.

subcutaneous implantation of the (VEGF) encapsulated Gel RGD into the dorsal side of mice (Figure 6.2).

6.3.3 Wound Healing

Short peptide hydrogels have emerged as excellent wound healing materials. In order to be applicable in wound healing, the gelator peptides should have good antibacterial properties. We reported self-assembled FF dipeptide as the minimal model for antibacterial supramolecular polymers [104]. The self-assembled nanostructures exhibited complete inhibition of bacterial growth, disrupted bacteria morphology, and caused membrane permeation and depolarization. These nanostructures were further integrated with tissue scaffolds for the development of antibacterial materials.

Self-assembled α/γ hybrid peptide hydrogels exhibited antibacterial activity against Gram-negative and Gram-positive bacteria [105]. Banerjee and coworkers discovered a series of peptide amphiphile-based hydrogelators that formed nanofibrous hydrogels [106]. These gels exhibited antimicrobial activity against Gram-positive bacteria (*Staphylococcus aureus*, *Bacillus subtilis*) and Gram-negative bacteria (*Escherichia coli*). Xu and coworkers designed an amphiphilic peptide

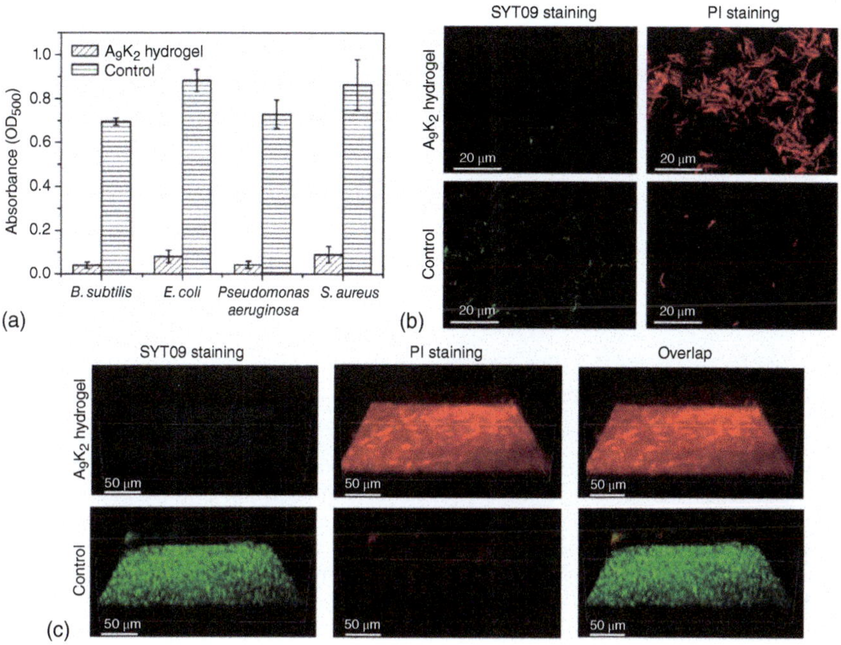

Figure 6.3 (a) The growth of bacteria in the solution above the A_9K_2 hydrogel surface after incubation for 24 hours. (b) Live dead staining of the bacteria (*B. subtilis* 168) in the solution above the A_9K_2 hydrogel surface after incubation for 24 hours. (c) Confocal laser scanning microscopy images of the bacteria (*B. subtilis* 168) on the A_9K_2 hydrogel surface after incubation for 24 hours and live/dead staining, concluding most of the bacteria are deposited on the gel surface. In all the cases, the bacteria incubated in the TCPS plates acted as a control and the live dead staining was performed with SYTO 9 and PI. Source: Bai, J. et al (2016) [107] / Figure5c / with permission from American Chemical Society.

A_9K_2 to prevent bacterial growth through membrane permeabilization [107]. The sol–gel transition was accomplished by the addition of fetal bovine serum or plasma amine oxidase. The hydrogels exhibited high antibacterial ability against both Gram-negative and Gram-positive bacterial strains and very low cytotoxicity (Figure 6.3). Interestingly, the hydrogel exhibited selective killing of bacteria when co-cultured with mammalian cells. In a similar work, design of another amphiphilic peptide I_4K_2, its enzymatic hydrogelation, and antibacterial activity is reported by Wang and coworkers [108]. From the above examples, it is obvious that judiciously designed peptide hydrogels exhibit inhibition of bacterial growth, which is highly desirable for wound healing applications. Additionally, peptide hydrogels are endowed with other excellent attributes including high gas permeability, hydrated environment, and ability to act as drug delivery vehicles. These qualities allow wound closure and recovery with minimum scars.

Hartgerink and coworkers reported multidomain peptide (MDP) hydrogels for wound healing applications (Figure 6.4) [109]. The hydrogels were composed of nanofibrous network and were syringe deliverable. The hydrogel exhibited accelerated wound healing in comparison with a clinically used hydrogel, after

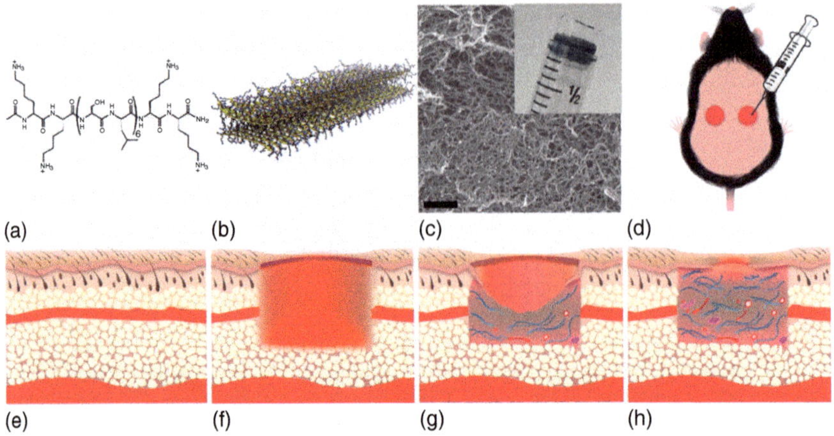

Figure 6.4 Nanofibrous hydrogel formation of MDP and its application in wound healing. (a) 16-amino acid MDP, $K_2(SL)_6K_2$ forms (b) nanofibers through non-covalent interactions. (c) The hydrogel formation occurs via cross-linking of nanofibers entangle after the addition of multivalent salts. Scale bar = 500 nm. (d) Application of the hydrogel to wounds retaining their shape. (e–h) Cartoon representation of the time course of wound healing. (e) The subcutaneous tissue is filled with adipose tissue and the panniculus carnosus muscle layer, prior to the creation of the wound. (f) Removal of epithelium, adipose tissue, and the panniculus carnosus due to the wounding of the dorsal tissue. (g) Granulation tissue, collagen, blood vessels, and neural fascicles fill the wound bed, and epithelial cells migrate across the granulation tissue creating epithelial tongues during the course of wound healing. (h) An increment in the amount of granulation tissue, collagen, blood vessels, and neural fascicles is observed over time, and the epithelial tongues extend to close the wound. Source: Carrejo, et al (2018) [109] / Figure1 / with permission from American Chemical Society.

its application to full-thickness dermal wounds in genetically diabetic mice. The MDP hydrogel promoted wound closure in 14 days, along with the formation of thick granulation tissue. Short aliphatic peptides, Ac-ILVAGK-NH_2 and Ac-LIVAGK-NH_2, were utilized to produce self-assembled hydrogels composed of helical fibers by Hauser and coworkers [110]. These hydrogel scaffolds were utilized for the healing of burn wounds. The hydrogels were observed to attain 86.2% and 92.9% wound closure after 14 days, along with epithelial and dermal regeneration in the absence of exogenous growth factors. In comparison, Mepitel, a silicone-coated polyamide net exhibited only 62.8% of healing, demonstrating the higher efficiency of the peptide hydrogels.

Cysteine-containing short peptides that produced hydrogels through disulfide cross-linking were later demonstrated by the same research group [111]. Disulfide cross-linking bestowed stiffness and shape fidelity to the only peptide hydrogels. The enhanced stiffness enabled handling of the hydrogel scaffolds by forceps during surgical procedure thus offering an advantage over non-cross-linked hydrogels. The hydrogels exhibited accelerated re-epithelialization during its application as wound dressing materials. Guler, Tekinay, and coworkers reported heparin-mimetic peptide nanofiber (HM-PA, lauryl-VVAGEGD(K-psb)S-Am) gels and their utilization in burn wound healing [112]. Histological observations, immunostaining, and marker

RNA/protein analysis were used to assess the wound healing process after 7, 14, and 21 days following injury. Formation of well-organized and collagen-rich granulation tissue layers, production of highly dense blood vessels, and an increase in re-epithelialization and skin appendage development with minimal crust formation, was observed in the heparin-mimetic peptide nanofiber treated burn wounds.

6.3.4 Drug Delivery

Hydrogels are endowed with many excellent attributes which make them a desirable candidate for drug delivery applications [113–117]. Their tunable mechanical property, hydrated environment, controllable degradability, and ability to protect drugs from degradation allow the hydrogels' application in drug delivery. Short peptide self-assembled hydrogels are particularly intriguing as they combine intrinsic biocompatibility with the above-mentioned attributes of other hydrogels and therefore are used by many research groups as efficient drug carriers.

A biocompatible hydrogel produced from the self-assembly of the peptide Ac-$(RADA)_4$-$CONH_2$ was appraised for the encapsulation and delivery of the chemotherapeutic drug DOX and the anticancer agent curcumin (CUR) [118]. It was observed that drug encapsulation did not affect the mechanical strength of the hydrogel. In another study, the self-assembling peptide, RADA16, was used to encapsulate hydrophobic antitumor drug paclitaxel (PTX) by virtue of the interactions between the peptide and the drug [119]. Drug release measurements revealed a longer half-release time in the hydrogels containing higher peptide concentration. The RADA16-PTX hydrogel inhibited the growth of the breast cancer cell line, MDA-MB-435S, *in vitro*.

In a very interesting study, Xu and coworkers reported the hydrogelation of two peptides, Ac-I_3SLKG-NH_2 and Ac-I_3SLGK-NH_2 [120]. They observed that the Ac-I_3SLKG-NH_2 hydrogels degraded in response to the enzyme MMP-2 due to the cleavage of Ac-I_3SLKG-NH_2 into Ac-I_3S and LKG-NH_2, while the Ac-I_3SLGK-NH_2 hydrogel did not. The MMP-2 enzyme, which is overexpressed by HeLa tumor cells, disturbed the entanglement of the fibers leading to the decreased mechanical strength of the hydrogels. This allowed its utilization as a platform for sustained drug release (Figure 6.5). They further entrapped an anticancer peptide $G(IIKK)_3I$-NH_2 (G3) into the Ac-I_3SLKG-NH_2 hydrogels and obtained its controlled release in a "cell-demanded" manner in the presence of HeLa cells. This resulted in an inhibitory effect on the growth of HeLa cells on the hydrogels.

Topical administration of anticancer drugs, though being very effective, has its own limitations. The efficiency of drug delivery is often limited by the physiological barriers from the skin to the tumor. To tackle this problem, He, Mo, and coworkers developed a paintable oligopeptide hydrogel which encapsulated cell-penetrating peptide-modified transfersomes (PTX-CT) that were loaded with the antitumor drug PTX [121]. The PTX-CTs-embedded hydrogel when plastered on the skin above the melanoma tumor offered excellent retention capacity. Furthermore, the hydrogels were also capable of improved skin and tumor stroma penetration and tumor growth inhibition (Figure 6.6).

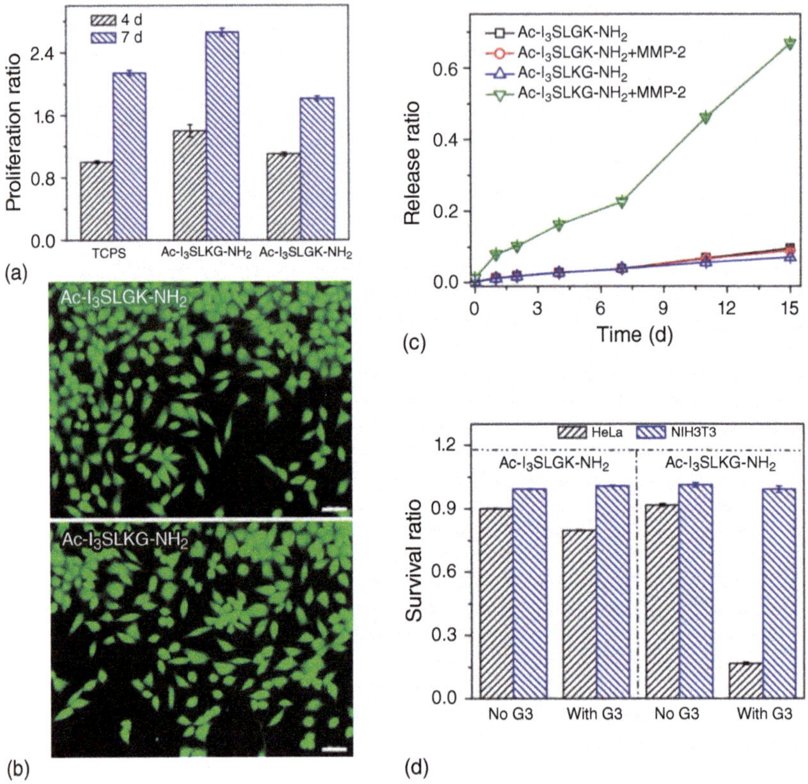

Figure 6.5 (a) MTT assay determining the cytotoxicity of the Ac-I_3SLKG-NH_2 and Ac-I_3SLGK-NH_2 hydrogels against NIH 3T3 cells. (b) Fluorescence images of NIH 3T3 cells on the hydrogels (calcein-AM staining). (c) G3 (G(IIKK)$_3$-NH_2) release from the G3-loaded Ac-I_3SLGK-NH2+MMP2 and Ac-I_3SLGK-NH_2 gels in the presence and absence of MMP-2. (d) MTT assay determining the viability of NIH 3T3 and HeLa cells on the two peptide gels with and without G3 loading after 24 hours. Source: Chen, C., et al. (2017) [120] / Figure6b / with permission American Chemical Society.

Yan and coworkers reported an injectable composite hydrogel composed of Fmoc-FF and poly-L-lysine possessing excellent therapeutic attributes including shear-thinning and self-healing properties, biocompatibility, and perfect biodegradability [122]. A photosensitive drug Chlorin e6 was entrapped within the composite hydrogels, and photodynamic antitumor therapy was conducted, where effective inhibition of tumor growth was observed.

Another strategy for drug delivery is developing new hydrogelators by chemically attaching drugs with peptides [123–125]. Xu and coworkers reported a hydrogel precursor bases on PTX chemically attached to a peptide [123]. The precursor produced hydrogel under the catalysis of alkaline phosphatase. The hydrogels were also observed to exhibit equal antitumor efficiency. Cui and coworkers developed an amphiphilic PTX-peptide conjugate that self-assembles into hydrogels [125].

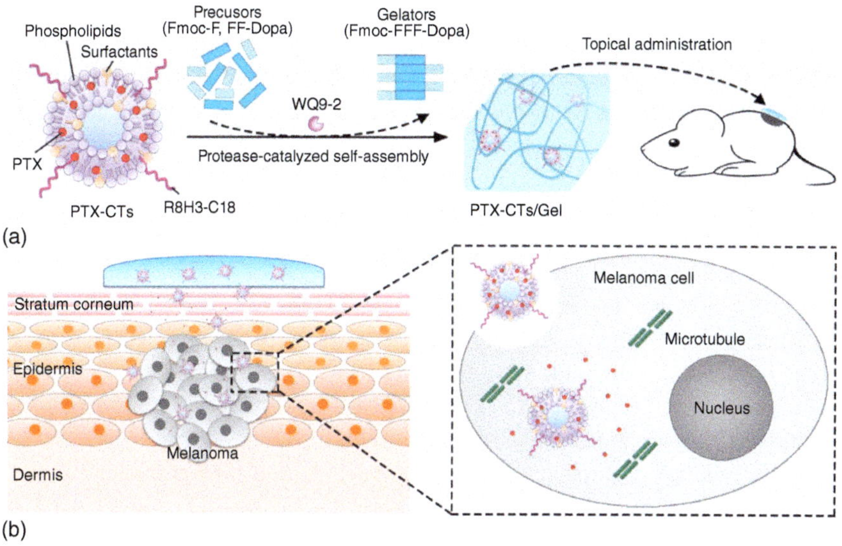

Figure 6.6 (a) Schematic representation of preparation and application of PTX-CTs/Gel as a paintable patch for topical drug delivery. (b) Schematic illustration depicting the enhancement on the transdermal efficiency of PTX by the PTX-CTs/Gel for noninvasive chemotherapy of Melanoma. Source: From Jiang et al. [121]/with permission of American Chemical Society.

The hydrogels were glutathione responsive and released PTX upon its addition. The *in vitro* cell experiments demonstrated the ability of the system to inhibit cancer cell growth.

6.4 Conclusions and Outlook

Peptides being fragments of proteins inherit their biocompatibility. Self-aggregation of peptides into supramolecular hydrogels is very important from the perspective of applications. In fact, short peptide-based supramolecular hydrogels recognize the manifestation of peptide nanotechnology into biomedical products. Interestingly, peptide self-assembled hydrogels have already been commercialized, one example being PuraMatrix™, a protected synthetic 16-mer peptide which is used for tissue regeneration. Not belittling the plethora of polymer gels and their excellent biomedical aptitudes, short peptides are the next-generation materials for commercial biomedical products.

This chapter sheds light on different biomedical applications of short peptide hydrogel. At first, we presented a brief introduction on different categories of peptide hydrogels and then discussed their relevant usage. We have included significant references demonstrating the cell scaffolding, wound healing, tissue engineering, and drug delivery applications of these hydrogels.

The design of functional peptide hydrogels with tunable physical, chemical, and biological properties is a blooming subject, and there is still plenty of room for further progress. Development of *de novo* peptides flanked with bioactive ligands in very intriguing, as is the discovery of hybrid gels with biopolymer and conductive polymers. These new discoveries will enhance the use of these wonderful materials in biomedical applications.

References

1 Chakraborty, P., Das, S., and Nandi, A.K. (2019). Conducting gels: a chronicle of technological advances. *Prog. Polym. Sci.* 88: 189–219.

2 Seow, W.Y. and Hauser, C.A.E. (2014). Short to ultrashort peptide hydrogels for biomedical uses. *Mater. Today* 17 (8): 381–388.

3 Trappmann, B., Gautrot, J.E., Connelly, J.T. et al. (2012). Extracellular-matrix tethering regulates stem-cell fate. *Nat. Mater.* 11 (7): 642–649.

4 Shin, J.W. and Discher, D.E. (2012). Soft gels select tumorigenic cells. *Nat. Mater.* 11 (8): 662–663.

5 Gelain, F., Bottai, D., Vescovi, A., and Zhang, S. (2006). Designer self-assembling peptide nanofiber scaffolds for adult mouse neural stem cell 3-dimensional cultures. *PLoS One* 1 (1): e119.

6 Zoldan, J., Karagiannis, E.D., Lee, C.Y. et al. (2011). The influence of scaffold elasticity on germ layer specification of human embryonic stem cells. *Biomaterials* 32 (36): 9612–9621.

7 Moreira Teixeira, L.S., Feijen, J., van Blitterswijk, C.A. et al. (2012). Enzyme-catalyzed crosslinkable hydrogels: emerging strategies for tissue engineering. *Biomaterials* 33 (5): 1281–1290.

8 Lee, K.Y. and Mooney, D.J. (2001). Hydrogels for tissue engineering. *Chem. Rev.* 101 (7): 1869–1881.

9 Shpaisman, N., Sheihet, L., Bushman, J. et al. (2012). One-step synthesis of biodegradable curcumin-derived hydrogels as potential soft tissue fillers after breast cancer surgery. *Biomacromolecules* 13 (8): 2279–2286.

10 Davis, M.E., Hsieh, P.C.H., Takahashi, T. et al. (2006). Local myocardial insulin-like growth factor 1 (IGF-1) delivery with biotinylated peptide nanofibers improves cell therapy for myocardial infarction. *Proc. Natl. Acad. Sci. U.S.A.* 103 (21): 8155–8160.

11 Milani, A.H., Freemont, A.J., Hoyland, J.A. et al. (2012). Injectable doubly cross-linked microgels for improving the mechanical properties of degenerated intervertebral discs. *Biomacromolecules* 13 (9): 2793–2801.

12 Bodugoz-Senturk, H., Macias, C.E., Kung, J.H., and Muratoglu, O.K. (2009). Poly(vinyl alcohol)-acrylamide hydrogels as load-bearing cartilage substitute. *Biomaterials* 30 (4): 589–596.

13 Takei, T., Nakahara, H., Ijima, H., and Kawakami, K. (2012). Synthesis of a chitosan derivative soluble at neutral pH and gellable by freeze-thawing, and its application in wound care. *Acta Biomater.* 8 (2): 686–693.

14 Tran, N.Q., Joung, Y.K., Lih, E., and Park, K.D. (2011). In situ forming and rutin-releasing chitosan hydrogels as injectable dressings for dermal wound healing. *Biomacromolecules* 12 (8): 2872–2880.
15 Nafea, E.H., Poole-Warren, A.M.L.A., and Martens, P.J. (2011). Immunoisolating semi-permeable membranes for cell encapsulation: focus on hydrogels. *J. Controlled Release* 154 (2): 110–122.
16 Adler-Abramovich, L. and Gazit, E. (2014). Correction: the physical properties of supramolecular peptide assemblies: from building block association to technological applications. *Chem. Soc. Rev.* 43 (20): 7236–7236.
17 Yemini, M., Reches, M., Rishpon, J., and Gazit, E. (2005). Novel electrochemical biosensing platform using self-assembled peptide nanotubes. *Nano Lett.* 5 (1): 183–186.
18 Rosenman, G., Amdursky, N., Molotskii, M. et al. (2009). Blue luminescence based on quantum confinement at peptide nanotubes. *Nano Lett.* 9 (9): 3111–3115.
19 Kholkin, A., Amdursky, N., Bdikin, I. et al. (2010). Strong piezoelectricity in bioinspired peptide nanotubes. *ACS Nano* 4 (2): 610–614.
20 Adler-Abramovich, L., Aronov, D., Beker, P. et al. (2009). Self-assembled arrays of peptide nanotubes by vapour deposition. *Nat. Nanotechnol.* 4 (12): 849–854.
21 Li, J., Xing, R., Bai, S., and Yan, X. (2019). Recent advances of self-assembling peptide-based hydrogels for biomedical applications. *Soft Matter* 15 (8): 1704–1715.
22 Mezzenga, R. and Fischer, P. (2013). The self-assembly, aggregation and phase transitions of food protein systems in one, two and three dimensions. *Rep. Prog. Phys.* 76 (4): 046601.
23 Bera, S., Mondal, S., Xue, B. et al. (2019). Rigid helical-like assemblies from a self-aggregating tripeptide. *Nat. Mater.* 18 (5): 503–509.
24 Reches, M. and Gazit, E. (2003). Casting metal nanowires within discrete self-assembled peptide nanotubes. *Science* 300: 625–628.
25 Zhang, S. (2003). Fabrication of novel biomaterials through molecular self-assembly. *Nat. Biotechnol.* 21 (10): 1171–1178.
26 Knowles, T.P.J., Oppenheim, T.W., Buell, A.K. et al. (2010). Nanostructured films from hierarchical self-assembly of amyloidogenic proteins. *Nat. Nanotechnol.* 5 (3): 204–207.
27 Fuentes-Caparrós, A.M., Dietrich, B., Thomson, L. et al. (2019). Using cavitation rheology to understand dipeptide-based low molecular weight gels. *Soft Matter* 15: 6340–6347.
28 Nolan, M.C., Fuentes Caparrós, A.M., Dietrich, B. et al. (2017). Optimising low molecular weight hydrogels for automated 3D printing. *Soft Matter* 13 (45): 8426–8432.
29 Fleming, S. and Ulijn, R.V. (2014). Design of nanostructures based on aromatic peptide amphiphiles. *Chem. Soc. Rev.* 43 (23): 8150–8177.
30 Fleming, S., Frederix, P.W.J.M., Ramos Sasselli, I. et al. (2013). Assessing the utility of infrared spectroscopy as a structural diagnostic tool for β-sheets in self-assembling aromatic peptide amphiphiles. *Langmuir* 29 (30): 9510–9515.

31 Smith, A.M., Williams, R.J., Tang, C. et al. (2008). Fmoc-diphenylalanine self assembles to a hydrogel via a novel architecture based on π–π interlocked β-sheets. *Adv. Mater.* 20 (1): 37–41.

32 Ulijn, R.V. and Smith, A.M. (2008). Designing peptide based nanomaterials. *Chem. Soc. Rev.* 37 (4): 664–675.

33 Adams, D.J., Butler, M.F., Frith, W.J. et al. (2009). A new method for maintaining homogeneity during liquid-hydrogel transitions using low molecular weight hydrogelators. *Soft Matter* 5 (9): 1856–1862.

34 Rughani, R.V., Salick, D.A., Lamm, M.S. et al. (2009). Folding, self-assembly, and bulk material properties of a de novo designed three-stranded β-sheet hydrogel. *Biomacromolecules* 10 (5): 1295–1304.

35 Adams, D.J. (2011). Dipeptide and tripeptide conjugates as low-molecular-weight hydrogelators. *Macromol. Biosci.* 11 (2): 160–173.

36 Basavalingappa, V., Guterman, T., Tang, Y. et al. (2019). Expanding the functional scope of the Fmoc-diphenylalanine hydrogelator by introducing a rigidifying and chemically active urea backbone modification. *Adv. Sci.* 6: 1900218.

37 Dasgupta, A., Mondal, J.H., and Das, D. (2013). Peptide hydrogels. *RSC Adv.* 3 (24): 9117–9149.

38 Frederix, P.W.J.M., Scott, G.G., Abul-Haija, Y.M. et al. (2015). Exploring the sequence space for (tri-)peptide self-assembly to design and discover new hydrogels. *Nat. Chem.* 7 (1): 30–37.

39 Toledano, S., Williams, R.J., Jayawarna, V., and Ulijn, R.V. (2006). Enzyme-triggered self-assembly of peptide hydrogels via reversed hydrolysis. *J. Am. Chem. Soc.* 128 (4): 1070–1071.

40 Frederix, P.W.J.M., Ulijn, R.V., Hunt, N.T., and Tuttle, T. (2011). Virtual screening for dipeptide aggregation: toward predictive tools for peptide self-assembly. *J. Phys. Chem. Lett.* 2 (19): 2380–2384.

41 Chakraborty, P., Guterman, T., Adadi, N. et al. (2019). A self-healing, all-organic, conducting, composite peptide hydrogel as pressure sensor and electrogenic cell soft substrate. *ACS Nano* 13 (1): 163–175.

42 Conte, M.P., Singh, N., Sasselli, I.R. et al. (2016). Metastable hydrogels from aromatic dipeptides. *Chem. Commun.* 52 (96): 13889–13892.

43 Mahler, A., Reches, M., Rechter, M. et al. (2006). Rigid, self-assembled hydrogel composed of a modified aromatic dipeptide. *Adv. Mater.* 18 (11): 1365–1370.

44 Jayawarna, V., Ali, M., Jowitt, T.A. et al. (2006). Nanostructured hydrogels for three-dimensional cell culture through self-assembly of fluorenylmethoxycarbonyl-dipeptides. *Adv. Mater.* 18: 611–614.

45 Tao, K., Levin, A., Adler-Abramovich, L., and Gazit, E. (2016). Fmoc-modified amino acids and short peptides: simple bio-inspired building blocks for the fabrication of functional materials. *Chem. Soc. Rev.* 45 (14): 3935–3953.

46 Mu, X., Eckes, K.M., Nguyen, M.M. et al. (2012). Experimental and computational studies reveal an alternative supramolecular structure for Fmoc-dipeptide self-assembly. *Biomacromolecules* 13 (11): 3562–3571.

47 Zhang, Y., Gu, H., Yang, Z., and Xu, B. (2003). Supramolecular hydrogels respond to ligand-receptor interaction. *J. Am. Chem. Soc.* 125 (45): 13680–13681.

48 Zhou, M., Smith, A.M., Das, A.K. et al. (2009). Self-assembled peptide-based hydrogels as scaffolds for anchorage-dependent cells. *Biomaterials* 30 (13): 2523–2530.

49 Cheng, G., Castelletto, V., Jones, R.R. et al. (2011). Hydrogelation of self-assembling RGD-based peptides. *Soft Matter* 7 (4): 1326–1333.

50 López-Pérez, D.E., Revilla-López, G., Hamley, I.W., and Alemán, C. (2013). Molecular insights into aggregates made of amphiphilic Fmoc-tetrapeptides. *Soft Matter* 9 (46): 11021–11032.

51 Zou, Y., Razmkhah, K., Chmel, N.P. et al. (2013). Spectroscopic signatures of an Fmoc-tetrapeptide, Fmoc and fluorene. *RSC Adv.* 3 (27): 10854–10858.

52 Gouveia, R.M., Jones, R.R., Hamley, I.W., and Connon, C.J. (2014). The bioactivity of composite Fmoc-RGDS-collagen gels. *Biomater. Sci.* 2 (9): 1222–1229.

53 Castelletto, V., Moulton, C.M., Cheng, G. et al. (2011). Self-assembly of Fmoc-tetrapeptides based on the RGDS cell adhesion motif. *Soft Matter* 7 (24): 11405–11415.

54 Orbach, R., Adler-Abramovich, L., Zigerson, S. et al. (2009). Self-assembled Fmoc-peptides as a platform for the formation of nanostructures and hydrogels. *Biomacromolecules* 10 (9): 2646–2651.

55 Ma, M., Kuang, Y., Gao, Y. et al. (2010). Aromatic-aromatic interactions induce the self-assembly of pentapeptidic derivatives in water to form nanofibers and supramolecular hydrogels. *J. Am. Chem. Soc.* 132 (8): 2719–2728.

56 Chakraborty, P., Ghosh, M., Schnaider, L. et al. (2019). Composite of peptide-supramolecular polymer and covalent polymer comprises a new multifunctional, bio-inspired soft material. *Macromol. Rapid Commun* 40: 1900175.

57 Zhang, S., Holmest, T., Lockshin, C., and Rich, A. (1993). Spontaneous assembly of a self-complementary oligopeptide to form a stable macroscopic membrane (B-sheet/insoluble filaments/ionic bonds/origin of life/zuotin). *Chemistry* 90 (April): 3334–3338.

58 Kisiday, J., Jin, M., Kurz, B. et al. (2002). Self-assembling peptide hydrogel fosters chondrocyte extracellular matrix production and cell division: implications for cartilage tissue repair. *Proc. Natl. Acad. Sci. U.S.A.* 99: 9996–10001.

59 Zhang, S., Holmes, T.C., Dipersio, C.M. et al. (1995). Self-complementary oligopeptide matrices support mammalian cell attachment. *Biomaterials* 16 (18): 1385–1393.

60 Yokoi, H., Kinoshita, T., and Zhang, S. (2005). Dynamic reassembly of peptide RADA16 nanofiber scaffold. *Proc. Natl. Acad. Sci. U.S.A.* 102 (24): 8414–8419.

61 Ozbas, B., Kretsinger, J., Rajagopal, K. et al. (2004). Salt-triggered peptide folding and consequent self-assembly into hydrogels with tunable modulus. *Macromolecules* 37 (19): 7331–7337.

62 Nagy, K.J., Giano, M.C., Jin, A. et al. (2011). Enhanced mechanical rigidity of hydrogels formed from enantiomeric peptide assemblies. *J. Am. Chem. Soc.* 133 (38): 14975–14977.

63 Haines-Butterick, L., Rajagopal, K., Branco, M. et al. (2007). Controlling hydrogelation kinetics by peptide design for three-dimensional encapsulation and injectable delivery of cells. *Proc. Natl. Acad. Sci. U.S.A.* 104 (19): 7791–7796.

64 Veiga, A.S., Sinthuvanich, C., Gaspar, D. et al. (2012). Arginine-rich self-assembling peptides as potent antibacterial gels. *Biomaterials* 33 (35): 8907–8916.

65 Hauser, C.A.E., Deng, R., Mishra, A. et al. (2011). Natural tri- to hexapeptides self-assemble in water to amyloid β-type fiber aggregates by unexpected α-helical intermediate structures. *Proc. Natl. Acad. Sci. U.S.A.* 108 (4): 1361–1366.

66 Mishra, A., Loo, Y., Deng, R. et al. (2011). Ultrasmall natural peptides self-assemble to strong temperature-resistant helical fibers in scaffolds suitable for tissue engineering. *Nano Today* 6 (3): 232–239.

67 Mishra, A., Chan, K.H., Reithofer, M.R., and Hauser, C.A.E. (2013). Influence of metal salts on the hydrogelation properties of ultrashort aliphatic peptides. *RSC Adv.* 3 (25): 9985–9993.

68 Seow, W.Y. and Hauser, C.A.E. (2013). Tunable mechanical properties of ultrasmall peptide hydrogels by crosslinking and functionalization to achieve the 3D distribution of cells. *Adv. Healthc. Mater.* 2 (9): 1219–1223.

69 Kaivosoja, E., Barreto, G., Levón, K. et al. (2012). Chemical and physical properties of regenerative medicine materials controlling stem cell fate. *Ann. Med.* 44 (7): 635–650.

70 Goldberg, M., Langer, R., and Jia, X. (2007). Nanostructured materials for applications in drug delivery and tissue engineering. *J. Biomater. Sci., Polym. Ed.* 18 (3): 241–268.

71 Diaferia, C., Ghosh, M., Sibillano, T. et al. (2019). Fmoc-FF and hexapeptide-based multicomponent hydrogels as scaffold materials. *Soft Matter* 15 (3): 487–496.

72 Discher, D.E., Janmey, P., and Wang, Y.L. (2005). Tissue cells feel and respond to the stiffness of their substrate. *Science* 310 (5751): 1139–1143.

73 Dvir, T., Timko, B.P., Kohane, D.S., and Langer, R. (2011). Nanotechnological strategies for engineering complex tissues. *Nat. Nanotechnol.* 6 (1): 13–22.

74 Dou, X.Q. and Feng, C.L. (2017). Amino acids and peptide-based supramolecular hydrogels for three-dimensional cell culture. *Adv. Mater.* 29 (16): 1604062.

75 Yang, Z. and Zhao, X. (2011). A 3D model of ovarian cancer cell lines on peptide nanofiber scaffold to explore the cell-scaffold interaction and chemotherapeutic resistance of anticancer drugs. *Int. J. Nanomed.* 6: 303–310.

76 Smith, D.J., Brat, G.A., Medina, S.H. et al. (2016). A multiphase transitioning peptide hydrogel for suturing ultrasmall vessels. *Nat. Nanotechnol.* 11 (1): 95–102.

77 Medina, S.H., Miller, S.E., Keim, A.I. et al. (2016). An intrinsically disordered peptide facilitates non-endosomal cell entry. *Angew. Chem. Int. Ed.* 55 (10): 3369–3372.

78 Medina, S.H., Li, S., Howard, O.M.Z. et al. (2015). Enhanced immunostimulatory effects of DNA-encapsulated peptide hydrogels. *Biomaterials* 53: 545–553.

79 Galler, K.M., Hartgerink, J.D., Cavender, A.C. et al. (2012). A customized self-assembling peptide hydrogel for dental pulp tissue engineering. *Tissue Eng. Part A* 18 (1, 2): 176–184.

80 Huang, H., Ding, Y., Sun, X.S., and Nguyen, T.A. (2013). Peptide hydrogelation and cell encapsulation for 3D culture of MCF-7 breast cancer cells. *PLoS One* 8 (3): e59482.

81 Huang, H., Herrera, A.I., Luo, Z. et al. (2012). Structural transformation and physical properties of a hydrogel-forming peptide studied by NMR, transmission electron microscopy, and dynamic rheometer. *Biophys. J.* 103 (5): 979–988.

82 Mujeeb, A., Miller, A.F., Saiani, A., and Gough, J.E. (2013). Self-assembled octapeptide scaffolds for in vitro chondrocyte culture. *Acta Biomater.* 9 (1): 4609–4617.

83 Marchesan, S., Qu, Y., Waddington, L.J. et al. (2013). Self-assembly of ciprofloxacin and a tripeptide into an antimicrobial nanostructured hydrogel. *Biomaterials* 34 (14): 3678–3687.

84 Ghosh, M., Halperin-Sternfeld, M., Grigoriants, I. et al. (2017). Arginine-presenting peptide hydrogels decorated with hydroxyapatite as biomimetic scaffolds for bone regeneration. *Biomacromolecules* 18 (11): 3541–3550.

85 Chen, G., Chen, J., Liu, Q. et al. (2015). Enzymatic formation of a meta-stable supramolecular hydrogel for 3D cell culture. *RSC Adv.* 5 (39): 30675–30678.

86 Qin, X., Xie, W., Tian, S. et al. (2013). Enzyme-triggered hydrogelation via self-assembly of alternating peptides. *Chem. Commun.* 49 (42): 4839–4841.

87 Chronopoulou, L., Lorenzoni, S., Masci, G. et al. (2010). Lipase-supported synthesis of peptidic hydrogels. *Soft Matter* 6 (11): 2525–2532.

88 Chronopoulou, L., Togna, A.R., Guarguaglini, G. et al. (2012). Self-assembling peptide hydrogels promote microglial cells proliferation and NGF production. *Soft Matter* 8 (21): 5784–5790.

89 Gao, Y., Shi, J., Yuan, D., and Xu, B. (2012). Imaging enzyme-triggered self-assembly of small molecules inside live cells. *Nat. Commun.* 3: 1033–1038.

90 Yang, Z., Liang, G., and Xu, B. (2008). Enzymatic hydrogelation of small molecules. *Acc. Chem. Res.* 41 (2): 315–326.

91 Shi, J., Du, X., Yuan, D. et al. (2014). D-amino acids modulate the cellular response of enzymatic-instructed supramolecular nanofibers of small peptides. *Biomacromolecules* 15 (10): 3559–3568.

92 Zhou, J., Du, X., Yamagata, N., and Xu, B. (2016). Enzyme-instructed self-assembly of small d-peptides as a multiple-step process for selectively killing cancer cells. *J. Am. Chem. Soc.* 138 (11): 3813–3823.

93 Kuang, Y., Long, M.J.C., Zhou, J. et al. (2014). Prion-like nanofibrils of small molecules (PriSM) selectively inhibit cancer cells by impeding cytoskeleton dynamics. *J. Biol. Chem.* 289 (42): 29208–29218.

94 Shi, J. and Xu, B. (2015). Nanoscale assemblies of small molecules control the fate of cells. *Nano Today* 10 (5): 615–630.

95 Loo, Y., Goktas, M., Tekinay, A.B. et al. (2015). Self-assembled proteins and peptides as scaffolds for tissue regeneration. *Adv. Healthc. Mater.* 4 (16): 2557–2586.

96 Knowles, T.P.J. and Mezzenga, R. (2016). Amyloid fibrils as building blocks for natural and artificial functional materials. *Adv. Mater.* 28 (31): 6546–6561.

97 Semino, C.E. (2008) Critical reviews in oral biology & medicine). Self-assembling peptides: from bio-inspired materials to bone regeneration. *J. Dent. Res.* 87 (7): 606–616.

98 Wei, G., Su, Z., Reynolds, N.P. et al. (2017). Self-assembling peptide and protein amyloids: from structure to tailored function in nanotechnology. *Chem. Soc. Rev.* 46 (15): 4661–4708.

99 Ghosh, M., Halperin-Sternfeld, M., Grinberg, I., and Adler-Abramovich, L. (2019). Injectable alginate-peptide composite hydrogel as a scaffold for bone tissue regeneration. *Nanomaterials* 9 (4): 497.

100 Sheikholeslam, M., Wheeler, S.D., Duke, K.G. et al. (2018). Peptide and peptide-carbon nanotube hydrogels as scaffolds for tissue & 3D tumor engineering. *Acta Biomater.* 69: 107–119.

101 Sleep, E., Cosgrove, B.D., McClendon, M.T. et al. (2017). Injectable biomimetic liquid crystalline scaffolds enhance muscle stem cell transplantation. *Proc. Natl. Acad. Sci. U.S.A.* 114 (38): E7919–E7928.

102 Ji, W., Álvarez, Z., Edelbrock, A.N. et al. (2018). Bioactive nanofibers induce neural transdifferentiation of human bone marrow mesenchymal stem cells. *ACS Appl. Mater. Interfaces* 10 (48): 41046–41055.

103 Cheng, B., Yan, Y., Qi, J. et al. (2018). Cooperative assembly of a peptide gelator and silk fibroin afford an injectable hydrogel for tissue engineering. *ACS Appl. Mater. Interfaces* 10 (15): 12474–12484.

104 Schnaider, L., Brahmachari, S., Schmidt, N.W. et al. (2017). Self-assembling dipeptide antibacterial nanostructures with membrane disrupting activity. *Nat. Commun.* 8 (1): 1365.

105 Malhotra, K., Shankar, S., Rai, R., and Singh, Y. (2018). Broad-spectrum antibacterial activity of proteolytically stable self-assembled αγ-hybrid peptide gels. *Biomacromolecules* 19 (3): 782–792.

106 Nandi, N., Gayen, K., Ghosh, S. et al. (2017). Amphiphilic peptide-based supramolecular, noncytotoxic, stimuli-responsive hydrogels with antibacterial activity. *Biomacromolecules* 18 (11): 3621–3629.

107 Bai, J., Chen, C., Wang, J. et al. (2016). Enzymatic regulation of self-assembling peptide A_9K_2 nanostructures and hydrogelation with highly selective antibacterial activities. *ACS Appl. Mater. Interfaces* 8 (24): 15093–15102.

108 Bai, J., Gong, Z., Wang, J., and Wang, C. (2017). Enzymatic hydrogelation of self-assembling peptide I_4K_2 and its antibacterial and drug sustained-release activities. *RSC Adv.* 7 (77): 48631–48638.

109 Carrejo, N.C., Moore, A.N., Lopez Silva, T.L. et al. (2018). Multidomain peptide hydrogel accelerates healing of full-thickness wounds in diabetic mice. *ACS Biomater. Sci. Eng.* 4 (4): 1386–1396.

110 Loo, Y., Wong, Y.C., Cai, E.Z. et al. (2014). Ultrashort peptide nanofibrous hydrogels for the acceleration of healing of burn wounds. *Biomaterials* 35 (17): 4805–4814.

111 Seow, W.Y., Salgado, G., Lane, E.B., and Hauser, C.A.E. (2016). Transparent crosslinked ultrashort peptide hydrogel dressing with high shape-fidelity accelerates healing of full-thickness excision wounds. *Sci. Rep.* 6 (August): 1–12.
112 Yergoz, F., Hastar, N., Cimenci, C.E. et al. (2017). Heparin mimetic peptide nanofiber gel promotes regeneration of full thickness burn injury. *Biomaterials* 134: 117–127.
113 Eskandari, S., Guerin, T., Toth, I., and Stephenson, R.J. (2017). Recent advances in self-assembled peptides: implications for targeted drug delivery and vaccine engineering. *Adv. Drug Delivery Rev.* 110, 111: 169–187.
114 Altunbas, A., Lee, S.J., Rajasekaran, S.A. et al. (2011). Encapsulation of curcumin in self-assembling peptide hydrogels as injectable drug delivery vehicles. *Biomaterials* 32 (25): 5906–5914.
115 Li, J.K., Wang, N., and Wu, X.S. (1998). Poly(vinyl alcohol) nanoparticles prepared by freezing-thawing process for protein/peptide drug delivery. *J. Controlled Release* 56 (1–3): 117–126.
116 Peppas, N.A. (1997). Hydrogels and drug delivery. *Curr. Opin. Colloid Interface Sci.* 2 (5): 531–537.
117 Chung, H.J. and Park, T.G. (2009). Self-assembled and nanostructured hydrogels for drug delivery and tissue engineering. *Nano Today* 4 (5): 429–437.
118 Karavasili, C., Panteris, E., Vizirianakis, I.S. et al. (2018). Chemotherapeutic delivery from a self-assembling peptide nanofiber hydrogel for the management of glioblastoma. *Pharm. Res.* 35 (8): 1–13.
119 Liu, J., Zhang, L., Yang, Z., and Zhao, X. (2011). Controlled release of paclitaxel from a self-assembling peptide hydrogel formed in situ and antitumor study in vitro. *Int. J. Nanomed.* 6: 2143–2153.
120 Chen, C., Zhang, Y., Hou, Z. et al. (2017). Rational design of short peptide-based hydrogels with MMP-2 responsiveness for controlled anticancer peptide delivery. *Biomacromolecules* 18 (11): 3563–3571.
121 Jiang, T., Wang, T., Li, T. et al. (2018). Enhanced transdermal drug delivery by transfersome-embedded oligopeptide hydrogel for topical chemotherapy of melanoma. *ACS Nano* 12: 9693–9701.
122 Abbas, M., Xing, R., Zhang, N. et al. (2018). Antitumor photodynamic therapy based on dipeptide fibrous hydrogels with incorporation of photosensitive drugs. *ACS Biomater. Sci. Eng.* 4 (6): 2046–2052.
123 Gao, Y., Kuang, Y., Guo, Z.F. et al. (2009). Enzyme-instructed molecular self-assembly confers nanofibers and a supramolecular hydrogel of taxol derivative. *J. Am. Chem. Soc.* 131 (38): 13576–13577.
124 Li, J., Li, X., Kuang, Y. et al. (2013). Self-delivery multifunctional anti-HIV hydrogels for sustained release. *Adv. Healthc. Mater.* 2 (12): 1586–1590.
125 Lin, R., Cheetham, A.G., Zhang, P. et al. (2013). Supramolecular filaments containing a fixed 41% paclitaxel loading. *Chem. Commun.* 49 (43): 4968–4970.

7

Supramolecular Assemblies of Glycopeptides as Mimics of the Extracellular Matrix

Diana Soares da Costa[1,2], Alexandra Brito[1,2], Rui L. Reis[1,2], and Iva Pashkuleva[1,2]

[1] 3B's Research Group, I3Bs – Research Institute on Biomaterials, Biodegradables and Biomimetics, University of Minho, Headquarters of the European Institute of Excellence on Tissue Engineering and Regenerative Medicine, AvePark, Parque de Ciência e Tecnologia, Zona Industrial da Gandra, Barco, Guimaraes, 4805-017, Portugal
[2] ICVS/3Bs – PT Government Associate Laboratory, Braga, Guimaraes, Portugal

7.1 Introduction

The extracellular matrix (ECM) is a key player in the regulation of cell function, development, and homeostasis [1–5]. Besides providing structural and mechanical support for cell attachment and growth, it also modulates the cellular behavior by activating and mediating biological processes that are fundamental for tissue development and function [3, 4, 6]. The dynamic crosstalk between different cells and their microenvironment generates ECM with unique biochemical composition and biophysical framework. Such specific ECM signatures are built by the supramolecular hierarchical assembly of different biomolecules. The understanding of cell–ECM interactions and the role of different ECM components in the regulation of cell behavior have driven the development of biomaterials that copycat different elements of the native cellular environment. Among these, supramolecular materials have received increasing attention over the past two decades [7, 8]. Main asset of these materials is their inherent responsiveness to external stimuli, which makes them an excellent choice for mimicking the ECM dynamic remodeling in response to environmental stimuli and physiological cues, such as stress and disease, and thus enables homeostasis [3]. The possibility to conduct the self-assembly process toward the formation of nanofibrous networks that resembles the structural organization of the native ECM is another benefit of supramolecular materials [9–13]. Finally, these materials can code different bioactivities by embedding specific sequences in the structure of the assembling block. Proteins and carbohydrates are main components in the ECM build up. Alone or as conjugates, i.e. proteoglycans and glycoproteins, these biomolecules are

Diana Soares da Costa and Alexandra Brito were contributed equally.

Multifunctional Hydrogels for Biomedical Applications, First Edition.
Edited by Ricardo A. Pires, Iva Pashkuleva, and Rui L. Reis.

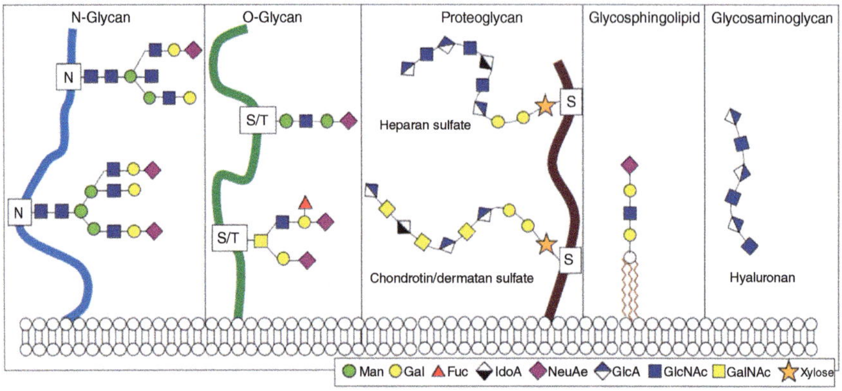

Figure 7.1 The main classes of carbohydrate components of the pericellular space: carbohydrates can be in free form, e.g. hyaluronan or as conjugates with proteins and lipids.

central to cell–cell and ECM–cell communication (Figure 7.1). They participate in different multivalent noncovalent interactions (e.g. van der Waals, π–π, hydrophobic and electrostatic interactions, metal coordination, and hydrogen bonding) with soluble bioactives, such as growth factors and cytokines, secreted by cells to enhance their stability, distribution, and availability to the cells. Self-assembling peptides with different length and bioactivity are usually used as simpler analogs of proteins to generate functionals supports for proliferation, differentiation, and delivery of cells in the context of regenerative medicine [14–17]. The important functions of glycoproteins and proteoglycans in the ECM have motivated the use of carbohydrate-functionalized blocks for the assembly of bioactive materials. In this chapter, we will discuss different designs of self-assembling blocks based on peptides and carbohydrates and approaches to obtain supramolecular biomaterials that mimic the ECM using these blocks.

7.2 Glycoproteins and Proteoglycans in the ECM

In the ECM and at the basement cellular membrane, most carbohydrates are presented as glycoconjugates (Figure 7.1). Among these conjugates, glycoproteins, in which the carbohydrate (glycan) is covalently bound to a core protein, are central to ECM–cell communication and involved in most signaling pathways that control fundamental biological processes as cellular differentiation, proliferation, and apoptosis. Proteoglycans are a subclass of glycoproteins that are heavily glycosylated with long, negatively charged glycosaminoglycan (GAG) chains. They are main structural elements of ECM where together with other components assemble into nanostructured hydrogel that has multiple roles, e.g. provides physical support for cell adhesion that can also resists compressive forces and serves as a reservoir of soluble bioactive molecules secreted by cells, such as growth factors. To create biofunctional ECM mimics, several supramolecular approaches that involve carbohydrates and proteins or their simpler analogs peptides have been developed to copycat key features of proteoglycans and glycoproteins signaling.

7.3 Design of Self-assembling Peptide–Saccharide Conjugates

The synthetic self-assembling glycopeptides contain two main elements: a peptide sequence (usually with a known bioactivity) and mono- or disaccharide that can be recognized by lectins. These two elements can be co-assembled (Figure 7.2b, c) or conjugated to obtain a single self-assembling molecule (Figure 7.2d, e, f, g, h, i) [16, 18–21]. In these conjugates, the peptide portion is commonly designed to trigger the self-assembly, e.g. by incorporation of aromatic amino acids (most often phenylalanine but also tyrosine and tryptophan) that participate in π–π and CH–π interactions (Figure 7.2a, d, e, f, g) or by introductions of amino acids with complementary charges to trigger electrostatic interactions (Figure 7.2.d). Conjugation of this usually hydrophobic sequence to the hydrophilic carbohydrate moiety results in amphiphilic molecules that can self-organize and form nanostructures with different morphologies, e.g. nanofibers, nanoribbons, and nanoparticles. The carbohydrate moiety can also participate in supramolecular interactions, such as hydrogen bonding, electrostatic interactions with cations (e.g. Na^+, Ca^{2+}), and hydrophobic interactions, thus affecting the balance of the supramolecular forces that drive the assembly process. For example, the nonglycosylated Ac-QQKFQFQFEQQ-Am peptide (Q11, Figure 7.2c) self-assembles into nanofibers that tend to aggregate, while its glycosylated derivative (Figure 7.2d) forms nanofibers, which remain dispersed at low concentration and organize hierarchically in aligned anisotropic networks at crowded environment [22]. In the design of short glycopeptides for which di- and tripeptides are used, an additional element – aromatic or aliphatic chain – is often required to maintain the self-assembling propensity of the molecule. This element is introduced either as a linker between the peptide and carbohydrate portion [16, 23–25] or at the peptide end of the amphiphiles [18, 26–29]. An additional feature in the molecular design of self-assembling glycopeptides is the modification of the carbohydrate. In natural proteoglycans, the carbohydrate chains known as glycosaminoglycans (GAGs) are longer and sulfated. This additional functionalization introduces negative charge that is associated with GAGs bioactivities. Several supramolecular designs have considered this feature and used sulfated monosaccharides as carbohydrate moiety of the synthetic glycopeptides. The supramolecular systems generated by these glycopeptides mimic heparin sulfate proteoglycans, e.g. they can bind and protect growth factors such as bone morphogenic protein-2 (BMP2) [16] and basic fibroblast growth factor (FGF2) [18].

The first example of ECM mimics generated by self-assembly of synthetic short glycopeptides was proposed by Xu who used a conjugate of a nucleobase (adenine), an integrin binding peptide (RGD) and a glucosamine moiety (Figure 7.2a) [26]. After this pioneer work, different glycopeptides that contain mannose [23, 30], glucosamine [19, 26, 27, 31], or *N*-acetylglucosamine [16] incorporated via *S*-[24, 32],

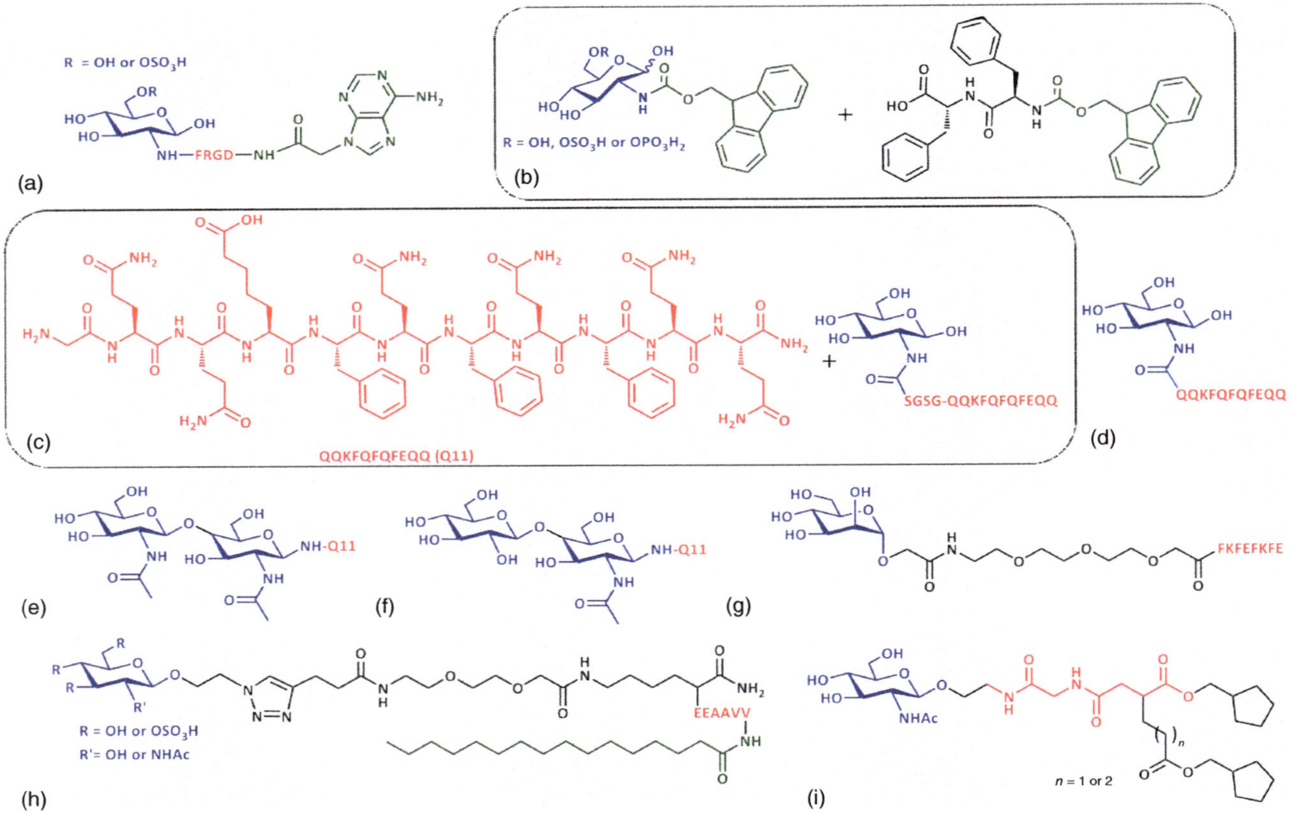

Figure 7.2 Examples of synthetic glycopeptides used to assemble extracellular matrix mimics. Different molecular functionalities are presented: carbohydrate in blue, peptide in red, linker in black, and amphiphile enhancer in green. Systems generated by co-assembly examples are gray-framed (b and d).

N-[25–28, 31], or *O*-[16, 19, 22, 23] glycosylation have been described. Supramolecular ECM mimics can be generated by self-assembly of single glycopeptide conjugate [16, 20–22] or via co-assembly with another, usually peptide component [18, 33–35]. In all these approaches, the unidirectional assembly leads to the formation of nanofibers with a peptide core and multivalent carbohydrate presentation on the shell, i.e. structural mimics of glycoproteins [16, 18, 20, 21]. Similarly to the native glycoproteins, the assembled nanofibers can further form hydrogels that mimic ECM structurally (hydrated nanomesh structure) and functionally because of the incorporated bioactive peptide sequences and carbohydrate moiety [36–38]. When compared to peptide ECM mimics, the glycosylated analogs usually promote higher cell adhesion, proliferation, and in some cases differentiation by engaging additional biospecific interactions with different proteins and cell receptors, e.g. lectins (Figure 7.3) [26, 28, 30, 38–40]. An example is the functionalization of the self-assembling peptide Q11 with *N*-acetylglucosamine (GlcNAc). This glycopeptide self-organizes into glycoclusters that resist to nonspecific interactions with proteins but encode selective recognition by lectins [22] – a family of soluble carbohydrate-binding proteins involved in regulation of fundamental physiological processes, such as cell adhesion, migration, inflammation, immune responses, and in different pathologies, e.g. cancers [19]. Among the lectins, galectins are unconventionally secreted into the ECM where they bind to galactose and lactose-containing glycoproteins and glycolipids [41]. The introduced GlcNAc group can be further converted into *N*-acetyllactosamine (LacNAc, Figure 7.2e) via glycosyltransferase, and the assembled nanofibers are specifically recognized by galectin-1 [42] or replaced with *N*,*N*′-diacetyllactosamine (LacDiNAc, Figure 7.2f) to induce high affinity toward galectin-3 [43].

The effect of ECM mimics assembled from glycopeptides on cellular behavior has been clearly demonstrated. An example is the nanofibrous gel generated by the glycopeptide Lauryl-VVAGKS(β-Glc)-Am that interacts with mesenchymal stem cells (MSCs) through CD44 receptors and induce their differentiation into the chondrogenic lineage [34, 44]. The extent of the differentiation depends on the degree of epitope density on the nanofiber system. It is well known that the glycosylation degree can affect the bioactivity of the glycoproteins [45]. In supramolecular systems, the co-assembly of glycopeptides with peptides at different ratios can be used to develop nanonetworks with different degree and spatial organization of the carbohydrate in the system [33, 46]. Such approach has been applied to the above-mentioned glycopeptide Lauryl-VVAGKS(β-Glc)-Am: its co-assembly with the sulfonated peptide (Lauryl-VVAGEK(*p*-sulfobenzoate)-Am) guides the MSCs differentiation toward adipogenic lineage [47], while the co-assembly with Lauryl-VVAGK induce MSCs differentiation into brown adipocytes [46]. Another example is the co-assembly of Q11 and its glycosylated analog (Figure 7.2c) at different ratios that demonstrates very elegant how the bioactivity can be optimized by maximizing the multivalent avidity effects and minimizing the steric hindrance [33]. In a different than co-assembly approach, the carbohydrate density can be tailored to specific protein binding by post-assembly functionalization of peptide nanostructures. Peptoid nanosheets can be functionalized before or after assembly

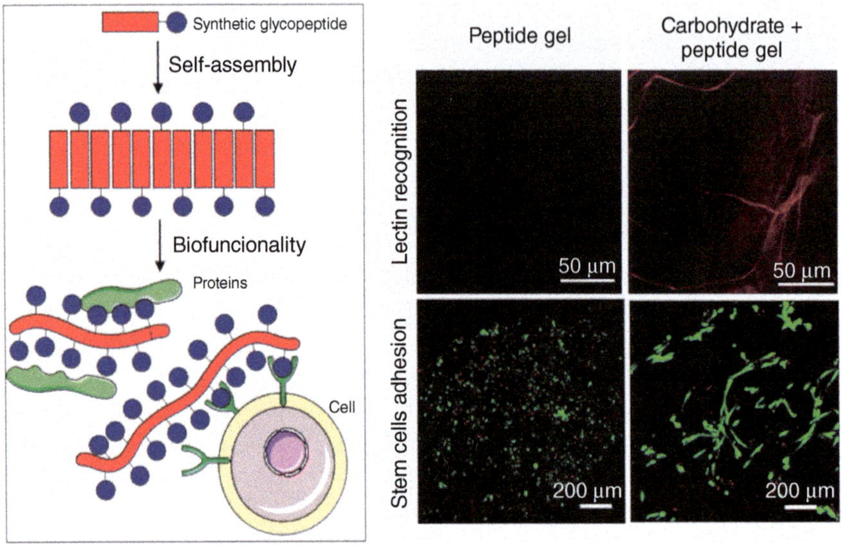

Figure 7.3 (a) Schematic presentation of glycopeptides (carbohydrate portion shown in blue and peptide moiety in red) and their self-assembly into supramolecular systems in which the carbohydrate participates in different biorecognition processes with, e.g. proteins and cells receptors; (b) confocal images showing interactions of the lectin Wheat German Agglutinin and adipose stem cells with supramolecular gels assembled from Fmoc-diphenylalanin (peptide gel) and its co-assembly with Fmoc-glucosamine-6-sulfate (carbohydrate + peptide gel). Chemical structures of gels components are presented in Figure 7.2b and details on their assembly can be found elsewhere [18].

by click chemistry using azido sugars that react with the alkanylated residues in the linkers and loop regions [48]. This approach is very convenient for the development of combinatorial libraries of carbohydrate-functionalized nanostructures.

All together these examples illustrate that the design of the self-assembling blocks can be tailored to the targeted application. In any of the above-mentioned systems, the avidity of carbohydrates dictates the interactions between the supramolecular systems and the targeted bioentity. While in conventional glycopolymers, the affinity is a direct consequence of the grafting density of the carbohydrate, in supramolecular systems an adjustment to the ligand can be achieved *in situ* by reorganization of the self-assembling blocks, therefore highlighting the advantages of these systems [42].

7.4 Supramolecular Systems Generated by Interfacial Co-assembly

In the ECM, proteoglycans that carry negatively charged GAGs interact with different classes of proteins through electrostatic interactions between the negatively charged groups (sulfate or carboxylate from uronic acids) and the positively charged amino acids (e.g. lysine and arginine) of the proteins. These interactions can be copycat to develop biofunctional nanomaterials by co-assembly of GAGs (e.g. hyaluronan, chondroitin sulfate, or heparin) and a self-assembling peptide or protein that contain a sequence recognizing these GAGs [35, 49–52]. Upon a contact of the two solutions, the GAG and the peptide form interfacial complex that prevents the mixing of the solutions and promote self-organization at the interface [35, 50, 53]. The hierarchically organized assemblies generated by this approach can be used as discrete cellular microenvironments such as sacs and membranes [50], release systems [49], or supports for cell adhesion [54, 55]. The specific molecular patterns and surface exposition/organization of the components promote specific interactions of the assembled systems with biologics that result in specific cell response such as differentiation [50]. Such systems also have enhanced mechanical properties and stability to enzymatic degradation as compared to GAG alone [49]. In a different approach heparin, a growth factor binding GAG was employed to promote nucleation and functionalization of self-assembled peptide–amphiphile nanofibers [35]. The assembled nanofibers display heparin on the surface and thus they can selectively bind and activate efficiently angiogenic growth factors such as vascular endothelial growth factor (VEGF) and FGF-2. As a result, this system stimulates angiogenesis and induces formation of new blood vessels *in vivo*. In a similar approach, heparin was co-assembled with a multidomain peptide (MDP) that comprises the cell adhesion RGD motif and an enzyme-cleavable site for cell-mediated degradation ($K(SL)_3RG(SL)_3KGRGDS$) to generate nanofibers [56]. MDPs are a new type of self-assembling peptides organized in ABA manner, where an amphiphilic core B (alternating hydrophilic S and hydrophobic L amino acids) is flanked by charged regions A [57]. The amphiphilic core drives the supramolecular assembly into a sandwich-like β-sheet nanofiber in which hydrogen bonding occurs parallel to the growing fiber axis. The flank charged regions A stabilize fiber assembly via electrostatic repulsion. These MDP-based hydrogels mimic the ECM nanostructure. The MDP can be functionalized with negatively charged GAGs, e.g. heparin at the A regions [56]. The generated construct allows entrapment and stabilization of heparin-binding growth factors, i.e. as ECM mimicking hydrogel, and can be used as controlled release systems.

7.5 Conclusions

The multifunctionality of glycoproteins in biological systems has inspired different approaches for the development of nanostructured responsive biomaterials using simpler glycopeptides. Density, valency, and position of the carbohydrates in the supramolecular structures interfere with the self-assembly and biofunctionality. The introduction of the carbohydrate moiety enhances the biofunctionality when compared with the respective peptide systems, even when simple monosaccharides are used. The recent developments in the field of supramolecular glycomaterials provide a toolbox of different building blocks to assemble structures with different shapes, sizes, and complexity. Such systems reproduce the most important properties of the

ECM – highly hydrated nanomesh that interacts specifically, directionally, and in responsive manner with different biologics.

Acknowledgments

We acknowledge the Portuguese Foundation for Science and Technology FCT for the financial support through the grants PTDC/NAN-MAT/28468/2017 CANCER_CAGE and PTDC/BTM-MAT/28327/2017 CardioHeal.

References

1 Frantz, C., Stewart, K.M., and Weaver, V.M. (2010). The extracellular matrix at a glance. *J. Cell Sci.* 123 (24): 4195.

2 Mecham, R.P. (2001). Overview of extracellular matrix. *Curr. Protoc. Cell. Biol.* 00: 10.1.1–10.1.14.

3 Lu, P., Takai, K., Weaver, V.M., and Werb, Z. (2011). Extracellular matrix degradation and remodeling in development and disease. *Cold Spring Harbor Perspect. Biol.* 3 (12): https://doi.org/10.1101/cshperspect.a005058 a005058.

4 Gattazzo, F., Urciuolo, A., and Bonaldo, P. (2014). Extracellular matrix: a dynamic microenvironment for stem cell niche. *Biochim. Biophys. Acta* 1840 (8): 2506–2519.

5 Malandrino, A., Mak, M., Kamm, R.D., and Moeendarbary, E. (2018). Complex mechanics of the heterogeneous extracellular matrix in cancer. *Extreme Mech. Lett.* 21: 25–34.

6 Muiznieks, L.D. and Keeley, F.W. (2013). Molecular assembly and mechanical properties of the extracellular matrix: a fibrous protein perspective. *Biochim. Biophys. Acta Mol. Basis Dis.* 1832 (7): 866–875.

7 Zhou, J., Li, J., Du, X., and Xu, B. (2017). Supramolecular biofunctional materials. *Biomaterials* 129: 1–27.

8 Hellmund, K.S. and Koksch, B. (2019). Self-assembling peptides as extracellular matrix mimics to influence stem cell's fate. *Front. Chem.* 7: 172.

9 Cui, H., Webber, M.J., and Stupp, S.I. (2010). Self-assembly of peptide amphiphiles: from molecules to nanostructures to biomaterials. *Biopolymers* 94 (1): 1–18.

10 Freeman, R., Boekhoven, J., Dickerson, M.B. et al. (2015). Biopolymers and supramolecular polymers as biomaterials for biomedical applications. *MRS Bull.* 40 (12): 1089–1101.

11 Hendricks, M.P., Sato, K., Palmer, L.C., and Stupp, S.I. (2017). Supramolecular assembly of peptide amphiphiles. *Acc. Chem. Res.* 50 (10): 2440–2448.

12 Matson, J.B. and Stupp, S.I. (2012). Self-assembling peptide scaffolds for regenerative medicine. *Chem. Commun.* 48 (1): 26–33.

13 Storrie, H., Guler, M.O., Abu-Amara, S.N. et al. (2007). Supramolecular crafting of cell adhesion. *Biomaterials* 28 (31): 4608–4618.

14 Aida, T., Meijer, E., and Stupp, S.I. (2012). Functional supramolecular polymers. *Science* 335 (6070): 813–817.

15 Webber, M.J., Appel, E.A., Meijer, E., and Langer, R. (2016). Supramolecular biomaterials. *Nat. Mater.* 15 (1): 13–26.

16 Lee, S.S., Fyrner, T., Chen, F. et al. (2017). Sulfated glycopeptide nanostructures for multipotent protein activation. *Nat. Nanotechnol.* 12 (8): 821–829.

17 Alakpa, E.V., Jayawarna, V., Lampel, A. et al. (2016). Tunable supramolecular hydrogels for selection of lineage-guiding metabolites in stem cell cultures. *Chem* 1 (2): 298–319.

18 Brito, A., Abul-Haija, Y.M., da Costa, D.S. et al. (2019). Minimalistic supramolecular proteoglycan mimics by co-assembly of aromatic peptide and carbohydrate amphiphiles. *Chem. Sci.* 10 (8): 2385–2390.

19 Restuccia, A., Tian, Y.F., Collier, J.H., and Hudalla, G.A. (2015). Self-assembled glycopeptide nanofibers as modulators of galectin-1 bioactivity. *Cell. Mol. Bioeng.* 8 (3): 471–487.

20 Yoshimura, I., Miyahara, Y., Kasagi, N. et al. (2004). Molecular recognition in a supramolecular hydrogel to afford a semi-wet sensor chip. *J. Am. Chem. Soc.* 126 (39): 12204–12205.

21 Kiyonaka, S., Sada, K., Yoshimura, I. et al. (2004). Semi-wet peptide/protein array using supramolecular hydrogel. *Nat. Mater.* 3 (1): 58–64.

22 Restuccia, A., Seroski, D.T., Kelley, K.L. et al. (2019). Hierarchical self-assembly and emergent function of densely glycosylated peptide nanofibers. *Commun. Chem.* 2 (1): 53.

23 Lim, Y.-b., Park, S., Lee, E. et al. (2007). Glycoconjugate nanoribbons from the self-assembly of carbohydrate-peptide block molecules for controllable bacterial cell cluster formation. *Biomacromolecules* 8 (5): 1404–1408.

24 Gour, N., Purohit, C.S., Verma, S. et al. (2009). Mannosylated self-assembled structures for molecular confinement and gene delivery applications. *Biochem. Biophys. Res. Commun.* 378 (3): 503–506.

25 Yang, J., Du, Q., Li, L. et al. (2020). Glycosyltransferase-induced morphology transition of glycopeptide self-assemblies with proteoglycan residues. *ACS Macro Lett.* 9: 929–936.

26 Du, X., Zhou, J., Guvench, O. et al. (2014). Supramolecular assemblies of a conjugate of nucleobase, amino acids, and saccharide act as agonists for proliferation of embryonic stem cells and development of zygotes. *Bioconjug. Chem.* 25 (6): 1031–1035.

27 Yuan, D., Shi, J., Du, X. et al. (2015). Supramolecular glycosylation accelerates proteolytic degradation of peptide nanofibrils. *J. Am. Chem. Soc.* 137 (32): 10092–10095.

28 Yang, Z., Liang, G., Ma, M. et al. (2007). D-Glucosamine-based supramolecular hydrogels to improve wound healing. *Chem. Commun.* 8: 843–845.

29 Zhao, F., Heesters, B.A., Chiu, I. et al. (2014). L-Rhamnose-containing supramolecular nanofibrils as potential immunosuppressive materials. *Org. Biomol. Chem.* 12 (35): 6816–6819.

30 Gunay, G., Sardan Ekiz, M., Ferhati, X. et al. (2017). Antigenic GM3 lactone mimetic molecule integrated mannosylated glycopeptide nanofibers for the activation and maturation of dendritic cells. *ACS Appl. Mater. Interfaces* 9 (19): 16035–16042.

31 Mahato, M., Arora, V., Pathak, R. et al. (2012). Fabrication of nanostructures through molecular self-assembly of small amphiphilic glyco-dehydropeptides. *Mol. BioSyst.* 8 (6): 1742–1749.

32 Roytman, R., Adler-Abramovich, L., Kumar, K.A. et al. (2011). Exploring the self-assembly of glycopeptides using a diphenylalanine scaffold. *Org. Biomol. Chem.* 9 (16): 5755–5761.

33 Restuccia, A. and Hudalla, G.A. (2018). Tuning carbohydrate density enhances protein binding and inhibition by glycosylated β-sheet peptide nanofibers. *Biomater. Sci.* 6 (9).

34 Yaylaci, S.U., Ekiz, M.S., Arslan, E. et al. (2016). Supramolecular GAG-like self-assembled glycopeptide nanofibers induce chondrogenesis and cartilage regeneration. *Biomacromolecules* 17 (2): 679–689.

35 Rajangam, K., Behanna, H.A., Hui, M.J. et al. (2006). Heparin binding nanostructures to promote growth of blood vessels. *Nano Lett.* 6 (9): 2086–2090.

36 Hudson, K.L., Bartlett, G.J., Diehl, R.C. et al. (2015). Carbohydrate-aromatic interactions in proteins. *J. Am. Chem. Soc.* 137 (48): 15152–15160.

37 McMahon, C.M., Isabella, C.R., Windsor, I.W. et al. (2020). Stereoelectronic effects impact glycan recognition. *J. Am. Chem. Soc.* 142 (5): 2386–2395.

38 Hakomori, S. (2004). Carbohydrate-to-carbohydrate interaction, through glycosynapse, as a basis of cell recognition and membrane organization. *Glycoconj. J.* 21 (3, 4): 125–137.

39 Liu, J., Sun, Z., Yuan, Y. et al. (2016). Peptide glycosylation generates supramolecular assemblies from glycopeptides as biomimetic scaffolds for cell adhesion and proliferation. *ACS Appl. Mater. Interfaces* 8 (11): 6917–6924.

40 Wang, W., Wang, H., Ren, C. et al. (2011). A saccharide-based supramolecular hydrogel for cell culture. *Carbohydr. Res.* 346 (8): 1013–1017.

41 Johannes, L., Jacob, R., and Leffler, H. (2018). Galectins at a glance. *J. Cell Sci.* 131 (9): jcs208884.

42 Liu, R. and Hudalla, G.A. (2019). Using self-assembling peptides to integrate biomolecules into functional supramolecular biomaterials. *Molecules* 24 (8): 1450.

43 Restuccia, A., Fettis, M.M., Farhadi, S.A. et al. (2018). Evaluation of self-assembled glycopeptide nanofibers modified with *N,N′*-diacetyllactosamine for selective galectin-3 recognition and inhibition. *ACS Biomater. Sci. Eng.* 4 (10): 3451–3459.

44 Yaylaci, S.U., Sen, M., Bulut, O. et al. (2016). Chondrogenic differentiation of mesenchymal stem cells on glycosaminoglycan-mimetic peptide nanofibers. *ACS Biomater. Sci. Eng.* 2 (5): 871–878.

45 Reily, C., Stewart, T.J., Renfrow, M.B., and Novak, J. (2019). Glycosylation in health and disease. *Nat. Rev. Nephrol.* 15 (6): 346–366.

46 Caliskan, O.S., Sardan Ekiz, M., Tekinay, A.B., and Guler, M.O. (2017). Spatial Organization of Functional Groups on bioactive supramolecular glycopeptide

nanofibers for differentiation of mesenchymal stem cells (MSCs) to brown adipogenesis. *Bioconjug. Chem.* 28 (3): 740–750.
47 Yasa, O., Uysal, O., Ekiz, M.S. et al. (2017). Presentation of functional groups on self-assembled supramolecular peptide nanofibers mimicking glycosaminoglycans for directed mesenchymal stem cell differentiation. *J. Mater. Chem. B* 5 (25): 4890–4900.
48 Battigelli, A., Kim, J.H., Dehigaspitiya, D.C. et al. (2018). Glycosylated peptoid nanosheets as a multivalent scaffold for protein recognition. *Acs Nano* 12 (3): 2455–2465.
49 Aviv, M., Halperin-Sternfeld, M., Grigoriants, I. et al. (2018). Improving the mechanical rigidity of hyaluronic acid by integration of a supramolecular peptide matrix. *ACS Appl. Mater. Interfaces* 10 (49): 41883–41891.
50 Capito, R.M., Azevedo, H.S., Velichko, Y.S. et al. (2008). Self-assembly of large and small molecules into hierarchically ordered sacs and membranes. *Science* 319 (5871): 1812–1816.
51 Mendes, A.C., Smith, K.H., Tejeda-Montes, E. et al. (2013). Co-assembled and microfabricated bioactive membranes. *Adv. Funct. Mater.* 23 (4): 430–438.
52 Abul-Haija, Y.M. and Ulijn, R.V. (2015). Sequence adaptive peptide-polysaccharide nanostructures by biocatalytic self-assembly. *Biomacromolecules* 16 (11): 3473–3479.
53 Carretero, A., da Costa, D.S., Reis, R.L., and Pashkuleva, I. (2017). Extracellular matrix-inspired assembly of glycosaminoglycan-collagen fibers. *J. Mater. Chem. B* 5 (17): 3103–3106.
54 Pang, X., O'Malley, C., Borges, J. et al. (2019). Supramolecular presentation of Hyaluronan onto model surfaces for studying the behavior of cancer stem cells. *Adv. Biosyst.* 3 (10): 1900017.
55 Pang, X., Li, W., Landwehr, E. et al. (2019). Mimicking the endothelial glycocalyx through the supramolecular presentation of hyaluronan on patterned surfaces. *Faraday Discuss.* 219: 168–182.
56 Galler, K.M., Hartgerink, J.D., Cavender, A.C. et al. (2012). A customized self-assembling peptide hydrogel for dental pulp tissue engineering. *Tissue Eng. Part A* 18 (1, 2): 176–184.
57 Dong, H., Paramonov, S.E., Aulisa, L. et al. (2007). Self-assembly of multidomain peptides: balancing molecular frustration controls conformation and nanostructure. *J. Am. Chem. Soc.* 129 (41): 12468–12472.

8

Supramolecular Assemblies for Cancer Diagnosis and Treatment

Shuang Liu[1,2] *and Bing Xu*[1]

[1] *Brandeis University, Department of Chemistry, 415 South Street, Waltham, MA 02454, USA*
[2] *Wuhan University of Technology, School of Materials Science and Engineering, 122 Luoshi Road, Wuhan, Hubei 430070, China*

8.1 Introduction

Molecular self-assembly is a process of spontaneous organization of disordered molecules into ordered supramolecular structures driven by non-covalent interactions [1]. This is an ubiquitous process in nature where macromolecules assemble into complex biological systems. Likewise, the assembly of small molecules (in the biological system) has profound biological implications [2]. Small molecules self-assemble into nanostructures or supramolecular assemblies in response to different physiological conditions. The generated supramolecular assemblies exhibit emergent properties that are not innate of the individual building blocks and offer a versatile platform for the development of biomedicine, including anticancer therapy.

Despite the continuing progresses in developing anticancer therapies, cancer remains as one of the biggest threats for human health. In 2018, 18.1 million new cases of cancer were diagnosed and 9.6 million people died from the disease. New methods for cancer diagnosis and treatment remain an urgent medical need. Supramolecular assemblies are emerging as a new approach for cancer diagnosis and treatment, and considerable amount of research activities have been carried out to explore them for potential cancer therapy. In this chapter, we review the progresses along this notion over the last two decades, with emphasis on the research performed in last five years. We discuss the exploration of supramolecular assemblies in two areas of cancer therapy: diagnosis and treatment. The section of diagnosis consists of optical imaging, magnetic resonance imaging (MRI), and photoacoustic imaging; the section of treatment contains supramolecular drug delivery and anticancer therapy. Particularly, we highlight the molecular design of probes or therapeutics that target cancer cells or tumors via enzyme-instructed self-assembly (EISA). In Section 8.4, we summarize the remaining problems and speculate on the new directions in the development of supramolecular assemblies for cancer therapy.

Multifunctional Hydrogels for Biomedical Applications, First Edition.
Edited by Ricardo A. Pires, Iva Pashkuleva, and Rui L. Reis.

8.2 Cancer Diagnosis

The early and accurate diagnosis of cancer can significantly improve cancer survival rates [3]. Among the cancer-related deaths, about 30% patients would have survived if their cancers were diagnosed earlier. Thus, it is necessary to develop novel diagnostic methods. In this section, we introduce three common methods, optical imaging, MRI, and photoacoustic imaging, that employ supramolecular assemblies for early diagnosis of cancers.

8.2.1 Optical Imaging

Optical imaging is one of the most popular diagnostic technologies because it offers multiple information with compact operation and low cost [4]. In optical imaging, the interaction between photon and biological matters leads to photophysical processes, such as absorption, photon scattering, and fluorescence emission. All of those processes can provide biological information [5]. Optical imaging probes that are preferentially uptaken by cancer cells or tumors can enhance the imaging signals for visualizing tumors in cancer diagnosis.

The design of supramolecular probes for tumor imaging relies on chromophores that show contrast for imaging before and after self-assembly, that is, they should display low fluorescence when existing as monomers but fluoresce brightly after the self-assembly. Nitrobenzofurazan (NBD) exhibits brighter fluorescence in hydrophobic environment and acts as a bright fluorophore inside self-assembled nanofibers. Xu and coworkers designed a NBD-modified precursor, which allowed the fluorescent imaging of phosphatase activity in cancer cells [6]. The conjugation of NBD to a phosphorylated peptidic self-assembling motif, Nap-FFK$_p$Y, produces the precursor **1P** (Figure 8.1a). Containing a phosphotyrosine residue, **1P** acts as a substrate of alkaline phosphatase (ALP), an enzyme expressed at higher levels in some cancer cells (e.g. HeLa cell) than in normal cells. ALP catalytically dephosphorylates **1P** to form **1**, which self-assembles to form nanofibers. Thus, after being incubated with **1P**, live HeLa cells show continuing increase of fluorescent intensity over time (Figure 8.1b). As most of the fluorescence occurred in the region of endoplasmic reticulum (ER), the authors proposed that a protein tyrosine phosphatase (PTP1B), a phosphatase at the cytoplasmic face of the ER, is likely the major phosphatase to catalyze the dephosphorylation of **1P** inside cells. Other phosphatases also likely contribute to the dephosphorylation. Nevertheless, this work, combining EISA and fluorophores, illustrates the use of EISA for imaging cancer cells.

Lipid rafts are subdomains of the plasma membrane containing high concentration of cholesterols. With a variety of membrane proteins involved in cell signaling, lipid rafts play an important role in the process of signal transduction [7]. To develop an approach for the imaging of lipid rafts and explore the dynamics of live cells membrane over large area and extended time, Xu and coworkers designed a raft-affinitive and enzyme-responsive probe **2P** (Figure 8.2a) [8]. Since lipid rafts enrich cholesterols and GPI-anchored enzymes, the probe contains a cholesterol, an

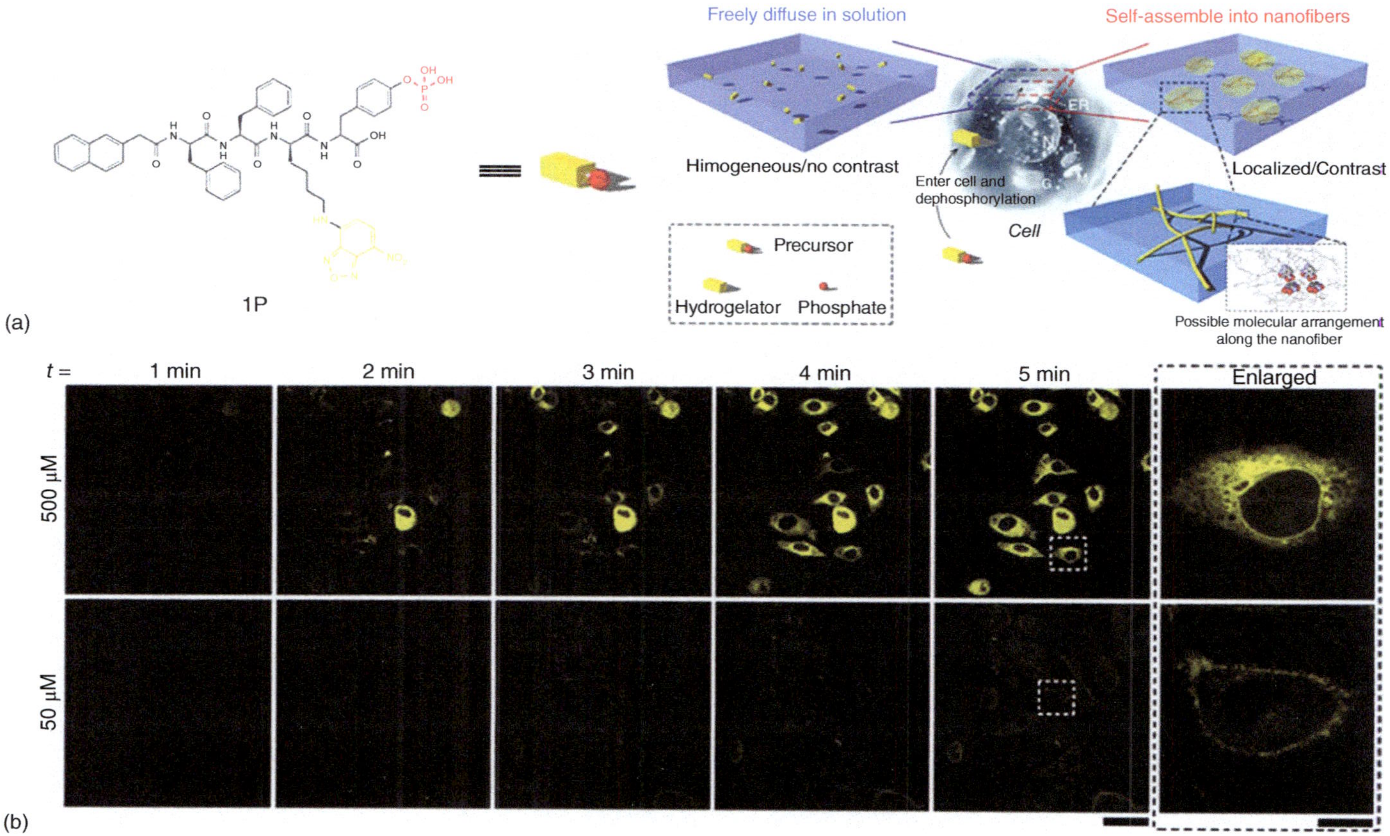

Figure 8.1 (a) The structure of compound **1P** and the principle of imaging enzyme-triggered self-assembly inside cells. (b) Time-dependent fluorescent confocal microscope images of HeLa cells after incubation with 500 or 50 μM of **1P** in PBS buffer. Scale bar is 50 μm. Source: Gao, Y., et al. (2012), [16], Figure 04, Pg 05/ with permission of Springer Nature.

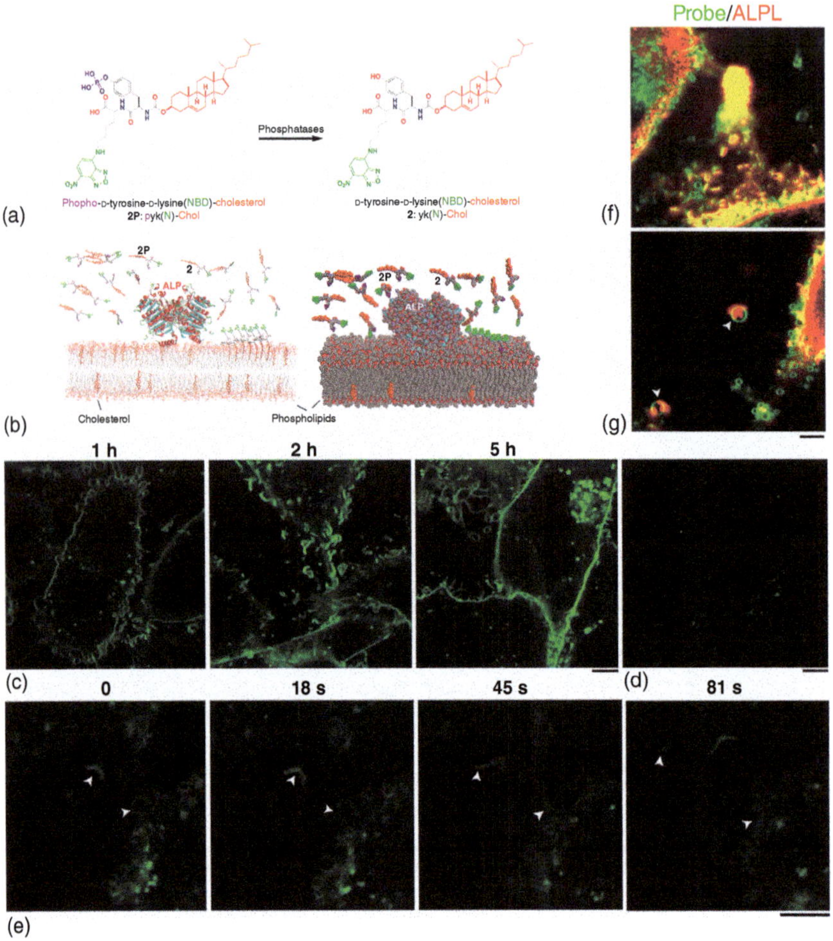

Figure 8.2 (a) Molecular structure of **2P**. Illustrations of EISA of **2P** to form assemblies of **2** that anchor in cell membranes in (b) stick and CPK models. (c and d) CLSM images of Saos2 cells treated with (c) **2P** for one, two, and five hours and (d) **2** (25 μM) for five hours, scale bar is 5 μm. (e) Time-dependent CLSM to show changes of membrane domains within 90 seconds, after treating Saos2 cells with **2P** (10 μM) for one hour, scale bar is 5 μm, the white arrow indicates the membrane domains of Saos2 cells. (f) Saos2 cells treated with **2P** (25 μM, two hours) and then analyzed by immunofluorescence for ALPL (red represents antibodies), Pearson's *R* value is 0.65 from 20 cells. (g) Matrix vesicles secreted by Saos2 cells containing ALPL, scale bar is 5 μm. Source: Wang, H., et al. (2018), [8], Figure 02, Pg 02/ with permission of American Chemical Society.

enzymatic trigger (phosphotyrosine), and a fluorophore (NBD). Tissue nonspecific alkaline phosphatase (ALPL), an ectoenzyme presumably co-localized with lipid rafts, converts **2P** to **2** to form strong fluorescent assemblies (Figure 8.2b), which reveals the membrane of Saos2 cells (Figure 8.2c) and indicates that the assembly of the probe tends to distribute in the cell membrane. Live cell imaging confirms the lateral mobility of membrane domains or the fluctuation of membrane domains, which is clearly observed over 100 seconds (Figure 8.2e). Immunofluorescence assay confirmed that GPI-anchored ALPL co-localizes with self-assemblies of probe (Figure 8.2f) and showed the matrix vesicles extruded from plasma membrane.

The probes even reveal the process of exosomes encapsulating ALPL (Figure 8.2g), illustrating the enzyme-responsive imaging probe for revealing the dynamics and the heterogeneity of cell membrane in highly heterogeneous cellular environment.

In biomedical application, fluorescence imaging may suffer several problems, such as photobleaching of fluorophores, background fluorescence, and autofluorescence. Chemiluminescence (CL) can address those issues. Liang and coworkers designed a multicomponent system consisting of an EISA gelation precursor and an CL agent (3-(2′-spiroadamantyl)-4-methoxy-4-(3″-phosphoryloxyphenyl)-1,2-dioxetane [AMPPD]) that emits a CL photon at 470 nm in the presence of ALP [9]. After ALP cleavage, the multicomponent system self-assembles into long, wide, regular nanofibers and forms a hydrogel. During the formation of the hydrogel, the system shows CL emissions. Polymers can also deliver small molecular dyes into cancer cells via supramolecular interactions. Rao et al. encapsulated small molecular near-infrared dyes by semiconducting polymer nanoparticles (SPNs) and used those nanoparticles for *in vivo* imaging [10].

8.2.2 Magnetic Resonance Imaging (MRI)

MRI, a clinical imaging modality, has found wide applications in cancer diagnosis. Although MRI is one of the most sensitive imaging techniques for cancer diagnosis and for revealing the position of tumors, it usually requires contrast agents (CAs) to improve the visibility of anatomical structure. There are two kinds of MRI CA: T_1 CAs and T_2 CAs. T_1 CAs reduce the spin-lattice relaxation times of nearby water, which leads to an increase of the signal from these protons, and makes the effected voxel seem "brighter" in T_1-weighted image. T_2 CAs make a "negative" contrast effect in T_2*/T_2-weighted image, by reducing the spin–spin relaxation time of water [11]. The main advantage of MRI is its superb spatial resolution and exquisite image contrast. However, compared to other imaging modalities, MRI still has relatively poor sensitivity so that considerable research efforts have centered on the development of "smart" and "activatable" probes for enhancing the signal-to-noise ratio of MRI [12]. Supramolecular assemblies may offer a new solution for developing MRI CAs because self-assembly increases the local concentration of CAs, thus enhancing the MRI signals. With proper targeting groups, the probes should be sensitive to reveal specific diseases.

Rao and coworkers reported the self-assembly of the molecules made by a new and effective click reaction, the reaction between 2-cyanobenzothiazole (CBT) and cysteine [13, 14]. According to the authors, the second-order rate constant of this reaction is significantly higher than the value reported for the conventional biocompatible click reaction [15]. This click reaction resembles the last step in the synthesis of luciferin, a common substrate of firefly luciferase, and allows researchers to design the probes that contain both CBT and cysteine residue. Such probe can undergo condensation reaction to generate relatively more hydrophobic and oligomeric products that self-assemble to form nanoparticles.

Using the CBT-based click reactions, Rao and coworkers designed a MRI probe **3-Gd**, which contains the DOTA-Gd complex for MRI (Figure 8.3a) [16]. Tris(2-carboxyethyl)phosphine (TCEP) as the reductant *in vitro* or glutathione (GSH) *in vivo* deprotects the disulfide bond to generate the thiol group. The free 1,2-aminothiol group condensates with CBT to form cyclized oligomers (dimeric, trimeric, tetrameric, and higher-order oligomers), as detected by matrix-assisted laser desorption/ionization (MALDI) mass spectrometry. The authors used nuclear magnetic relaxation dispersion (NMRD) to study the longitudinal relaxation rate R_1 of water protons in solution of probes. In the presence of TCEP at 35 °C, relaxation rate of **3-Gd** shows significant increase. At 25.6 MHz (0.6 T) and at 64 MHz (1.5 T), the relaxation rates increase by 160% and 110%, respectively (Figure 8.3b). T_1-weighted MRI of probe **3** clearly exhibits a shortened T_1 relaxation time after TCEP reduction, while the control probe does not. Since the replacement of Gd^{3+} in **3-Gd** unlikely would affect its cell uptake, the authors synthesized **3-Eu**, a fluorescent europium analog **3-Gd** (Figure 8.3c). After incubation with **3-Eu**, MDA-MB-468 cells fluorescence strongly (Figure 8.3d), suggesting that MDA-MB-468 cells uptake **3-Gd**. After being incubated with **3-Gd**, the pellet of MDA-MB-468 cells shows significant higher relaxivity than that incubated with the control probe. The condensation between cysteine and CBT induces the self-assembly of Gd-based MRI CA, and the self-assembly enhances T_1 relaxivity *in vitro* and in living cells. Besides, this probe has a good cell permeability. Such supramolecular assemblies illustrate a new platform approach for developing MRI probes via fast condensation reactions.

In addition to being a common T_1 MRI CA, gadolinium complex also enhances the T_2-weighted MRI. Based on the CBT-Cys click reaction, Liang and coworkers designed a Gd-based MRI probe **4** that underwent proteolysis catalyzed by γ-glutamyltranspeptidase (GGT), a cell surface-associated enzyme for cleaving the glutamyl bond of GSH (Figure 8.4a, b). After the enzymatic reaction catalyzed by GGT, the resulting molecule self-assembles to form nanoparticles [17]. The probe **4** exhibits three features: (i) Glu–Cys is the substrate of GGT so that GGT-cleavage releases the amino group of cysteine; (ii) GSH reduces the thiol group (protected by disulfide bond) to form free thiol, and the 1,2-aminothiol group can click react with CBT; (iii) DOTA-Gd is the Gd-based MRI CA moiety. After being incubated with GGT and GSH for cleavage and reduction, respectively, **4** forms dimers that self-assemble into **4-NPs**. The authors used a 9.4 T MR scanner to generate T_2- and T_1-weighted MR phantom images for studying the ability of **4-NPs** to enhance MRI. Figure 8.4c,d show that the formation of **4-NPs** *in vitro* enhances the r_2 value by 4.34-fold, while it hardly affects the r_1. Thus, the r_2/r_1 of **4** increases as the formation of **4-NPs**, suggesting that **4** could act as a T_2-dominated CA. A similar process occurs on GGT-overexpressing HeLa cells. TEM shows **4-NPs** on the HeLa cells treated by **4**, but few nanoparticles on the HeLa cell treated by the controls (Figure 8.4e,f). T_2- and T_1-weighted MR phantom images provide similar results to *in vitro* experiment: the HeLa cells treated **4** show significant enhancement of r_2, while little difference observed for r_1 (Figure 8.4g,h). Having the enhanced r_2/r_1 ratio, **4** acts as an T_2-dominated CA. After being subcutaneously xenografted

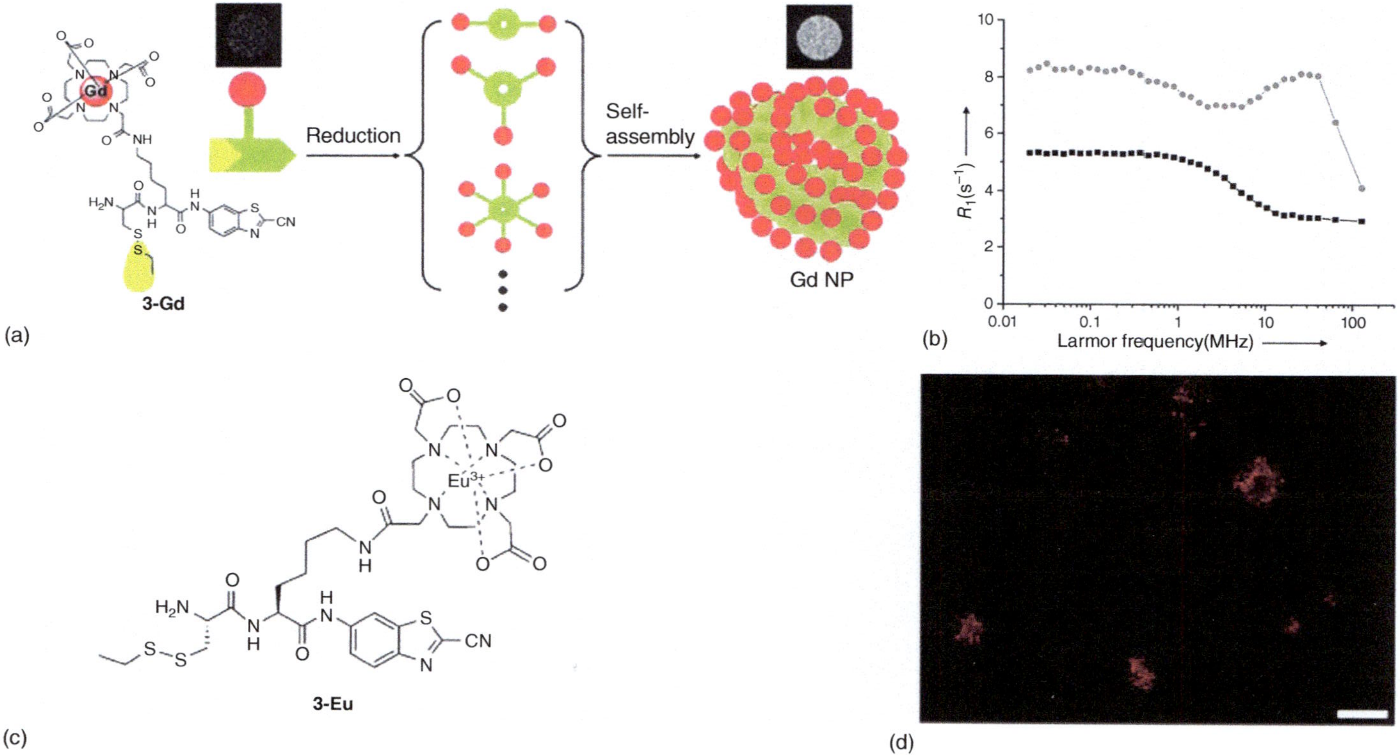

Figure 8.3 (a) Reduction-controlled condensation of **3-Gd** to assemble gadolinium-containing nanoparticles (GdNPs) to enhance MRI signal. (b) NMRD profiles of **3-Gd** (768 μM in 0.2 M phosphate buffer, pH 7.4) treated with (solid circle) and without (solid square) 4 mM of TCEP at 35 °C, R_1 = longitudinal relaxation rate. (c) Structure of **3-Eu**. (d) Two-photon laser microscopy image (λ_{ex} = 725 nm, λ_{em} = 565–615 nm) of MDA-MB-468 cells incubated with **3-Eu** at 192 μM for eight hours and then rinsed and fixed prior to imaging, scale bar is 20 mm. Source: Liang, G., et al. (2012), [16], Figure 03, Pg 03 / with permission of Wiley-VCH.

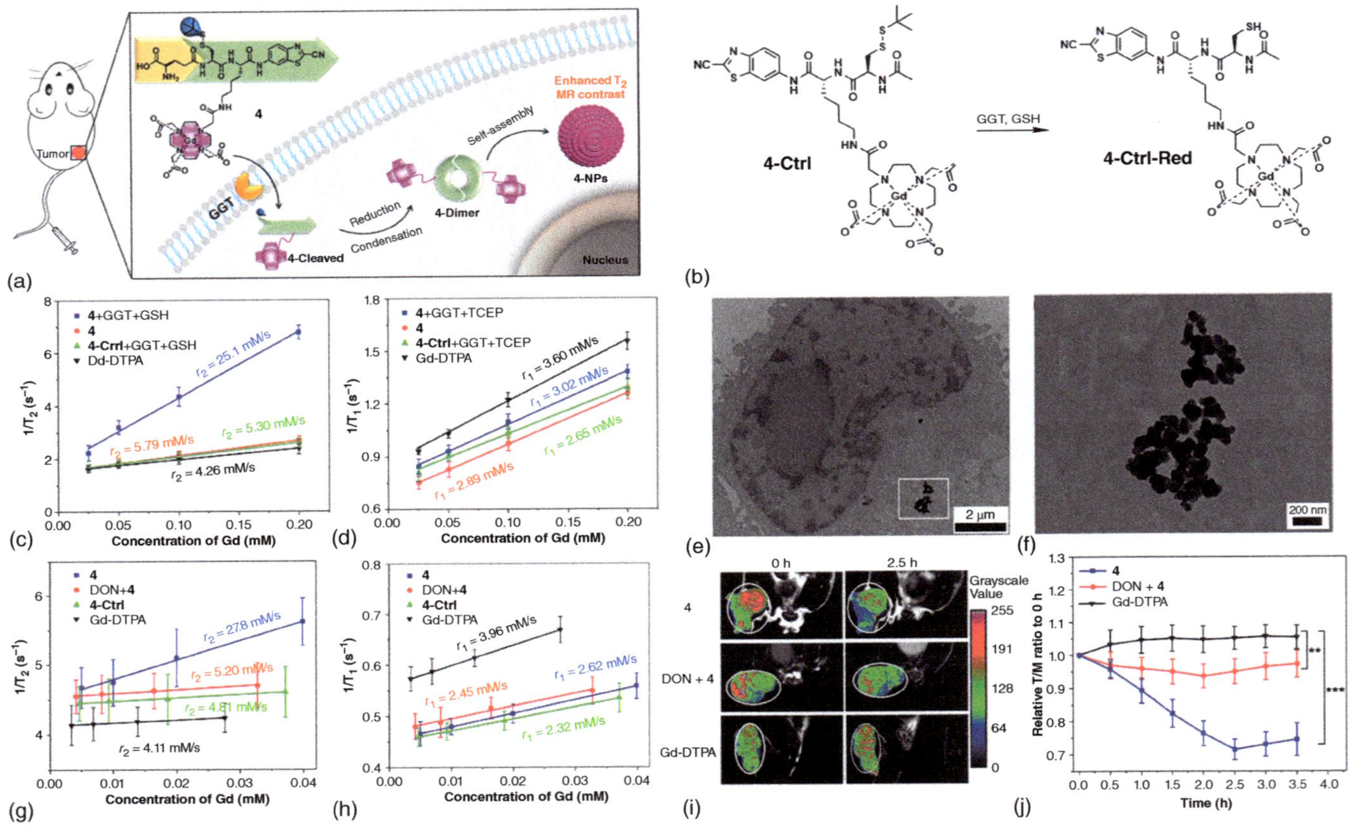

Figure 8.4 (a) Schematic illustrations of the GGT- and reduction-triggered condensation of **4** to form **4-NPs** for enhancement of T_2 MR contrast. (b) Schematic illustrations of the GSH-triggered reduction of **4-Ctrl** to yield **1-Ctrl-Red**. (c) Transverse relaxation rates ($1/T_2$) and (d) longitudinal relaxation rates ($1/T_1$) of **4**+GGT+GSH, **4**, **4**-Ctrl+GGT+GSH, or Gd-DTPA in PBS at different Gd concentrations. Each error bar represents the standard deviation of three independent experiments. (e) Low-magnification TEM image of HeLa cells after incubation with 200 μM **4** for four hours. (f) High-magnification TEM image of the white rectangle area in (e). (g) $1/T_2$ and (h) $1/T_1$ of HeLa cells after treated at different Gd concentrations. Each error bar represents the standard deviation of three independent experiments. (i) T_2-weighted coronal MR images of HeLa tumor bearing mice intravenously injected with 0.08 mmol/kg **4** (top row), 0.25 mmol/kg DON for 0.5 hour and then 0.08 mmol/kg **4**, and 0.08 mmol/kg Gd-DTPA at 0 and 2.5 hours. (j) Normalized time course tumor-to-muscle (T/M) contrast ratios of T_2 values in (i). Each error bar represents the standard deviation of three independent experiments. $^{**}p < 0.01$, $^{***}p < 0.001$; analyzed by Student's *t*-test. White circles indicate the tumors. Source: Wang, H., et al., (2018) [17] / with permission of American

with GGT-overexpressing HeLa tumor, nude mouse received the injection of **4**, GGT inhibitor+**4**, or Gd-DTPA. In **4**-injected mouse, the tumor-to-muscle (T/M) contrast ratios of T_2 values decrease to 71.4% after 2.5 hours, while the other control groups showed almost no change (Figure 8.4j). Although these results illustrate the potential of **4** as a "smart" probe for T_2-weighted MRI of GGT-related cancers, the high magnetic field remains a concern for clinical translation.

Fe_3O_4 is another T_2 MRI CA. Liang et al. designed Ac-Asp-Glu-Val-Asp-Cys(StBu)-Lys-CBT (**5**) (Figure 8.5a) that undergoes caspase (Casp3/7)-controlled condensation because Asp-Glu-Val-Asp is a substrate of Casp3/7 [18]. The authors also designed the scrambled compound of **5**, Ac-Lys-Asp-Glu-Asp-Val-Cys(StBu)-CBT (**5-Scr**) as the control. The Lys residues of those two small molecules react with Fe_3O_4 NPs to provide Fe_3O_4@**5** NPs and Fe_3O_4@**5-Scr** NPs. After GSH reduction and the enzymatic reaction catalyzed by Casp3/7, the resulting 1,2-aminothiol groups of Fe_3O_4@**5** NPs react with CBT to form nanoparticle aggregates (Figure 8.5b), while Fe_3O_4@**5-Scr** NPs show little difference. This aggregation also leads to a significant increase of transverse relaxation rate (R_2) (Figure 8.5c). After the incubation of apoptotic HepG2 cells and healthy HepG2 cells with Fe_3O_4@**5** NPs and Fe_3O_4@**5-Scr** NPs, respectively, TEM shows that many NPs aggregate in the Fe_3O_4@**5** NPs-treated apoptotic cells (Figure 8.5e,f), but few in the other three groups. T_2-weighted MR phantom image of HepG2 cells on a 9.4 T MR scanner indicated that, compared to 61.5 ms (the T_2 relaxation time of Fe_3O_4@**5** NPs incubated with healthy HepG2 cells), the T_2 value of Fe_3O_4@**5** NPs incubated with apoptotic HepG2 cells decreased to 42.5 ms. However, the apoptotic and healthy HepG2 cells treated with Fe_3O_4@**5-Scr** NPs showed similar T_2 values, 57.2 and 57.6 ms, respectively. This result implies that Casp3/7 enzymes in apoptotic cells induce the aggregation of NPs. With a decreased T_2 value, the Fe_3O_4@**5** NPs incubated with apoptotic HepG2 also have an increased R_2 (Figure 8.5d). After being subcutaneously xenografted with HepG2 tumor and the injection of doxorubicin (DOX) or saline, nude mouse received the injection of Fe_3O_4@**5** NPs or Fe_3O_4@**5-Scr** NPs. The DOX-treated tumor in Fe_3O_4@**5** NPs-injected mouse showed strong enhancement of T_2 signal than saline-treated tumor in Fe_3O_4@**5** NPs-injected mouse (Figure 8.5g). The apoptotic tumors in Fe_3O_4@**5** NPs injected mice also showed a larger average contrast change than nonapoptotic tumors. As an example of enzyme-induced intracellular covalent aggregation, this work illustrates the importance of NPs in the design of T_2 MR probes.

8.2.3 Photoacoustic Imaging

Photoacoustic imaging is a multimodality imaging method based on the photoacoustic effect. Integrating optical excitation and ultrasonic detection, photoacoustic imaging provides deeper tissue imaging penetration and higher spatial resolution. Supramolecular assemblies allow the aggregation of imaging probes, thus enhancing photoacoustic signals.

Rao and coworkers SPN-based probe, **6-SPN**, which exhibited significant stronger photoacoustic signal than the photoacoustic probes based on single-walled

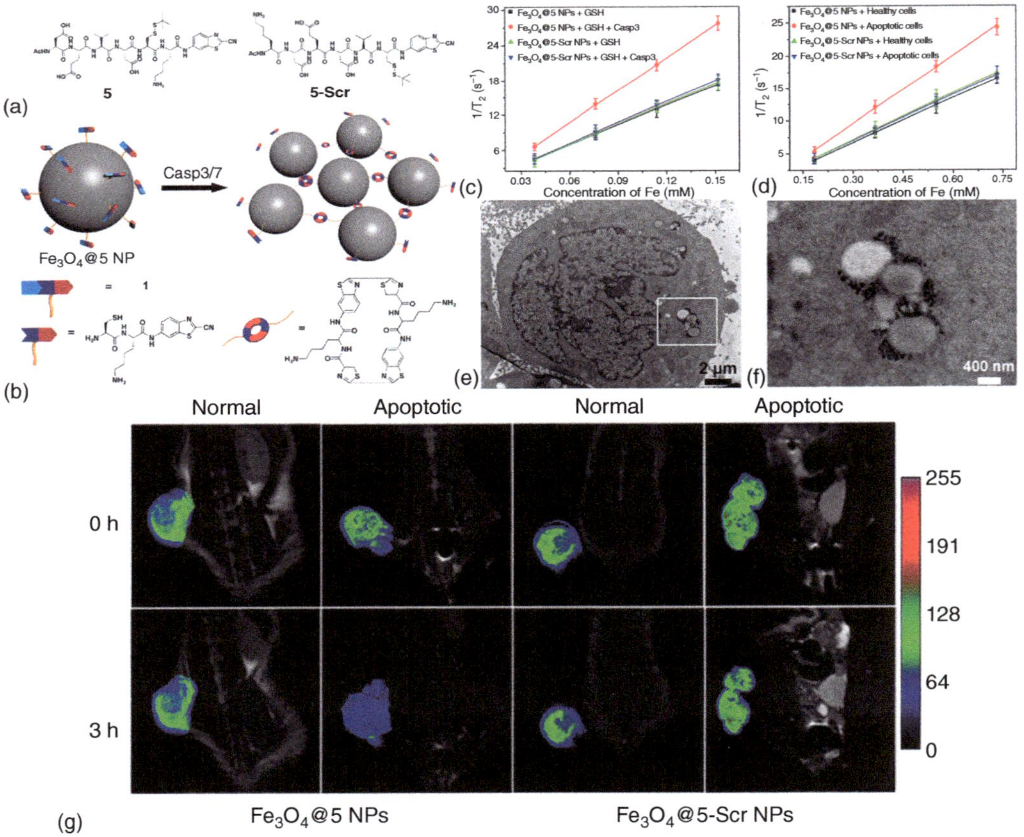

Figure 8.5 (a) Chemical structures of **5** and **5-Scr**. (b) Schematic illustration of intracellular Casp3/7-instructed aggregation of Fe_3O_4@**5** NPs. Transverse relaxation rates ($1/T_2$) of Fe_3O_4@**5** NPs or Fe_3O_4@**5-Scr** NPs at different concentrations in the (c) presence/absence of Casp3, (d) healthy/apoptotic HepG2 cells. Each error bar represents the standard deviation of three parallel experiments. (e) Low-magnification TEM image of apoptotic HepG2 cells after incubation with Fe_3O_4@**5** NPs at 37 °C for 1.5 hours. (f) High-magnification TEM image of the white rectangle area in (e). (g) *In vivo* T_2-weighted coronal MR images of Fe_3O_4@**5** NPs-injected saline-treated mice, Fe_3O_4@**5** NPs-injected DOX-treated mice, Fe_3O_4@**5-Scr** NPs-injected saline-treated mice, and Fe_3O_4@**5-Scr** NPs-injected DOX-treated mice at 0 or 3 hours post injection. Source: Yuan, Y., et al. (2016), [18], Figure 03, Pg 04 / with permission of American Chemical Society.

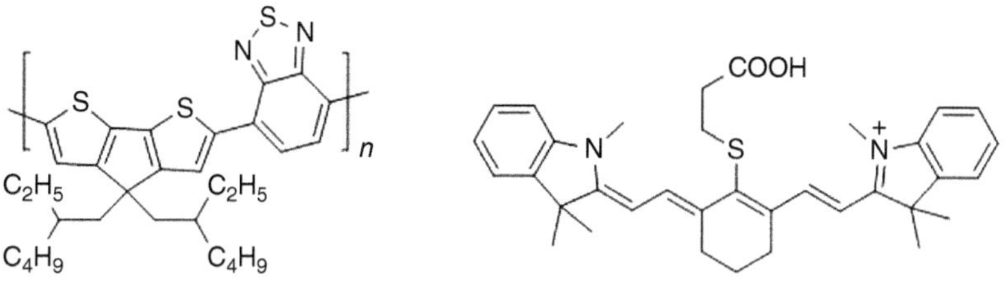

Figure 8.6 Structure of **6-SP** and IR775S [19].

carbon nanotubes (SWNTs) or gold nanorods (GNRs) [19]. The precipitation with poly(cyclopentadithiophene-*alt*-benzothiadiazole) (**6-SP**) (Figure 8.6) and 1,2-dipalmitoyl-*sn*-glycero-3-phosphocholine (DPPC) provides water-soluble micelles of **6-SPN**.

At the same mass concentrations, the **6-SPN** shows 5.2- and 7.1-times higher photoacoustic amplitude than those of SWNTs and GNRs do. With diameters of 20–50 nm, **6-SPN** favors to accumulate in lymph nodes (LNs). After intravenous injection, both photoacoustic and fluorescence imaging of living mice show the accumulation of **6-SPN** in brachial lymph nodes (BLNs), inguinal lymph nodes (ILNs), and superficial cervical lymph nodes (SCLNs). To process ROS imaging, the authors synthesized a ratiometric photoacoustic probe **6-RSPN** by coupling IR775S (a cyanine dye derivative) to **6-SPN**. The photoacoustic spectrum of **6-RSPN** shows three peaks at 700, 735, and 820 nm with similar amplitude. The addition of $ONOO^-$ significantly decreases the signal at 820 nm but changes little at 700 nm. Further research has proved that, among all the ROS, only $ONOO^-$ and ClO^- decrease PA_{700}/PA_{820}. After the treatment by lipopolysaccharide (LPS) and interferon-γ (INF-γ), the absorption ratio (PA_{700}/PA_{820}) in RAW264.7 cells increases significantly and it decreases after reducing ROS. The authors next used zymosan to generate ROS in mouse model. After the treatment of saline or zymosan, the photoacoustic amplitude at 700 nm remains unchanged, but the photoacoustic amplitude at 820 nm decreases, which leads to an increase of PA_{700}/PA_{820}. According to the authors, this study represents the first demonstration of a photoacoustic imaging probe for ROS detection and may offer a new approach for advanced photoacoustic imaging in clinical applications.

Using low-bandgap diketopyrrolopyrrole (DPP)-based SPs, Rao and coworkers designed a series of SPNs (Figure 8.7b) for *in vivo* PA to compare with **6-SPN**. Adding the solution of SPNs in tetrahydrofuran (THF) into poor solvent (water) under sonication affords water-soluble SPNs (Figure 8.7a) [20]. The PA amplitudes of the four SPNs at 710 nm displayed a linear relationship between PA signal and concentration. Among those four SPNs investigated, **7-SPN3** exhibited the highest PA signal. The *in vivo* imaging of **7-SPN3** shows a linear correlation between concentration and PA signal (Figure 8.7c,d). With the tissue background signal of 25 ± 6 a.u., **7-SPN3** has a detection of limit of 0.60 μg/ml, which is 3.3-times lower than **6-SPN** (2 μg/ml). **7-SPN3** also shows high photostability, almost no intensity

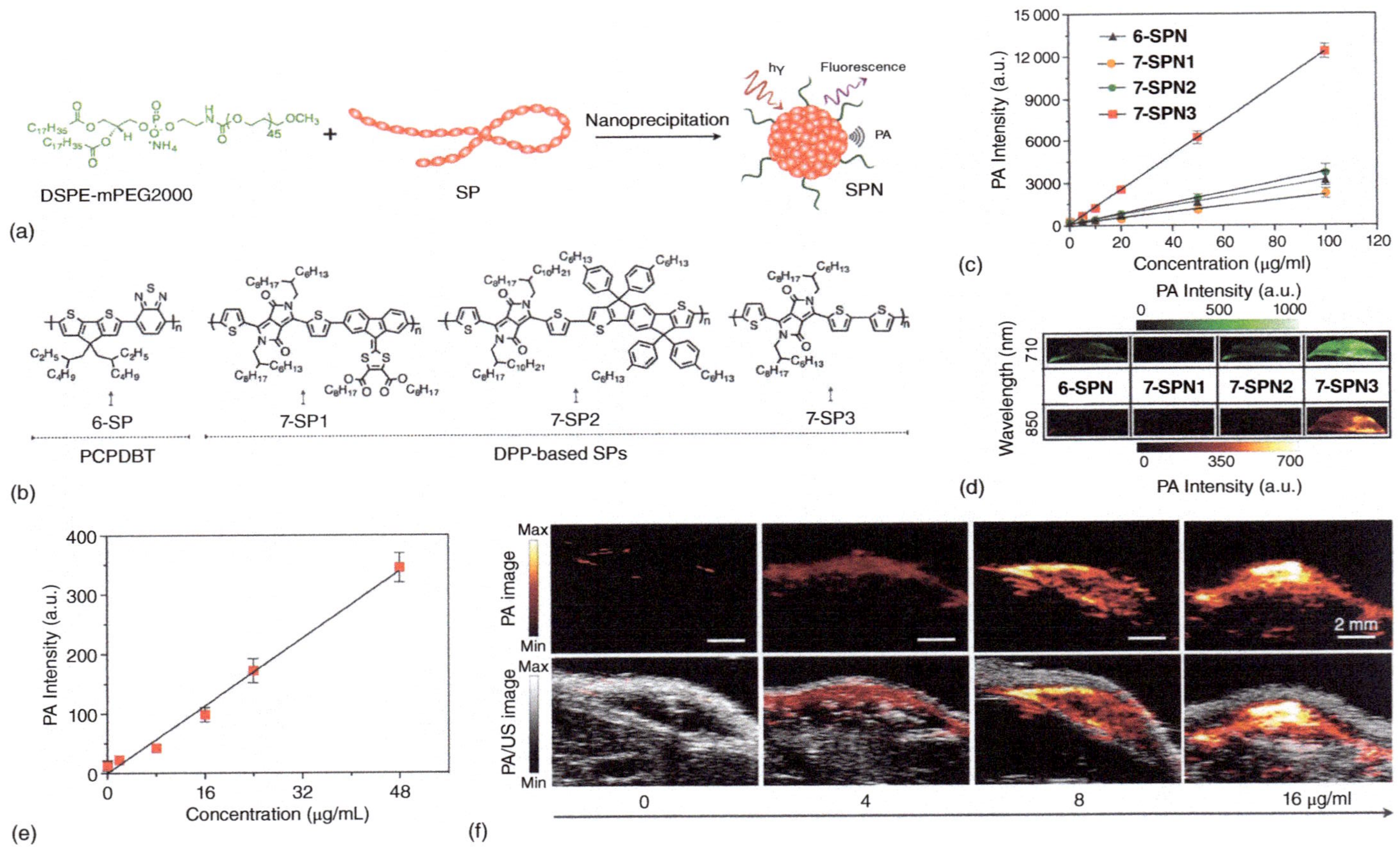

Figure 8.7 (a) Scheme illustration of preparation of SPNs via nanoprecipitation. (b) Chemical structures of **6-SP** and DPP-based SPs (**7-SP1**, **7-SP2**, and **7-SP3**). (c) PA intensities of SPNs as a function of nanoparticle concentration in PBS. $R^2 = 0.997, 0.996, 0.997, 0.993$ for **6-SPN**, **7-SPN1**, **7-SPN2**, and **7-SPN3**, respectively. (d) Representative PA images of SPNs solution at the concentration of 2 μg/ml each excited by pulsed laser at 710 and 850 nm, respectively. Error bars represent standard deviations of three separate measurements. (e) PA intensities of **7-SPN3**-matrigel inclusions (30 μl) in the subcutaneous dorsal space of living mice as a function of nanoparticle mass concentration. The tissue background signal, calculated as the average PA signal in areas where no nanoparticles were injected, was 25 ± 6 a.u. $R^2 = 0.991$. (f) PA (upper) and PA/ultrasound co-registered (lower) images of the nanoparticle–matrigel inclusions in mice at indicated concentrations. The images represent transverse slices through the subcutaneous inclusions. A single laser pulse at 750 nm with a laser fluence of 9 mJ/cm^2 and a pulse repetition rate of 20 Hz was used for all experiments. Error bars represent

loss after being exposed to 2700 laser pulses. For tumor imaging, the PA signal of **7-SPN3** is 5.3-fold of the background signal after its intravenous injection into mice.

8.3 Cancer Treatment

In addition to being applied for cancer diagnosis, self-assembly of small molecules is an emerging approach for developing anticancer therapy [21–24]. Formed by self-assembly, supramolecular assemblies may exhibit emergent properties for new physical, chemical, and biological functions [25, 26]. As a type of higher-order structures (in comparison to individual molecules), supramolecular assemblies can exhibit multiple functions and simultaneously act on more than one target, which should provide a chance to reduce acquired drug resistance in cancer therapy [27]. In the following sections, we introduce supramolecular assemblies for cancer treatment in two parts: drug delivery and EISA for developing anticancer therapy.

8.3.1 Drug Delivery

Chemotherapy remains as one of the major strategies for cancer therapy. It relies on the cytotoxicity of chemotherapeutic agents. However, the inherent properties of these agents, such as the nonspecific distribution, poor bioavailability, rapid blood clearance, and poor solubility, often limit the efficiency of the therapy [28]. Using supramolecular assemblies for drug delivery may offer a new way to address those issues, especially when the molecular assemblies are able to target special subcellular compartments of cancer cells.

Cisplatin and camptothecin are two first-line anticancer drugs [29, 30]. To inhibit cancer cells, cisplatin cross-links double-stranded DNA, and camptothecin inhibits a DNA-associated enzyme, topoisomerase I. However, it is hard to deliver negatively charged 10-hydroxycamptothecine (HCPT) into nucleus, and cisplatin can hardly accumulate in cisplatin-resistant cells. To address these issues, Yang and coworkers designed a HCPT-based molecule **8** (Figure 8.8b), which chelates with cisplatin and self-assembles to form nanostructures (Figure 8.8a) [31]. Compound **8** consists of HCPT and peptide sequence FFERGD, and it forms short nanofibers in water. In the presence of 1 equiv of cisplatin, **8** co-assembles with the cisplatin to form thicker and longer nanofibers, named **Complex 8-1**. In the presence of 1.5 equiv of cisplatin, **8** co-assembles with the cisplatin into nanoparticles, named **Complex 8-2**. Those two complexes can release HCPT and cisplatin, showing "S" release curves (Figure 8.8c). After releasing of cisplatin, the complexes dissociate, thus further accelerating the release rate. The formation of the complexes enhances the uptake of both HCPT and cisplatin in A549/DDP cells (Figure 8.8d,e) via endocytosis.

After the incubation with complexes, A549 shows significant stronger green fluorescence of HCPT (Figure 8.8f–i). Confocal laser scanning microscopy (CLSM) also shows green fluorescence in the nucleus of the complex-treated cells, but not in the nucleus of free HCPT or **8**-treated A549 cells. Cytotoxicity and *in vivo* experiments have confirmed that the formation of complexes significantly improves the efficiency

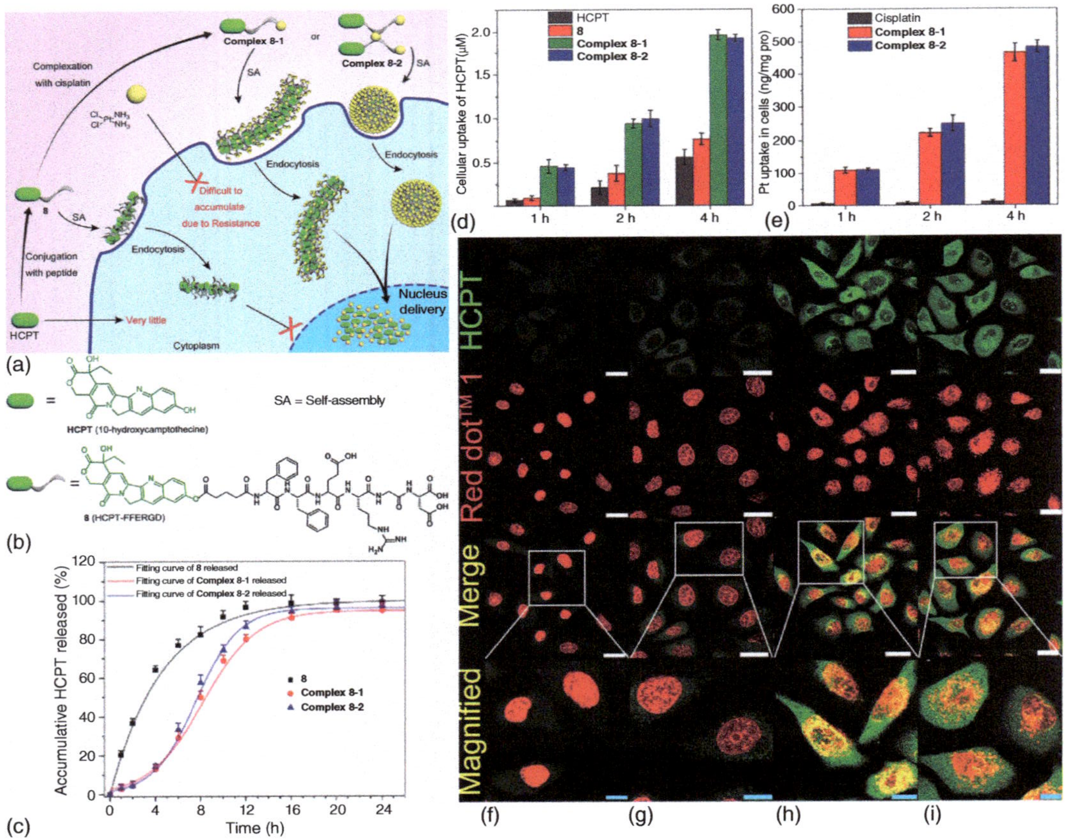

Figure 8.8 (a) Schematic illustration for preparation of dual-drug assemblies and the nuclear drug delivery. (b) Chemical structures of HCPT and **8**. (c) Accumulative release profile from solution containing 1 mg/ml of different compounds. Intracellular concentration of (d) HCPT and (e) Pt in A549 cells (SEM ± mean, $n = 3$). CLSM images of A549 cells treated with (f) HCPT, (g) **8**, (h) **Complex 8-1**, and (i) **Complex 8-2** (100 μM) for two hours, and then stained with 1× Red dot 1. Scale bar represent 25 and 10 μm at low and high magnification images, respectively. Source: Cai, Y., et al. (2017), [31], Figure 03, Pg 04 / with permission of American Chemical Society.

of cancer cell inhibition. This research illustrates a “Trojan Horse” approach that delivers two drugs to nucleus of cells for synergistic inhibition of cancer cells and tumors. It may ultimately offer a new method for the development of supramolecular delivery systems if the therapeutic index permits.

Besides nucleus, mitochondria are another important target for developing anticancer drugs because mitochondria play essential roles in many cellular processes. Xu and coworkers designed an amphipathic compound **9** (Figure 8.9a), which consists of a self-assembling peptide sequence (Nap-FFK), the FLAG-tag (DYKDDDDK), and a fluorophore (NBD) [32]. Among those three parts, FLAG-tag is a substrate of enterokinase (ENTK). **9** self-assembles to form micelles in H_2O but turns to nanofibers after its proteolytic cleavage catalyzed by ENTK. Being incubated with cells, **9** likely self-assembles to form micelles on the surface of cells. Then, the micelles enter cells via endocytosis. After escaping from lysosome, the micelles target mitochondria and self-assemble to form nanofibers on the outer membrane of mitochondria upon the action of ENTK. Cell viability assay confirmed that **9** exhibits little cytotoxicity to HeLa and U87MG cells. After the incubation of HeLa or U87MG cells for two hours, the cells exhibited strong fluorescence of **9**, indicating a rapid cellular uptake. The fluorescence from **9** overlaps with the fluorescence of MitoTracker, confirming the targeting of mitochondria. The mitochondria-targeting ability likely originates from the ENTK-catalyzed proteolysis and the electrostatic interaction between the negative-charged FLAG-tag moiety and the positive-charged intermembrane of mitochondria and enables an analog Compound **9-A** (Figure 8.9b) to deliver cargos. In molecule **9-A**, a tyrosine replaces the NBD. Incubating HeLa cells expressing GFP-Cyt c or Omi-mcherry with RPE protein or DOX in the presence of **9-A** results in overlap of RPE signal with the fluorescence of GFP-Cyt c (Figure 8.9c). Quantification of the overlap indicates that **9-A** significantly boost the localization of RPE or DOX in mitochondria (Figure 8.9d). Moreover, after mixing with **9-A**, DOX exhibits significantly increased cytotoxicity against HeLa cells (Figure 8.9e). Isolated mitochondria from HeLa cells also prove the self-assembly instructed by ENTK on the mitochondria. As the first report of mitochondria targeting and delivery via enzymatic self-assembly, this work highlights the promise of EISA for targeting subcellular organelles.

Despite traditional drugs, other anticancer agents can also be delivered by supramolecular assembling systems. Wang and coworkers used phosphatase-triggered self-assembly to prepare iron oxide-based nanogels, which deliver superoxide dismutase (SOD) and chloroperoxidase (CPO) into tumor cells and convert the endogenous ROS ($^{\cdot}O_2-$ and H_2O_2) into $^1O_2$ by the cascade reaction of SOD and CPO, subsequently cause the death of cancer cells [33].

8.3.2 Enzyme-Instructed Self-assembly (EISA for Cancer Therapy)

In addition to acting as a method for the preparation of supramolecular assemblies (see Chapter 4), EISA has shown promises in the development of novel cancer therapy [21, 34, 35] because it generates spatiotemporally controlled nanostructures in cellular environment. Inhibition of cancer cells by the self-assembled

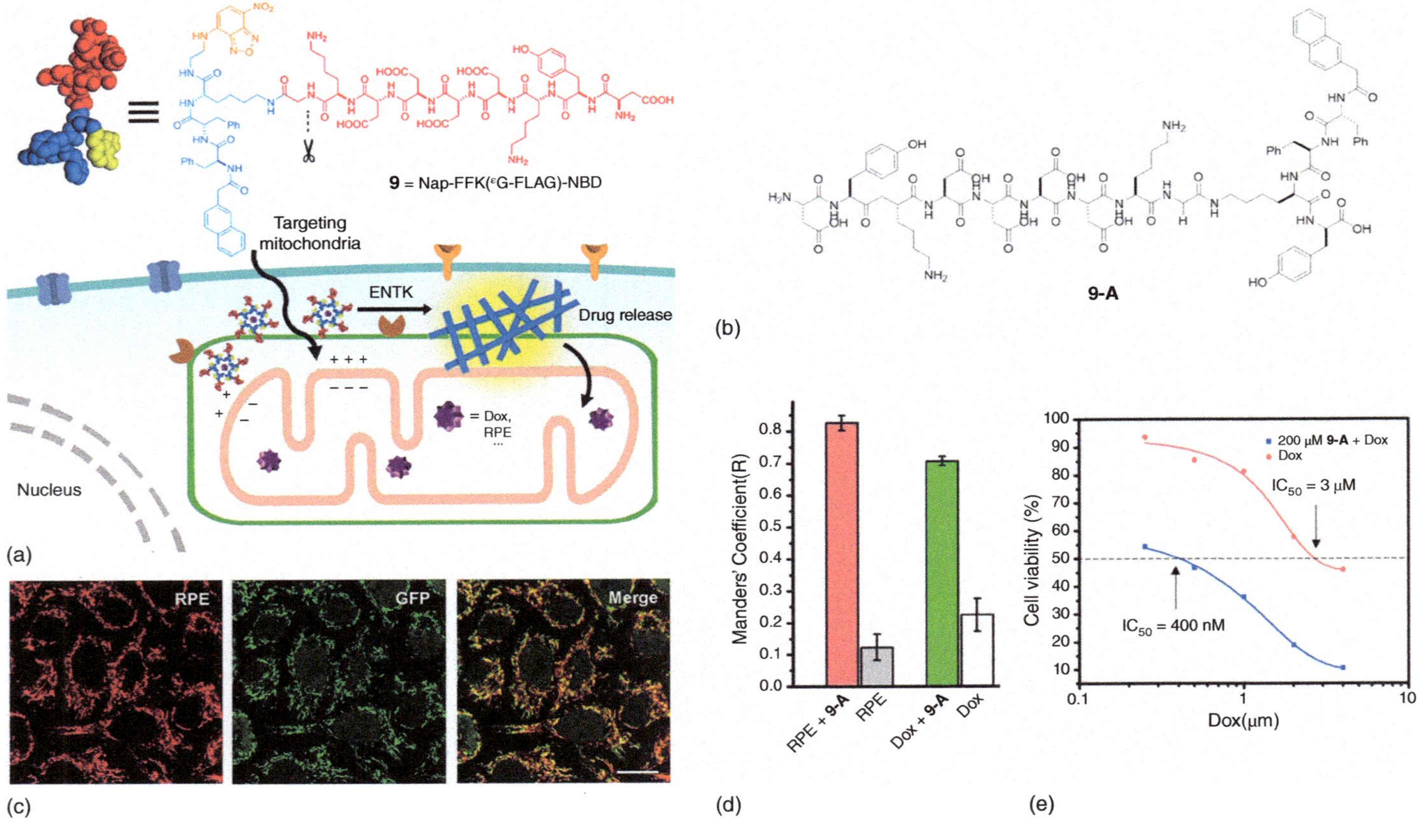

Figure 8.9 (a) Structure of **9** and ENTK cleaving **9** to convert micelles to nanofibers on mitochondria. (b) Chemical structure of **9-A**. (c) GFP-Cyt c HeLa cells treated by the mixture of RPE (1 μg/ml) and **9-A** (200 μM) for two hours. Scale bar = 30 μm. (d) Co-localization analysis of GFP-Cyt c and Omi-mcherry expressing HeLa cells treated by RPE or DOX in the presence of **9-A**. $R = 1$ indicates perfect co-localization. (e) The combination of DOX (2 μM) and **9-A** exhibit increased HeLa cell inhibition. Source: He, H. et al. (2018), [32], Figure 02, Pg 03 / with permission of American Chemical Society.

nanostructures has shown exceptional selectivity against cancer cells, which have stimulated considerable research activities for developing EISA of supramolecular assemblies for cancer therapy.

Following their earlier exploration of EISA for cancer therapy, [21] Xu and coworkers combined EISA with cisplatin for killing drug-resistant ovarian cancer. They designed two enantiomeric compounds, **10P-L** and **10P-D**, which could be hydrolyzed by carboxylesterases (CES) to turn into self-assembling hydrogelators, **10-L** and **10-D** (Figure 8.10a) [36]. Adding CES to the solution of **10P-L** or **10P-D** in PBS buffer results in hydrogels made of nanofibers of **10-L** or **10-D**, respectively. After being incubated with SKOV3 or A2780cis cells for four hours, more than 85% of the **10P-L** or **10P-D** turned into **10-L** or **10-D** and cellular uptake of **10P-L** is more efficient than that of **10P-D**. The incubation of three ovarian cancer cell lines with the mixture of **10P-L** or **10P-D** and cisplatin (CDDP) reduces the cell viability of the ovarian cancer cells (Figure 8.10b), indicating that **10P-L** or **10P-D** significantly increases the effect of CDDP. **10P-L** shows higher efficacy than **10P-D**, agreeing with the higher uptake of **10P-L**. After being treated by **10P-D**, SKOV3 cells exhibit far fewer well-defined, long actin filaments than control SKOV3 cells (without treatment), which agrees with hypothesis that the intracellular self-assembled nanofibers disrupt actin dynamics (Figure 8.10c). This research demonstrated that EISA of small molecules is an effective method to boost the effect of CDDP against drug resistant ovarian cancer cells, and it may lead to a new approach to develop combination therapy of cancer treatment.

Targeting an essential organelle is a promising approach for killing cancer cells without inducing drug resistance. Mitochondria play vital roles in many cellular processes, and disruption of mitochondria may be a useful method to cause death of cancer cells. Xu and coworkers designed Compounds **11P-L** and **11P-D** for mitochondria targeting and cancer cell death (Figure 8.11a) [37]. The molecules consist of a tetrapeptide (FFYK) as the self-assembling motif, tyrosine phosphate as an enzymatic trigger of ALP, NBD as a fluorophore, and triphenyl phosphinium (TPP) as the mitochondrial targeting motif. On the surface of Saos2 cancer cells, the overexpressing ALP hydrolyzes **11P-L/11P-D** to **11-L/11-D**, which self-assemble on cell plasma membrane and then get into cell via endocytosis. After escaping from the lysosomes of the cancer cells, the assemblies target and accumulate at mitochondria, finally lead to cell apoptosis. After being incubated with **11P-L/11P-D** for one hour, the Saos2 cells show significant fluorescence that overlaps well with that of Lyso-Tracker. After four hours incubation, the assemblies of **11P-L/11P-D** escape from the lysosome into cytosol and then merged with the fluorescence of Mito-Tracker (Figure 8.11b). To study the mechanism of cell apoptosis, the author used ELISA to detect the level of key signaling proteins in pathways controlling survival and apoptosis (Figure 8.11c). During the apoptosis of cells, the expression level of phosphorylated Bad increases first and then decreases quickly. The dropped expression level of phosphorylated Bad confirmed that Bad is activated by dephosphorylation under stress. This stress also activates the apoptosis and leads to the release of Cyt c from mitochondria. The time-dependent Western blot analysis also proves the release of Cyt c (Figure 8.11d). To prove that **11P-L** or **11P-D** minimizes

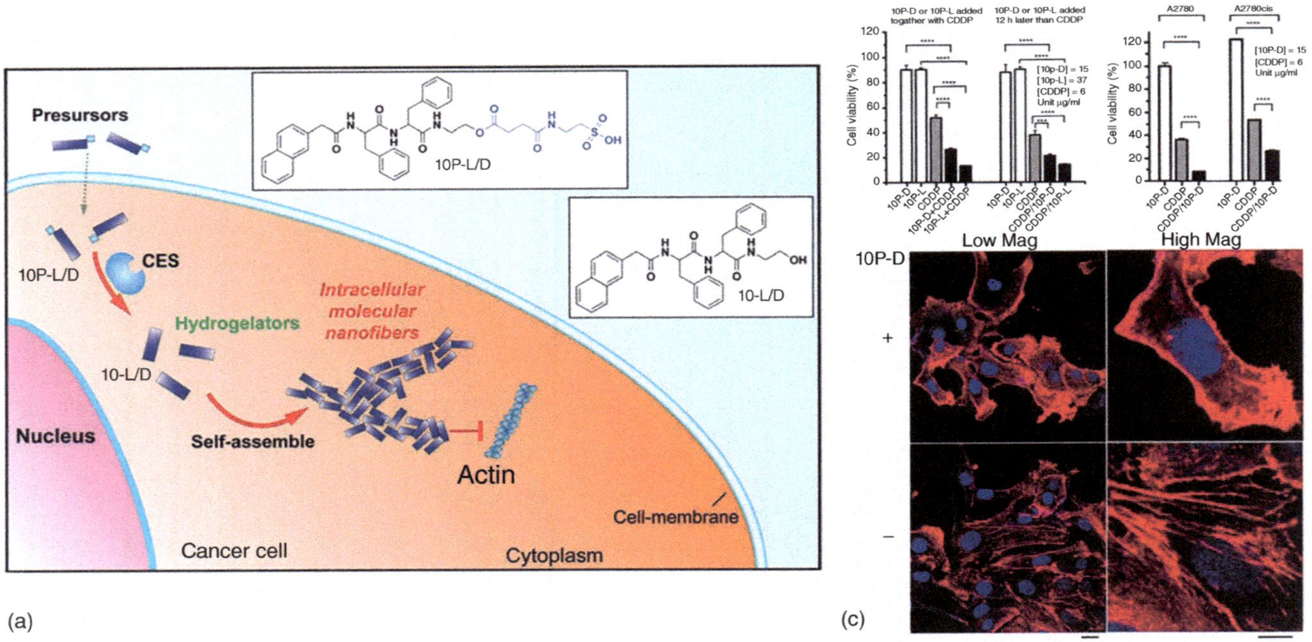

Figure 8.10 (a) Enzymatic transformation of the precursor (**10P-L/D**) as a substrate of carboxylesterase (CES) to the corresponding hydrogelator (**10-L/D**) for intracellular self-assembly. (b) The cell viability of SKOV3 cells incubated with the precursors **10P-D** or **10P-L** alone, or in combination with CDDP for 72 hours (left); the cell viability of A2780 cells and A2780cis cells incubated with the precursors **10P-D** alone, or in combination with CDDP for 72 hours (*** = $p \leq 0.001$, **** = $p \leq 0.0001$). (c) The fluorescence images of SKOV3 cells stained with Alexa Fluor 633 Phalloidin (F-actin) and Hoechst (nuclei) (upper) after treatment of **10P-D** at concentration of 20 μm for 20 hours or (bottom) without the treatment of **10P-D**. Scale bars: left = 20 μm, right = 10 μm. Source: Li, J., et al. (2015), [36], Figure 03, Pg 04 / with permission of Wiley-VCH.

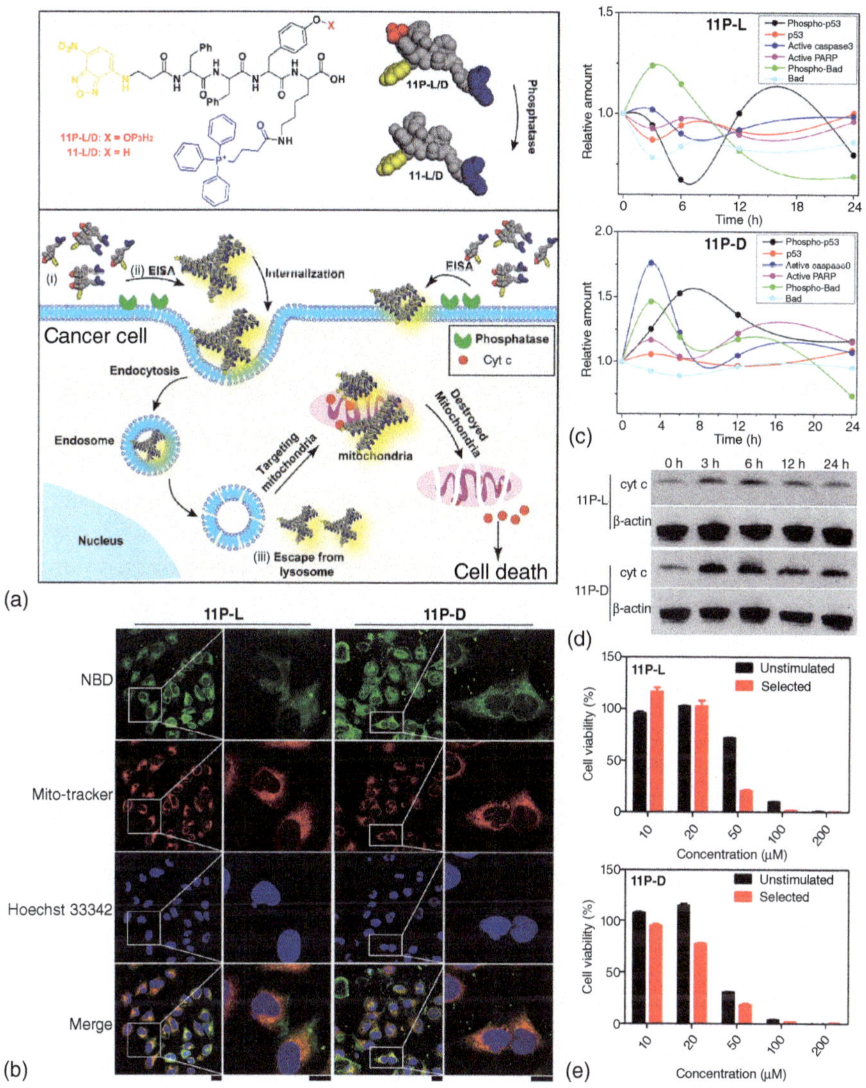

Figure 8.11 (a) Illustration of enzyme-instructed self-assembly for targeting mitochondria and inducing death of cancer cell. (b) Confocal laser scanning microscopy images of Saos2 cells treated with **11P-L** or **11P-D** (50 μM) for four hours and then stained with Mito-tracker. Scale bar for low magnification is 25 μm and for higher magnification is 15 μm. (c) Time-dependent activation of apoptotic proteins of Saos2 cell treated with **11P-L** or **11P-D** (50 μM). (d) Time-dependent Western blot analysis of Cyt c from the cytosolic fraction of Saos2 cells treated with **11P-L** or **11P-D** (50 μM). (e) Cell viability of unstimulated Saos2 cell line or selected Saos2 cell line (after five weeks treatment of the precursors with gradually increase concentrations) incubated with **11P-L** or **11P-D** at different concentrations for 48 hours. Source: Wang, H., et al. (2016), [37], Figure 05, Pg 06 / with permission of American Chemical Society.

acquired drug resistance, the authors selected cells by repeatedly stimulating Saos2 with **11P-L** or **11P-D** for five weeks. The cell viability experiments confirm that the selected cells and the unselected cells exhibit similar sensitivity to the **11P-L** or **11P-D**, indicating little drug resistance (Figure 8.11e). This research illustrates that the combination of EISA and organelle targeting is a promising strategy for minimizing acquired drug resistance.

Another molecule, as an substrate of EISA for organelle targeting, is **12P** (Figure 8.12a), which accumulates at ER [38]. Similar to **11P-L/D**, **12P** consists of self-assembling tripeptide (FFY), tyrosine phosphate as an enzymatic trigger of ALP, naphthyl group offering aromatic–aromatic interaction, and positive-charged L-homoarginine residue promoting membrane interaction. On the membrane of cells, some **12P** converts to **12** by ALP hydrolysis and self-assembles into crescent-shaped nanostructures. After getting into the cells by endocytosis, the assemblies accumulate at ER, increase the ER stress, and then lead to the cell death. In cell assays, **12P** shows significant higher toxicity to ALP expressing cancer cells than HS-5 cells (a stromal cell expresses little ALP) and **12** exhibits minimal toxicity to those cancer cells, which indicates the selectivity for the cancer cells that overexpress ALP (Figure 8.12c). As shown in time-lapse microscopy that studies the dynamic interaction of **12P** with membrane, membrane curvature and tabulation occur on the HeLa cells incubated with **12P**. By replacing the naphthyl group in molecule **12P** by NBD, the authors designed the fluorescent analog **12FP** (Figure 8.12b). Time-lapse microscopy shows the generation and distribution of the molecular assemblies by EISA: at the beginning, fluorescent spots appear on the surface of cell; after 40 minutes, cytoplasm exhibits fluorescence; and membrane blebs (white arrow) near the fluorescent spots during this change (Figure 8.12e). After one hour incubation with **12FP**, HeLa cells show significant fluorescence of NBD, which co-localizes well with the fluorescence of ER tracker (Figure 8.12f), indicating that most of the assemblies accumulate on the ER. Accumulation of assemblies may induce ER dysfunction and increase ER stress. The time-dependent Western blot shows that ER-stress markers (Bip, CHOP) expression of the HeLa cells increase after the incubation with **12P** (Figure 8.12d). Additional experiments indicate that EISA of **12P** can activate IRE1α and PERK pathway to induce ER stress and cell death. This work shows another EISA-based organelle targeting for killing cancer cells, which promises new applications for cancer treatment.

The membrane affinity and promiscuity of cholesterol allows it to serve as a molecular motif for targeting cancer cells via EISA. For example, Xu and coworkers used **13P** for inhibiting cancer cells (Figure 8.13a) [39]. The dosage of **13P** is much lower than cisplatin (Figure 8.13b,c) against A2780cis, an ovarian cancer cell line. The viability of A2780cis and HS-5 cells after 48 hours incubation with **13P** or **13** shows that **13P** can inhibit A2780cis but hardly inhibit HS-5 (Figure 8.13d), which indicates the selectivity of **13P** against cancer cells. With laurdan as fluorescent marker, **13P** treated A2780cis cells show increased inhomogeneity of the fluorescence (laurdan), indicating that **13P** increases the microheterogeneity of the cell membrane (Figure 8.13e). Besides, **13P**-treated A2780cis cells exhibit short, ill-defined actin filaments and the microtubules reorganized in the proximity of plasma membranes,

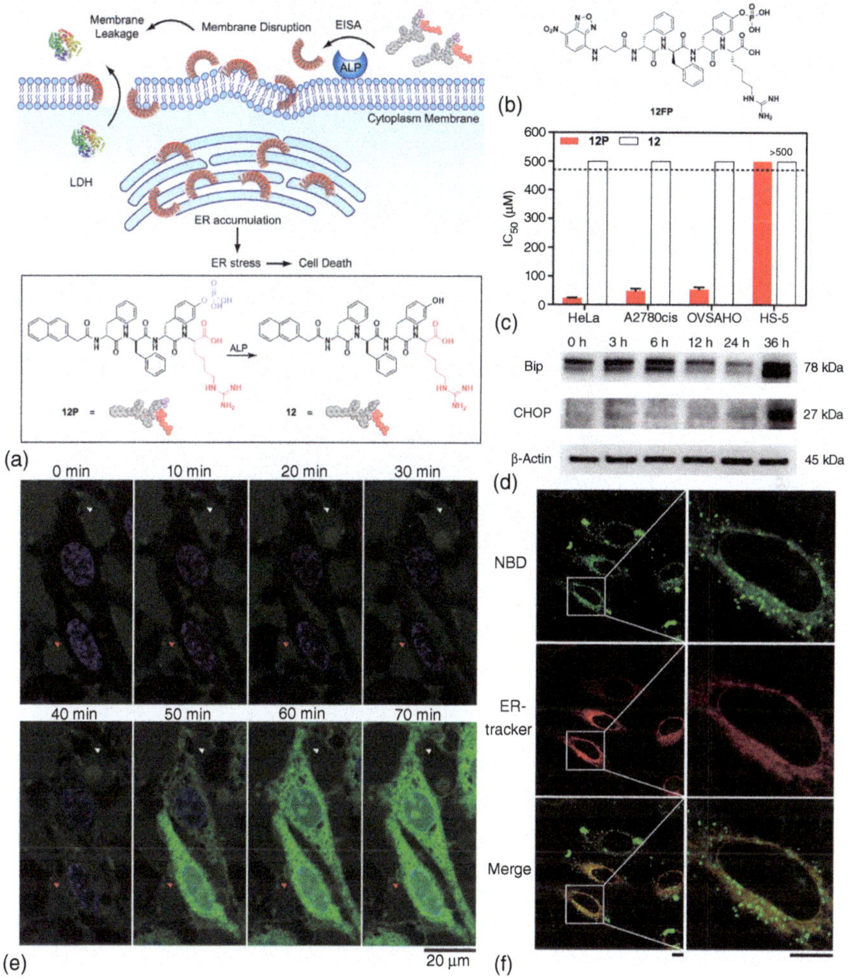

Figure 8.12 (a) Illustration of EISA assemblies to disrupt the cell membrane and to target the ER and molecular structure of an EISA precursor. (b) Chemical structure of **12FP**. (c) IC_{50} (24 hours) of **12P** or **12** against HeLa cells, A2780cis cells, OVSAHO cells, and HS-5 cells. (d) Western blot analysis of ER-stress marker (Bip, CHOP) after treating HeLa cells with **12P** (50 μM) at different times (i.e. 0, 3, 6, 12, 24, or 36 hours). (e) Time-lapse microscopy images of live HeLa cells incubated with **12FP** (200 μM) for 0–70 minutes, showing the *in situ* generation of assemblies of F1P on cell membrane (pink arrow), membrane disruption (white arrow), and real-time distribution in the HeLa cells. Before incubating with **12FP**, the nuclei of HeLa cells were stained with Hoechst 33342. (f) Confocal laser scanning microscopy images of HeLa cells treated with **12FP** (200 μM) for one hour and then stained with the ER tracker. Scale bar is 10 μm. Source: Feng, Z., et al. (2018), [38], Figure 08, Pg 08/ with permission of American Chemical Society.

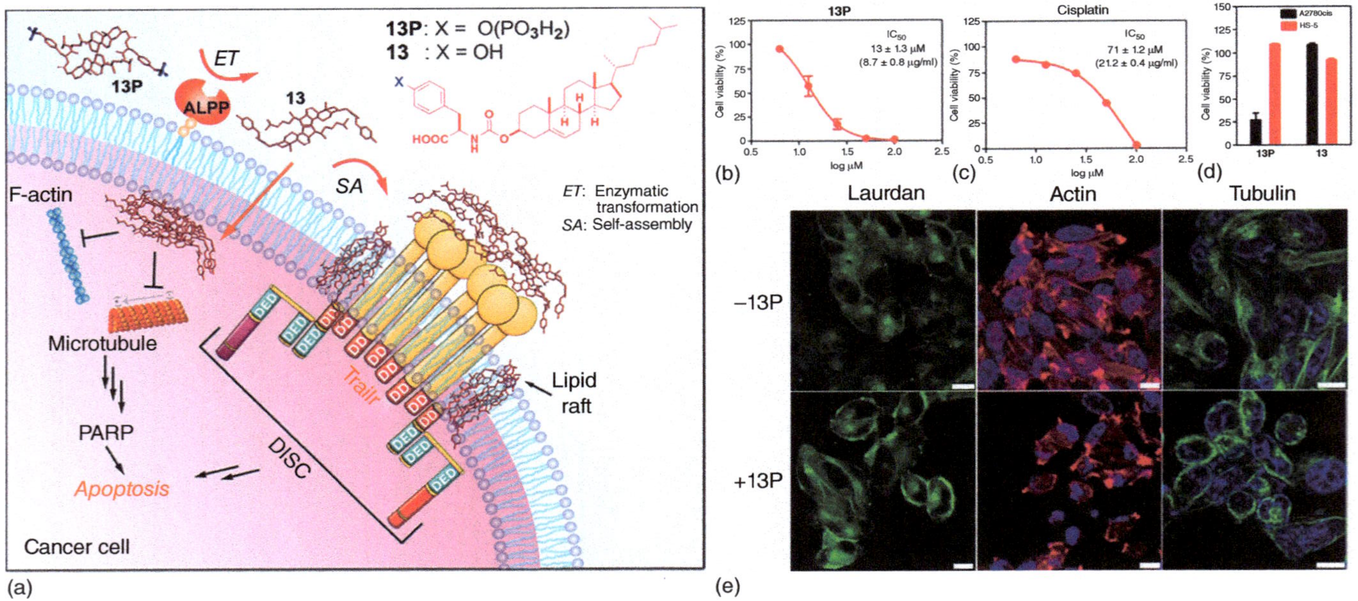

Figure 8.13 (a) EISA of the tyrosine cholesterol conjugate activates extrinsic and intrinsic cell death signaling (ALPP, Alkaline phosphatase, placental type; PARP, poly ADP-ribose polymerase; DISC, death-inducing signalling complex). Dosage curves of (b) **13P** and (c) cisplatin against A2780cis cells at 48 hours. (d) Viability of A2780cis or HS-5 cell lines incubated with 12.5 μM of **13P** or **13** for 48 hours. (e) Confocal images of A2780cis cells stained with laurdan (10 μM), Alexa Fluor 633 phalloidin (F-actin, red), and Hoechst (nuclei, blue) or tubulin tracker (green) without or with the addition of **13P** (12.5 μM) for 12 hours (scale bar is 10 μm). Source: Wang, H., et al. (2016), [39], Figure 04, Pg 04/ with permission of American Chemical Society.

indicating that the assemblies of **13P** interact with F-actin and disrupt the dynamics of F-actin, and promote the formation of apoptotic microtubule networks. This work illustrates a new approach to use EISA to target lipid rafts, and the assemblies may be used for counter anticancer drug resistance because there is little acquired drug resistance for **13P** [27].

Recently, Xu, Tang, and coworkers reported the first example of using EISA, without any other anticancer drugs, for inhibiting tumors in a mouse model [40]. As reported, on the membrane of ALP expressing cancer cells, **14P** (Figure 8.14a) is partly hydrolyzed by ALP and then enters into cells by endocytosis. The intracellular self-assembly of **14** further increases the cell stress and induces cell death. The IC_{50} of **14P** on the HepG2 cells is over two orders of magnitude higher than the IC_{50} on Saos2 cells (Figure 8.14b), which indicates that **14P** selectively inhibits the osteosarcoma cells without harming liver cells. After being subcutaneously xenografted with tumors of luciferase-labeled Saos2 cells (Saos2-luc) and its highly metastatic subtype (Saos2-lung) cells, the mice received intravenous injection of **14P** or saline. Treating with **14P** for four weeks results in the 8-fold and 25-fold reduction in tumor volume of Saos2-luc and Saos2-lung (Figure 8.14d,e), respectively, which agrees with the slightly lower expression level of ALP on Saso2-luc than Saos2-lung cells (Figure 8.14c). This result indicates that **14P** effectively inhibits the osteosarcoma tumors. By using the bioluminescence of luciferase-transfected tumor cells in real time to monitor the tumor growth, the authors further confirm that **14P** efficiently inhibits the growth of osteosarcoma tumor *in vivo*. This work demonstrates the ability of EISA for inhibition of osteosarcoma. The design principle used in this work may also be applicable to design molecules for inhibiting the tumors that overexpress other enzymes.

Uptake and retention of drugs are important for cancer therapy. Yang and coworkers designed the molecule **15P** (Figure 8.15a, b) [41], which turns into **15** to form nanoparticles upon the hydrolysis catalyzed by extracellular ALP. Subsequent intracellular GSH reduction converts **15** to **15-Thiol**, which forms nanofibers. CLSM images show yellow fluorescent dots around HepG2 cells after 0.5 hour incubation with **15P** (200 μM), and yellow fluorescent fibers inside the cells after the four hours (Figure 8.15c, d). The uptake experiments indicate that liver cancer cells uptake **15P** more efficiently than normal liver cells do (Figure 8.15e, f). Since nanoparticle-to-nanofiber transformations in cancer cells offer a better retention of nanomedicines in tumors [42], this work may provide a new strategy for designing supramolecular systems to improve drug uptake and retention.

Induced pluripotent stem cells (iPSCs) have immense potentials for treating diseases by cell therapy [43]. However, residual iPSCs may produce teratomas in animals [44]. Recently, Saito and coworkers use tri-D-phenylalanine-derived phospho-D-peptides **16** (Figure 8.16a) as a selective iPSC elimination agent, which shows strong toxicity against iPSCs, but has little effect on differentiated cells and normal cells [45]. Figure 8.16b shows that the viability of the cells treated by **16** negatively correlates with the amount of ALP expression, indicating that ALP-induced aggregation **16** causes death of cells. After the authors treated the co-cultured cells (201B7 cells/cardiomyocytes = 1/9) with 400 μM **16** for one hour,

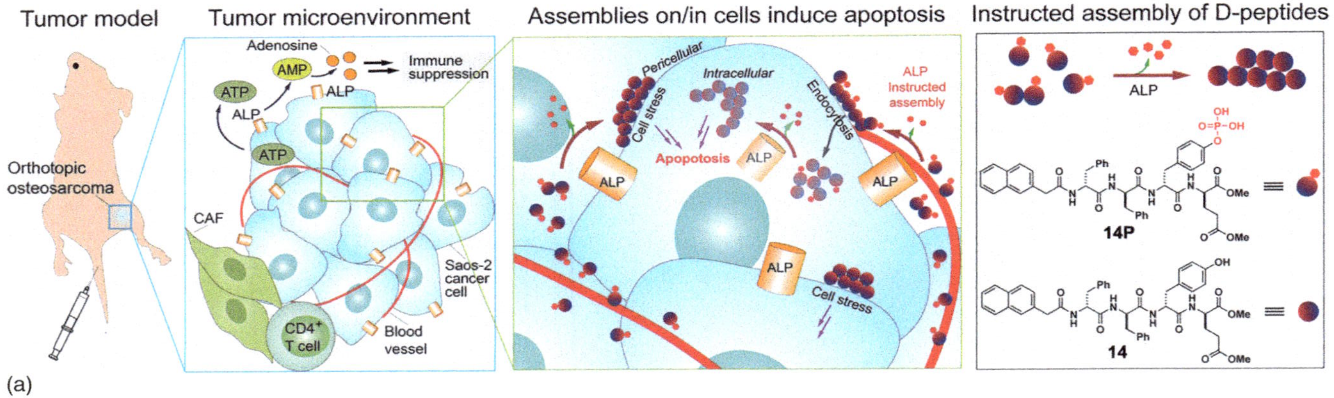

Figure 8.14 (a) Schematic representation of ALP-instructed assembly for inhibiting metastatic osteosarcoma within an immunosuppressive tumor microenvironment in an orthotopic mouse model and molecular structures of the precursor (**14P**) and hydrogelator [14]. (b) IC_{50} values of **14P** (24, 48, and 72 hours) against Saos2 or HepG2 cells. (c) ALP activities on Saso2-luc and Saos2-lung cells. Tumor volume of orthotopic osteosarcoma model established by Saos2-luc and Saos2-lung cells after tail intravenous injection of compound **14P** or saline for four weeks: the photos (d) and the measured volumes (e) of the tumors (***$p < 0.001$). (f) Images of osteosarcoma tumor growth using *in vivo* imaging system (IVIS) for orthotopic osteosarcoma model established by Saos2-luc and Saos2-lung cells at weeks one to four after **14P** or saline treatment. (D, F) Source: Feng, Z., et al. (2019), [40], Figure 03, Pg 06/ with permission of Elsevier.

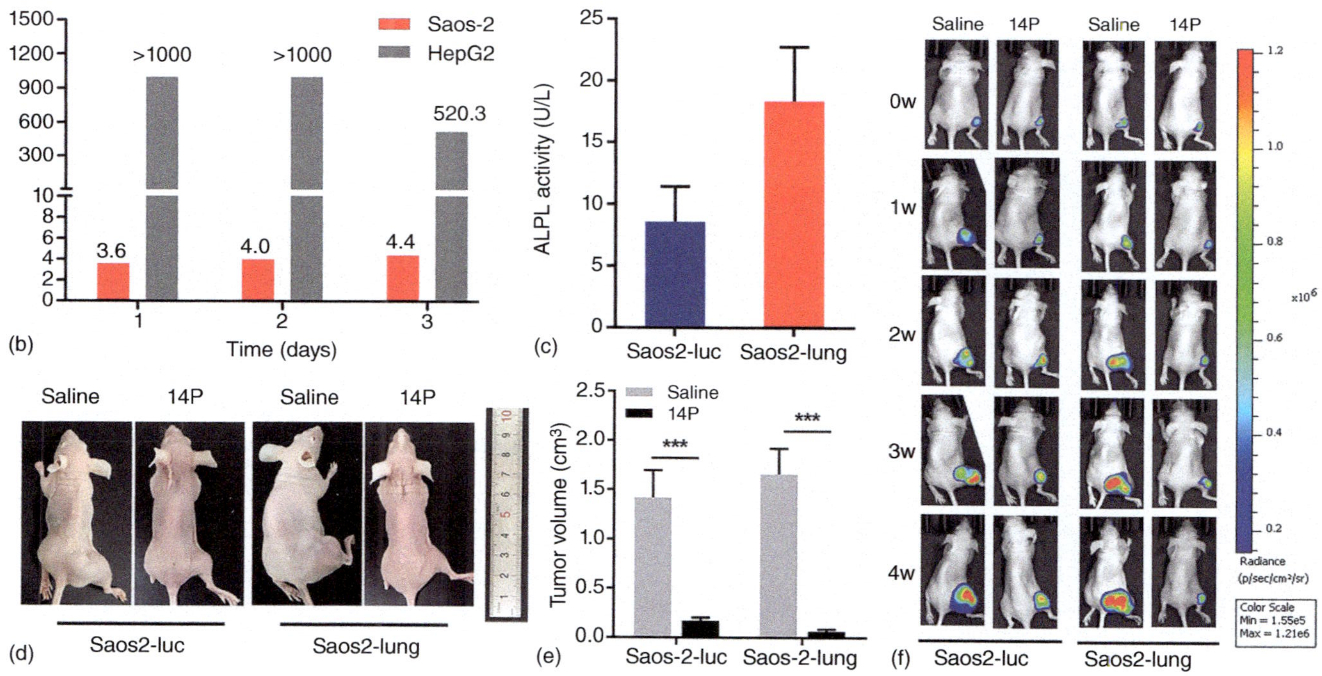

Figure 8.14 (*Continued*)

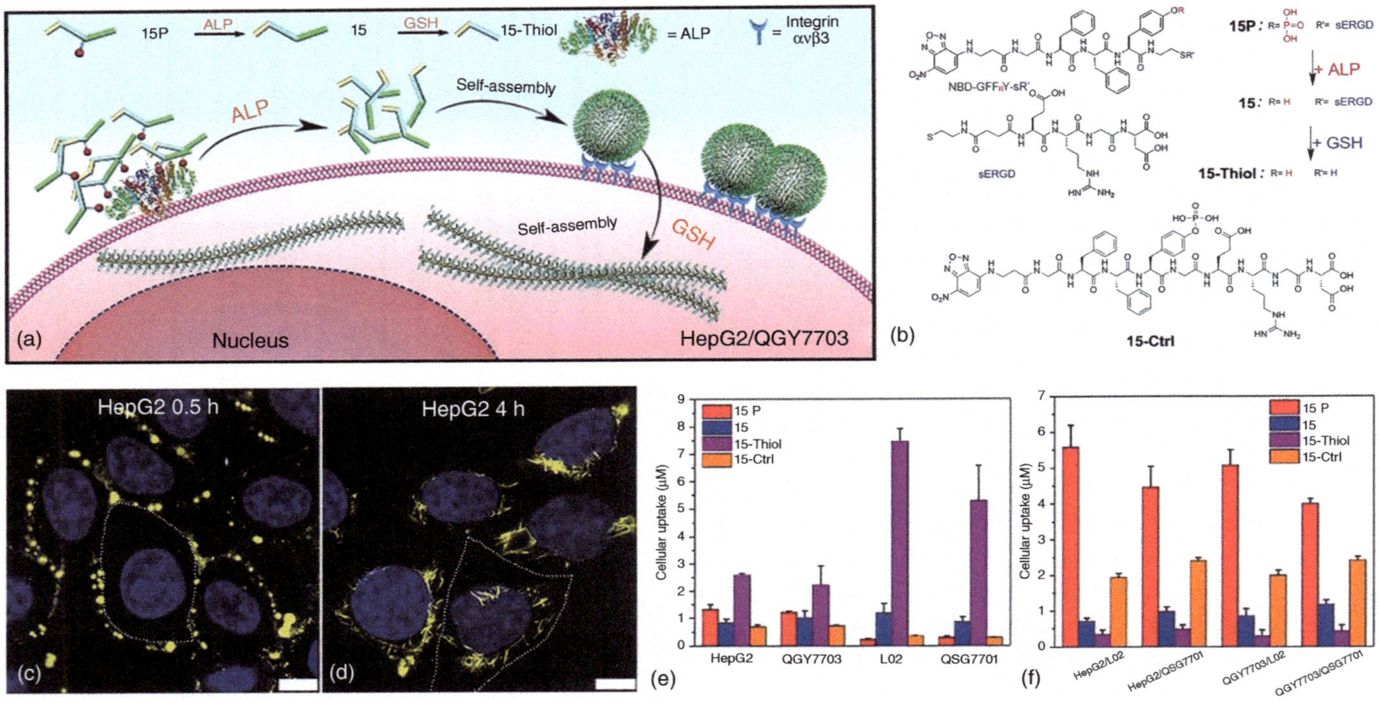

Figure 8.15 (a) Proposed mode of the tandem molecular self-assembly in the extra- and intracellular environment of liver cancer cells. (b) Chemical structures of **15P**, **15**, **15-Thiol**, and **15-Ctrl**, and schematic illustration of the conversion of **15P** into **15** by phosphatase (ALP) and then of **15** into **15-Ctrl** by glutathione (GSH). Merged confocal laser scanning microscopy images (blue fluorescence from Hoechst 33342 and yellow fluorescence from NBD represent the nucleus and NBD peptide, respectively) of HepG2 cells incubated with **15P** (200 μm) for (c) 0.5 hour and (d) 4 hours. Scale bars: 10 mm. The white dashed line indicates the boundary of a cell. (e) Cellular uptake and (f) cellular uptake ratios for **15P**, **15**, **15-Thiol**, and **15-Ctrl** by HepG2, QGY7703, L02, and QSG7701 cells at the four hours time point. Peptide concentration = 200 μm, mean ± SD, $N = 3$. Source: Zhan J, et al. (2018), [41], Figure 02, Pg 02/ with permission of Wiley-VCH.

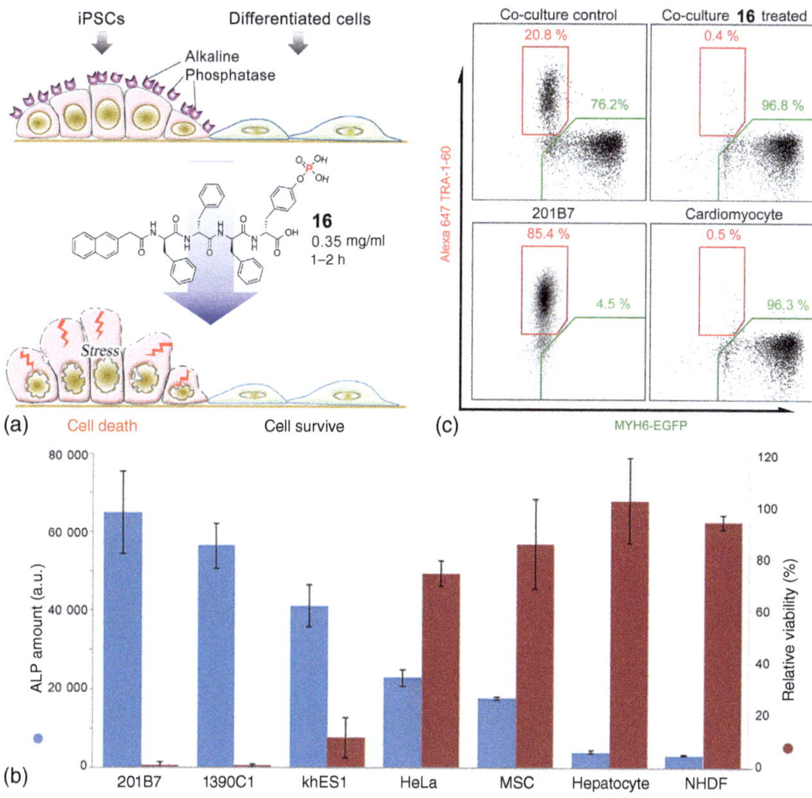

Figure 8.16 (a) Illustration of the possible mechanism by which **16** induces iPSC-selective cell death. (b) Alkaline phosphatase expression (antibody staining) and the viability (live cell count) after one hour treatment of **16** at 400 mM on different types of cells (iPSCs; 201B7 and 1390C1, ESCs; khES1, mesenchymal stem cells [MSCs]). For the viability test, the data are presented as the mean ± SD; $n = 3$. For the ALP amount, the data are presented as the mean ± SE; $n = 3$. (c) Flow cytometry analysis of co-cultured 201B7 cells and 201B7-derived MHY6-EGFP-expressing cardiomyocytes with or without one hour incubation with 400 mM **16**. The total seeding density was 5.3×10^4 cells/cm^2; the seeding ratio was 1 (201B7): 9 (cardiomyocytes). Source: From Kuang et al. [45] / with permission from Elsevier.

flow cytometry analysis showed that the **16**-treated co-culture contained only 0.4% 201B7 cells, while the untreated co-culture control contained 20.8% 201B7 cells (Figure 8.16c). After confirming that **16** selectively eliminates residual iPSCs, the researcher next transplanted co-cultures (treated or untreated with **16**) into immunodeficient (SCID) mice. Three months after transplantation, no teratoma was observed in **16**-treated co-culture injection groups, while seven of the eight untreated co-culture injections showed teratoma. Demonstrating the use of EISA to selectively remove iPSCs from a mixed culture with differentiated cells, this work also confirms the excellent selectivity of EISA for targeting ALP-overexpressing cancer cells.

As proteolytic enzymes, matrix metalloproteinases (MMPs) play important roles in tumor invasion [46] and various cancer cells overexpress and secrete matrix

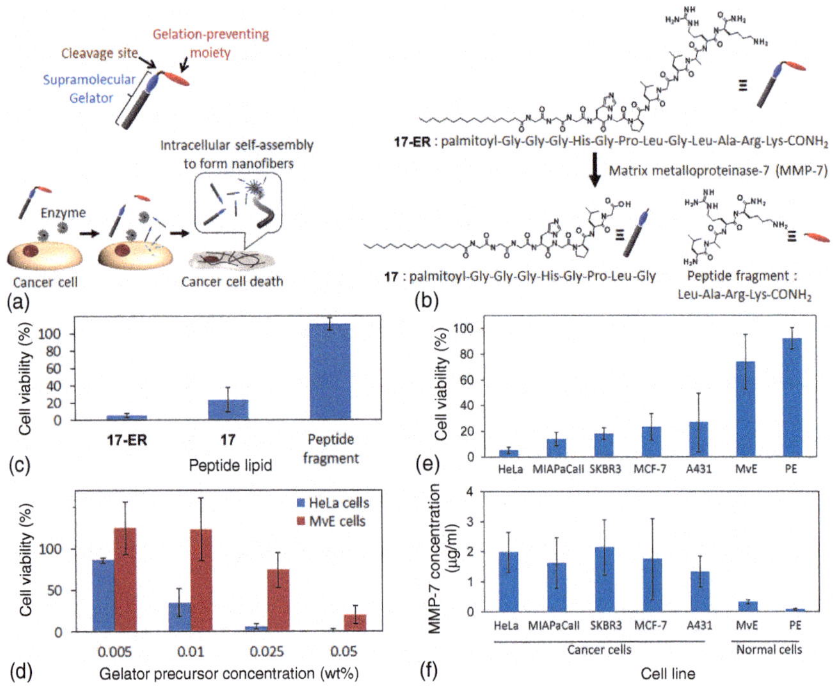

Figure 8.17 (a) Cancer cell death induced by molecular self-assembly of an enzyme-responsive supramolecular gelator. (b) Molecular structures of *N*-palmitoyl-Gly-Gly-Gly-His-Gly-Pro-Leu-Gly-Leu-Ala-Arg-Lys-CONH$_2$ (**17-ER**), *N*-palmitoylGly-Gly-Gly-His-Gly-Pro-Leu-Gly [17], and Leu-Ala-Arg-Lys-CONH$_2$ (Peptide fragment). (c) Effect of peptide lipids and a peptide (0.025 wt%) on the viability of HeLa cells. (d) Effect of **17-ER** concentration on the cell viability. MvE cells represent primary normal human dermal microvascular endothelial cells. Error bars represent standard deviations in 6 replicates for each sample. (e) Viability assays of cancer cells and normal human cells after incubation with **17-ER** (0.025 wt%). (f) MMP-7 concentration in the culture media after culturing the cells. PE represents primary human pancreatic epithelial cells. Source: From Tanaka et al. [47] / with permission from American Chemical Society.

metalloproteinase-7 (MMP-7). Maruyama and coworkers reported a precursor peptide-lipid (**17-ER**), which converts into supramolecular hydrogelator **17** after being hydrolyzed by MMP-7 (Figure 8.17b). The self-assemblies of **17** in cells impair cellular function and induce the death of cancer cells (Figure 8.17a) [47]. Incubation with **17-ER** or **17** results in <5.3% or <24% viability of HeLa cells, respectively, while the peptide fragment exhibits no cytotoxicity (Figure 8.17c). Viability assays show that **17-ER** exhibits significant higher cytotoxicity against cancer cells (HeLa cells) than normal cells (MvE cells) (Figure 8.17d), and the further examination on various cancer cells and normal cells also indicates that **17-ER** exhibits cytotoxicity to cancer cells while having a mild effect on normal cells (Figure 8.17e). The authors determined the MMP-7 concentration in the culture medium of these cells, and the result implies that cancer cells secrete significantly more MMP-7 than normal cells (Figure 8.17f), which indicates that the cytotoxicity of **17-ER** may correlate with the amount of MMP-7 secreted by cells. This work is another example of using EISA for anticancer applications.

Recently, Ulijn, Pires, and coworkers reported a precursor **18P** (Figure 8.18a), which selectively decreases the metabolic activity of Saos2 cells by forming the nanonet around the cancer cells (Figure 8.18b) [48]. Figure 8.18c–e implies that the metabolic activity of Saos2 cells decreases significantly after **18P**-treatment, while **18P** shows almost no effect on ATDC5 cells, and the addition of Pierce phosphatase inhibitor can remove the affect by **18P**. With brightfield microscopy, the authors observed a layer of gel covering the surface of the Saos2 cells cultured in the presence of **18P** (Figure 8.18f,g). SEM also showed a fibrous network in the pericellular space of Saos2 cells after being incubated with **18P** (Figure 8.18h,i). This work is an example for inhibition of metabolic activity by EISA, it may be particularly useful for developing anticancer strategies.

8.4 Future Perspectives

The research on supramolecular self-assembly for cancer diagnosis and treatment over the past two decades has furthered the fundamental understanding on how to develop new approaches for cancer diagnosis and treatment. A unique feature of supramolecular assemblies is that they exhibit emergent properties that can be modulated to improve the efficacy and the selectivity of anticancer nanomedicine. With the advantages mentioned in this chapter, supramolecular self-assembly is promised to be a powerful approach for cancer diagnosis and treatment. For example, the self-assemblies of probes enhance some imaging signals, such as MRI [49–52] and photoacoustic imaging [53, 54]; the self-assemblies of drugs lead to the accumulation of drugs in cancer cells [37, 55]; the selective self-assembles in cancer cells or tumors improve the selectivity of both diagnosis and treatment [56–58]. Moreover, intracellular self-assemblies can also interact with organelle, block cellular pathways, and inhibit cancer cells. Using enzymes that overexpress by cancer cell for EISA represents a fundamentally new way for developing cancer therapy. Differing from the traditional chemotherapeutic agents, the ESIA generated assemblies selectively accumulate in cancer cells, which reduce the side effects, enable multiple targeting, and reduce drug resistance [37, 39, 55]. Like any other approaches, there are still challenges to meet. While supramolecular assemblies exhibit anticancer activities, the mechanism of the actions is less understood. This drawback is partly resulted from the lack of structural and kinetic elucidation of the assemblies in cells and in animals. Currently, the concentration of EISA substrates for inhibiting cancer cells or tumors, still is relatively high, except for a few examples [40, 59, 60]. Future solutions may need to combine supramolecular assembly with other anticancer drugs, as recently demonstrated by Yang and coworkers [59] Overall, supramolecular assembly offer a versatile platform for the development of multifunctional therapeutics. With increasing research on supramolecular assemblies, we believe that they may lead to solutions of unsolved problems in cancer diagnosis and treatment.

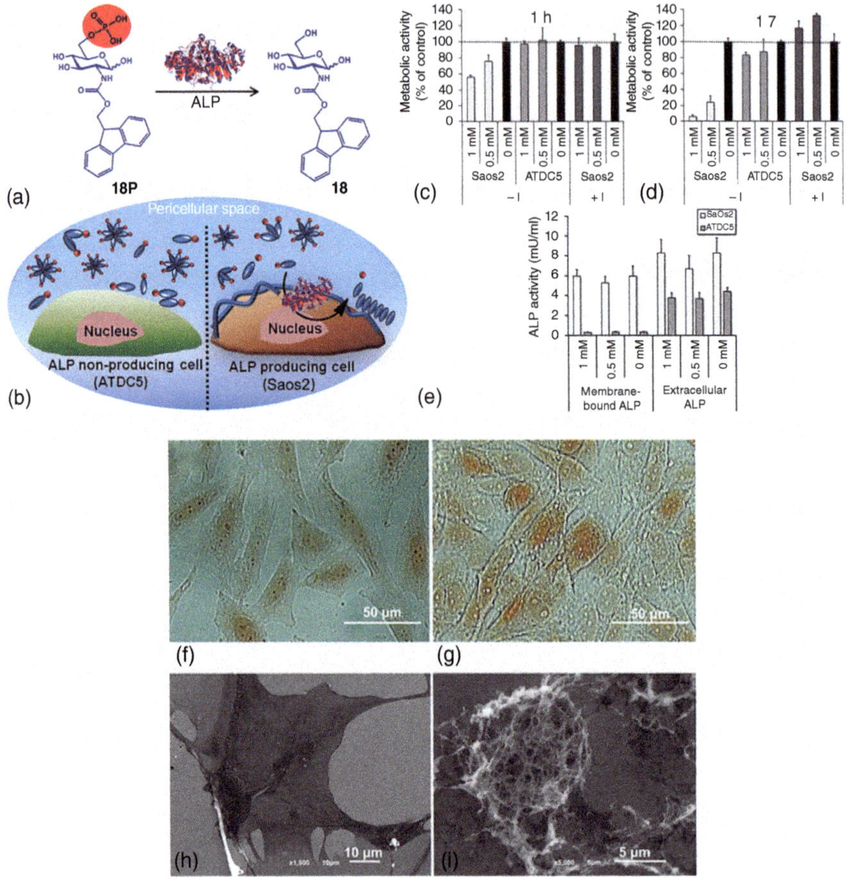

Figure 8.18 (a) Illustration of enzymatic transformation of **18P** to **18**. (b) *In situ* biocatalytic self-assembly. Metabolic activity of Saos2 and ATDC5 monolayer cultures in the presence of different concentrations of **18P** (control 0, 0.5, and 1 mM), without (−I) and with (+I) phosphatase inhibitor. Values refer to (c) one hour and (d) seven hours of cell culture. (e) Activity of the membrane bound and extracellular ALP in the Saos2 and ATDC5 cell cultures as a function of the concentration of **18P**. Quantification at seven hours of cell culture. (f and g) Brightfield and (h and i) SEM images of Saos2 cells, cultured during seven hours, in the (f and h) absence and (g and h) presence of **18P** (0.5 mM). Source: Pires, R. A., et al. (2015), [48], Figure 04, Pg 05/ with permission of American Chemical Society.

References

1 Whitesides, G., Mathias, J., and Seto, C. (1991). Molecular self-assembly and nanochemistry: a chemical strategy for the synthesis of nanostructures. *Science* 254 (5036): 1312–1319.

2 Du, X., Zhou, J., Shi, J., and Xu, B. (2015). Supramolecular hydrogelators and hydrogels: from soft matter to molecular biomaterials. *Chem. Rev.* 115 (24): 13165–13307.

3 Liu, H.W., Chen, L., Xu, C. et al. (2018). Recent progresses in small-molecule enzymatic fluorescent probes for cancer imaging. *Chem. Soc. Rev.* 47 (18): 7140–7180.

4 Sokolov, K., Follen, M., and Richards-Kortum, R. (2002). Optical spectroscopy for detection of neoplasia. *Curr. Opin. Chem. Biol.* 6 (5): 651–658.

5 Licha, K. and Olbrich, C. (2005). Optical imaging in drug discovery and diagnostic applications. *Adv. Drug Delivery Rev.* 57 (8): 1087–1108.

6 Gao, Y., Shi, J., Yuan, D., and Xu, B. (2012). Imaging enzyme-triggered self-assembly of small molecules inside live cells. *Nat. Commun.* 3: 1033.

7 Pike, L.J. (2003). Lipid rafts: bringing order to chaos. *J. Lipid Res.* 44 (4): 655–667.

8 Wang, H., Feng, Z., Del Signore, S.J. et al. (2018). Active probes for imaging membrane dynamics of live cells with high spatial and temporal resolution over extended time scales and areas. *J. Am. Chem. Soc.* 140 (10): 3505–3509.

9 Hai, Z., Li, J., Wu, J. et al. (2017). Alkaline phosphatase-triggered simultaneous hydrogelation and chemiluminescence. *J. Am. Chem. Soc.* 139 (3): 1041–1044.

10 Palner, M., Pu, K., Shao, S., and Rao, J. (2015). Semiconducting polymer nanoparticles with persistent near-infrared luminescence for in vivo optical imaging. *Angew. Chem. Int. Ed.* 54 (39): 11477–11480.

11 Cao, C.Y., Shen, Y.Y., Wang, J.D. et al. (2013). Controlled intracellular self-assembly of gadolinium nanoparticles as smart molecular MR contrast agents. *Sci. Rep.* 3: 1024.

12 Terreno, E., Castelli, D.D., Viale, A., and Aime, S. (2010). Challenges for molecular magnetic resonance imaging. *Chem. Rev.* 110 (5): 3019–3042.

13 Liang, G., Ren, H., and Rao, J. (2010). A biocompatible condensation reaction for controlled assembly of nanostructures in living cells. *Nat. Chem.* 2 (1): 54–60.

14 Yuan, Y. and Liang, G. (2014). A biocompatible, highly efficient click reaction and its applications. *Org. Biomol. Chem.* 12 (6): 865–871.

15 Ren, H., Xiao, F., Zhan, K. et al. (2009). A biocompatible condensation reaction for the labeling of terminal cysteine residues on proteins. *Angew. Chem. Int. Ed.* 48 (51): 9658–9662.

16 Liang, G., Ronald, J., Chen, Y. et al. (2011). Controlled self-assembling of gadolinium nanoparticles as smart molecular magnetic resonance imaging contrast agents. *Angew. Chem. Int. Ed.* 50 (28): 6283–6286.

17 Hai, Z., Ni, Y., Saimi, D. et al. (2019). γ-glutamyltranspeptidase-triggered intracellular gadolinium nanoparticle formation enhances the T_2-weighted MR contrast of tumor. *Nano Lett.* 19 (4): 2428–2433.

18 Yuan, Y., Ding, Z., Qian, J. et al. (2016). Casp3/7-instructed intracellular aggregation of Fe_3O_4 nanoparticles enhances T_2 MR imaging of tumor apoptosis. *Nano Lett.* 16 (4): 2686–2691.

19 Pu, K., Shuhendler, A.J., Jokerst, J.V. et al. (2014). Semiconducting polymer nanoparticles as photoacoustic molecular imaging probes in living mice. *Nat. Nanotechnol.* 9 (3): 233–239.

20 Pu, K., Mei, J., Jokerst, J.V. et al. (2015). Diketopyrrolopyrrole-based semiconducting polymer nanoparticles for in vivo photoacoustic imaging. *Adv. Mater.* 27 (35): 5184–5190.

21 Yang, Z.M., Xu, K.M., Guo, Z.F. et al. (2007). Intracellular enzymatic formation of nanofibers results in hydrogelation and regulated cell death. *Adv. Mater.* 19 (20): 3152–3156.

22 Gao, Y., Kuang, Y., Guo, Z.-F. et al. (2009). Enzyme-instructed molecular self-assembly confers nanofibers and a supramolecular hydrogel of taxol derivative. *J. Am. Chem. Soc.* 131 (38): 13576–13577.

23 Kuang, Y., Long, M.J., Zhou, J. et al. (2014). Prion-like nanofibrils of small molecules (PriSM) selectively inhibit cancer cells by impeding cytoskeleton dynamics. *J. Biol. Chem.* 289 (42): 29208–29218.

24 Kuang, Y. and Xu, B. (2013). Disruption of the dynamics of microtubules and selective inhibition of glioblastoma cells by nanofibers of small hydrophobic molecules. *Angew. Chem. Int. Ed.* 52 (27): 6944–6948.

25 Kim, B.J., Yang, D., and Xu, B. (2020). Emerging applications of supramolecular peptide assemblies. *Trends Chem.* 2: 71–83.

26 Shy, A.N., Kim, B.J., and Xu, B. (2019). Enzymatic noncovalent synthesis of supramolecular soft matter for biomedical applications. *Matter* 1 (5): 1127–1147.

27 Wang, H., Feng, Z., Yang, C. et al. (2019). Unraveling the cellular mechanism of assembling cholesterols for selective cancer cell death. *Mol. Cancer Res.* 17 (4): 907–917.

28 Qin, S.Y., Zhang, A.Q., Cheng, S.X. et al. (2017). Drug self-delivery systems for cancer therapy. *Biomaterials* 112: 234–247.

29 Sledge, G.W. Jr., Loehrer, P.J. Sr., Roth, B.J., and Einhorn, L.H. (1988). Cisplatin as first-line therapy for metastatic breast cancer. *J. Clin. Oncol.* 6 (12): 1811–1814.

30 Pizzolato, J.F. and Saltz, L.B. (2003). The camptothecins. *Lancet* 361 (9376): 2235–2242.

31 Cai, Y., Shen, H., Zhan, J. et al. (2017). Supramolecular "Trojan Horse" for nuclear delivery of dual anticancer drugs. *J. Am. Chem. Soc.* 139 (8): 2876–2879.

32 He, H., Wang, J., Wang, H. et al. (2018). Enzymatic cleavage of branched peptides for targeting mitochondria. *J. Am. Chem. Soc.* 140 (4): 1215–1218.

33 Wu, Q., He, Z., Wang, X. et al. (2019). Cascade enzymes within self-assembled hybrid nanogel mimicked neutrophil lysosomes for singlet oxygen elevated cancer therapy. *Nat. Commun.* 10 (1): 240.

34 Kuang, Y., Shi, J., Li, J. et al. (2014). Pericellular hydrogel/nanonets inhibit cancer cells. *Angew. Chem. Int. Ed.* 53 (31): 8104–8107.

35 Zhou, J. and Xu, B. (2015). Enzyme-instructed self-assembly: a multistep process for potential cancer therapy. *Bioconjugate Chem.* 26 (6): 987–999.

36 Li, J., Kuang, Y., Shi, J. et al. (2015). Enzyme-instructed intracellular molecular self-assembly to boost activity of cisplatin against drug-resistant ovarian cancer cells. *Angew. Chem. Int. Ed.* 54 (45): 13307–13311.

37 Wang, H., Feng, Z., Wang, Y. et al. (2016). Integrating enzymatic self-assembly and mitochondria targeting for selectively killing cancer cells without acquired drug resistance. *J. Am. Chem. Soc.* 138 (49): 16046–16055.

38 Feng, Z., Wang, H., Wang, S. et al. (2018). Enzymatic assemblies disrupt the membrane and target endoplasmic reticulum for selective cancer cell death. *J. Am. Chem. Soc.* 140 (30): 9566–9573.

39 Wang, H., Feng, Z., Wu, D. et al. (2016). Enzyme-regulated supramolecular assemblies of cholesterol conjugates against drug-resistant ovarian cancer cells. *J. Am. Chem. Soc.* 138 (34): 10758–10761.

40 Feng, Z., Han, X., Wang, H. et al. (2019). Enzyme-instructed peptide assemblies selectively inhibit bone tumors. *Chem* 5 (9): 2442–2449.

41 Zhan, J., Cai, Y., He, S. et al. (2018). Tandem molecular self-assembly in liver cancer cells. *Angew. Chem. Int. Ed.* 57 (7): 1813–1816.

42 Yang, P.P., Luo, Q., Qi, G.B. et al. (2017). Host materials transformable in tumor microenvironment for homing theranostics. *Adv. Mater.* 29 (15): 1605869.

43 Takahashi, K. and Yamanaka, S. (2006). Induction of pluripotent stem cells from mouse embryonic and adult fibroblast cultures by defined factors. *Cell* 126 (4): 663–676.

44 Liu, Z., Tang, Y., Lu, S. et al. (2013). The tumourigenicity of iPS cells and their differentiated derivates. *J. Cell. Mol. Med.* 17 (6): 782–791.

45 Kuang, Y., Miki, K., Parr, C.J.C. et al. (2017). Efficient, selective removal of human pluripotent stem cells via ecto-alkaline phosphatase-mediated aggregation of synthetic peptides. *Cell Chem. Biol.* 24 (6): 685–94 e4.

46 Polette, M., Nawrocki-Raby, B., Gilles, C. et al. (2004). Tumour invasion and matrix metalloproteinases. *Crit. Rev. Oncol. Hematol.* 49 (3): 179–186.

47 Tanaka, A., Fukuoka, Y., Morimoto, Y. et al. (2015). Cancer cell death induced by the intracellular self-assembly of an enzyme-responsive supramolecular gelator. *J. Am. Chem. Soc.* 137 (2): 770–775.

48 Pires, R.A., Abul-Haija, Y.M., Costa, D.S. et al. (2015). Controlling cancer cell fate using localized biocatalytic self-assembly of an aromatic carbohydrate amphiphile. *J. Am. Chem. Soc.* 137 (2): 576–579.

49 Ding, Z., Sun, H., Ge, S. et al. (2019). Furin-controlled Fe_3O_4 nanoparticle aggregation and ^{19}F signal "turn-on" for precise MR imaging of tumors. *Adv. Funct. Mater.* 29 (43): 1903860.

50 Zheng, Z., Sun, H., Hu, C. et al. (2016). Using "on/off" ^{19}F NMR/magnetic resonance imaging signals to sense tyrosine kinase/phosphatase activity in vitro and in cell lysates. *Anal. Chem.* 88 (6): 3363–3368.

51 Yan, R., Hu, Y., Liu, F. et al. (2019). Activatable NIR fluorescence/MRI bimodal probes for in vivo imaging by enzyme-mediated fluorogenic reaction and self-assembly. *J. Am. Chem. Soc.* 141 (26): 10331–10341.

52 Yuan, Y., Zhang, J., Qi, X. et al. (2019). Furin-mediated intracellular self-assembly of olsalazine nanoparticles for enhanced magnetic resonance imaging and tumour therapy. *Nat. Mater.* 18 (12): 1376–1383.

53 Jiang, Y., Upputuri, P.K., Xie, C. et al. (2019). Metabolizable semiconducting polymer nanoparticles for second near-infrared photoacoustic imaging. *Adv. Mater.* 31 (11): e1808166.

54 Zhen, X., Zhang, J., Huang, J. et al. (2018). Macrotheranostic probe with disease-activated near-infrared fluorescence, photoacoustic, and photothermal signals for imaging-guided therapy. *Angew. Chem. Int. Ed.* 57 (26): 7804–7808.

55 Yuan, Y., Wang, L., Du, W. et al. (2015). Intracellular self-assembly of taxol nanoparticles for overcoming multidrug resistance. *Angew. Chem. Int. Ed.* 54 (33): 9700–9704.

56 Zhou, J., Du, X., Yamagata, N., and Xu, B. (2016). Enzyme-instructed self-assembly of small D-peptides as a multiple-step process for selectively killing cancer cells. *J. Am. Chem. Soc.* 138 (11): 3813–3823.

57 Wang, H., Feng, Z., Qin, Y. et al. (2018). Nucleopeptide assemblies selectively sequester ATP in cancer cells to increase the efficacy of doxorubicin. *Angew. Chem. Int. Ed.* 57 (18): 4931–4935.

58 Zhou, J., Du, X., Chen, X. et al. (2018). Enzymatic self-assembly confers exceptionally strong synergism with NF-κB targeting for selective necroptosis of cancer cells. *J. Am. Chem. Soc.* 140 (6): 2301–2308.

59 Liang, C., Yan, X., Zhang, R. et al. (2019). Enhanced cellular uptake and nuclear accumulation of drug-peptide nanomedicines prepared by enzyme-instructed self-assembly. *J. Controlled Release* 317: 109–117.

60 Feng, Z., Wang, H., Zhou, R. et al. (2017). Enzyme-instructed assembly and disassembly processes for targeting downregulation in cancer cells. *J. Am. Chem. Soc.* 139 (11): 3950–3953.

9

Polyzwitterionic Hydrogels as Wound Dressing Materials

Konstans Ruseva and Elena Vassileva

Sofia University, Department of Pharmaceutical and Applied Organic Chemistry, Laboratory on Structure and Properties of Polymers, Faculty of Chemistry and Pharmacy, 1 James Bourchier Blvd, Sofia 1164, Bulgaria

9.1 Polyzwitterions

9.1.1 General Structure and Properties

Polyzwitterions (PZIs) are polymers that possess both negatively and positively charged functional groups in their pendant chains resulting into overall charge neutrality. The cationic group is usually ammonium, phosphonium, pyridinium, or imidazolium group, while the anionic moiety is commonly carboxylate, sulfonate, or phosphate group. The zwitterionic structure is a well-known motif from living nature, e.g. the phospholipids polar heads are built from positively charged ammonium groups covalently bonded to phosphate anions; the amino acid betaine has quaternary ammonium cation and negatively charged carboxylic groups. Thus, PZI are often referred to as biomimetic materials and this is considered to be the ground for their inherent biocompatibility.

The zwitterionic structure drives the formation of specific dipole–dipole self-assemblies, called zip clusters (Figure 9.1a) that are salt-responsive [1]. Upon addition of low-molecular weight salts (LMSs), PZI assemblies increase their swelling degree, i.e. expand in volume and gain weight, and this effect is increasing with the LMS concentration [2]. Such salt-philic behavior is due to the screening effect that LMS ions have on the zip clusters that play the role of physical junctions: their initial disintegration causes decrease in the physical network density, i.e. the swelling ability increases, ultimately leading to their disintegration and liberating the zwitterionic moieties (Figure 9.1b) [1].

9.1.2 Nonfouling Properties

Recently, PZIs have attracted an attention with their excellent nonfouling performance, which made them one of the strongest competitors of poly(ethylene glycols) (PEGs) – the golden standard in the field of nonfouling biomaterials. The nonfouling materials minimize or prevent the nonspecific protein adsorption onto their

Multifunctional Hydrogels for Biomedical Applications, First Edition.
Edited by Ricardo A. Pires, Iva Pashkuleva, and Rui L. Reis.

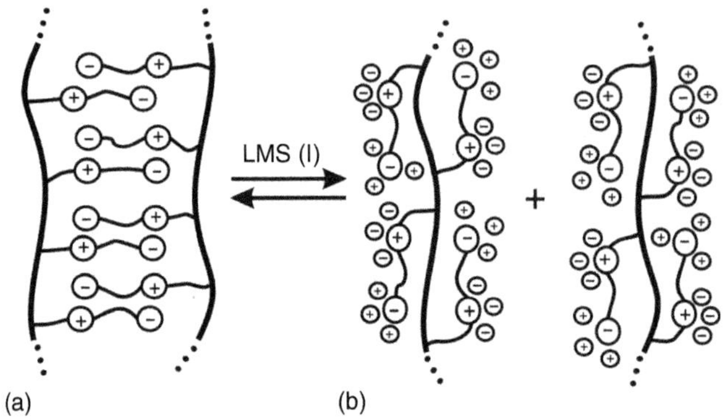

Figure 9.1 (a) Dipole–dipole self-assemblies of oppositely oriented dipoles (zip clusters) of polyzwitterions (PZI) and (b) disintegration of the zip clusters upon addition of low-molecular weight salt (LMS) into PZI aqueous solutions or hydrogels. Source: Georgiev et al. [1]/with Permission from American Chemical Society.

surfaces, which is the first stage of many complex biological processes such as cell attachment, bacterial biofilm formation, and marine biofouling. The very low non-specific protein adsorption of PZI (e.g. for plasma proteins it could be in the range of 1.65 ng/cm^2) [3] is explained by their affinity to water: molecule dynamics simulations have shown that the zwitterionic moieties strongly bind water molecules by electrostatic interactions. In contrast, the hydrophilic and neutral PEG chains interact with water molecules via hydrogen bonding [4, 5]. PZIs such as polycarboxybetaines (PCBs), polyphosphobetaines (PPBs), and polysulfobetaines (PSBs) bind water much tighter than PEGs, especially in the low water/polymer range. At stoichiometric water–polymer ratios, i.e. the added water is equal or close to the maximum available sites for binding on polymer chains, a hydrated monolayer is formed. In this fully hydrated layer, each PEG monomeric unit binds one water molecule, while one zwitterionic (e.g. sulfobetaine) moiety can bind 7–8 molecules of water [4]. When water is in excess, each zwitterionic moiety is isolated from the others by structured hydration shell, where the additional water acts just like free/bulk water. Thus, the unbound water molecules in PZI solutions or hydrogels are more mobile than those in PEG.

The nonfouling behavior of PZI materials is due to this high water affinity expressed by the formation of protective water layer at the water–material interface. The proteins bounce at this layer, avoiding a direct contact with the material [6]. Of note, this process does not affect the proteins' conformation contrary to the protein adsorption during which the protein conformation is changed, e.g. by releasing water molecule from its own hydration layer. The ability of PZI to prevent such triggering defines the wide range of biomedical applications of PZI.

9.2 Wound Management and Wound Dressings

Wound management is one of the most challenging and widely spread health care problem: 34% of the population suffer one or more wounds, of which 74% are being treated in community health care and 21% in acute care [7]. Thus, 27%–50% of acute hospital beds are occupied by patients with a wound – a phenomenon often called "Silent Epidemic" and whose management is estimated to account for 3% of all health care expenditure and covers spending on dressings, full-time nurses, and hospitalization.

Wounds can be classified depending on their cause and healing. Acute wounds can have different cause, e.g. surgical intervention, injury, or burns and they heal by a normal wound healing process, i.e. at rate that is expectable and predictable. Chronic wounds, such as leg ulcers, diabetic foot ulcers, and pressure ulcers, are usually associated with extrinsic factors (pressure, shear, and infection) or underlying conditions (diabetes and vascular diseases) and heal at slower rate [8]. While acute wounds are relatively inexpensive to manage, costs can increase tremendously in the case of chronic ones [8].

The wound management can be improved by (i) reducing healing time, (ii) optimizing the wound dressing (e.g. efficacy and change frequency), and (iii) preventing complications such as wound infection. On average, wound dressings are changed about three times per week, but some of the wounds (~20%) require daily change. Frequent dressing change increases the treatment costs and the risk of infections and complications. Therefore, many efforts are devoted to the improvement and development of wound dressing. The main requirements for wound dressing include but are not limited to:

- effective take up of the excess wound exudates and toxins from the wound surface;
- preserve the wound humidity because wound drying hampers the healing process;
- provide thermal and mechanical insulation of the wound;
- allow a gaseous exchange;
- provide protection against secondary infection;
- be nontoxic;
- be easily removable without damaging the newly formed tissue;
- be transparent to allow monitoring of the wound without need for dressing change;
- be flexible to provide efficient wound coverage that does not allow formation of niches for bacteria growth;
- possess antibiofouling and antibacterial functionality to prevent bacterial biofilm formation.

PZIs meet most of these requirements and their potential for the wound management will be discussed in this chapter.

9.3 PZIs as Dressings Materials for Acute Wounds

9.3.1 Polycarboxybetaines (PCBs)

The first attempt to use PZI-based material for wound management was reported by Fujishita et al. [9] who have studied the effect of a thin film of the random copolymer of carboxybetaine (1-carboxy-*N,N*-dimethyl-*N*-(2-methacryloyloxyethyl) methanaminium inner salt) (CMB, 30 mol%) and *n*-butyl methacrylate (BMA) (Figure 9.2a) on the healing of a full-thickness excisional and incisional wounds in hairless rats.

BMA was chosen as a co-monomer of CMB, because the copolymer had film-forming characteristics and the obtained coatings were stable in an aqueous environment [9]. In fact, BMA forms hydrophobic domains playing the role of physical junctions which make the physically cross-linked polymer stable in water. These copolymers have an excellent blood compatibility expressed by the suppression of platelet adhesion and complement activation on the polymer surface [10]. The poly(CMB-r-BMA) film significantly enhanced wound closure and complete healing of a full-thickness excisional wound when compared to the effect of poly(*n*-butyl methacrylate) (PBMA) and poly(ethylene terephthalate) (PET) films.

Their effect on the wound healing was compared to Tegaderm®, a commercially available wound dressing, consisting of thin polyurethane membrane coated with a layer of an acrylic adhesive. The poly(CMB-r-BMA) film significantly enhanced wound closure as compared to Tegaderm after day 7, and the time for achievement of complete healing was 1.8 day shorter for the copolymer than for the commercial control ($p < 0.05$). This effect of the poly(CMB-r-BMA) on the wound healing is comparable to the results obtained with medicines as basic fibroblast growth factor (bFGF), povidone iodine, lysozyme chloride ointment, solcoseryl ointment, and tocoretinate ointment, which are known to enhance the wound healing and to shorten the time for complete healing by ~two days. Poly(CMB-r-BMA) film also showed the lowest protein adsorption and amount of adherent neutrophiles as compared to PBMA,

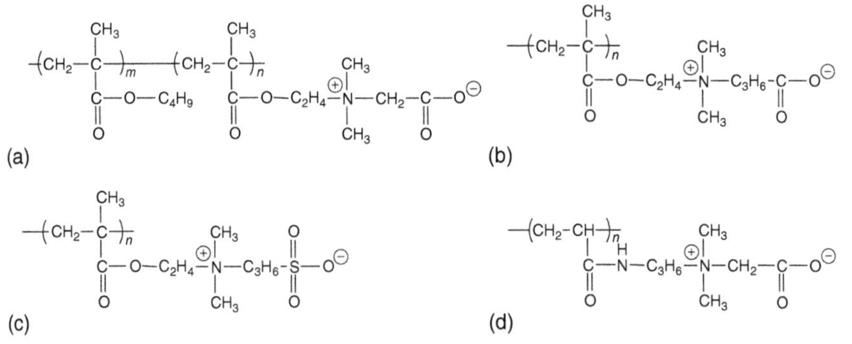

Figure 9.2 Chemical structure of (a) poly(carboxybetaine-*co*-butyl methacrylate) (poly(CMB-r-BMA)), (b) poly(carboxybetaine-*co*-methyl methacrylate) copolymer (CBMA), (c) poly(sulfobetaine methacrylate) (PSBMA), and (d) poly(carboxybetaine acrylamide) (PCBAA).

PET, and Tegaderm. This property of poly(CMB-r-BMA) is important for the wound healing, because cells such as platelets, macrophages, neutrophiles, lymphocytes, and proteins (bFGF, epidermal growth factor [EGF], platelet derived growth factor [PDGF], and transforming growth factor-β [TGF-b]) are maintained in the wound region covered with the copolymer and thus, the wound healing is more efficient.

Unnithan et al. [11] have prepared poly(carboxybetaine-co-methyl methacrylate) copolymer (CBMA, Figure 9.2b) nanomembranes via electrospinning for wound dressing application. As in the case of poly(CMB-r-BMA), the hydrophobic co-monomer, methyl methacrylate, forms physical network that makes the hydrogel stable in water. Electrospunned CBMA mats consisted in smooth and flexible nanofibers with 800–900 nm diameters and showed very low cell attachment. Lack of cell attachment is one of the requirements for the wound dressing as dressing change/removal must neither damage the regenerating skin layer nor cause pain to the patient. The platelet attachments on the surface of the CBMA mats was also minimal indicating low probability of blood clots formation, and hence, the CBMA wound dressings can be applied on large-area wounds. The CBMA nanofiber membranes were able to inhibit both Gram-positive and Gram-negative bacterial strains growth. When applied as dressings to incisional wounds in Wistar rats, the CBMA mats promoted faster healing than the control (bare wound) in the first and second weeks and faster wound closure after three weeks (Figure 9.3). Other benefits of the application of CBMA dressings were the presence of densely packed keratinocytes in the epidermis, significant vascularization after three weeks; the granulation layer thickness was comparable to that of nonwounded skin, indicating a perfect healing nature.

Nejad et al. [12] prepared poly(sulfobetaine methacrylate) (PSBMA, Figure 9.2c) hydrogels as wound dressing materials and incorporated silver nanoparticle (AgNPs) to impart antimicrobial functionality. In phosphate-buffered saline (PBS), 46 μg/l silver was released from PSBMA–AgNPs hydrogel ($5 \times 5\,cm^2$), which is comparable with SilvaSorb – a Ag releasing wound dressing, which is used currently in

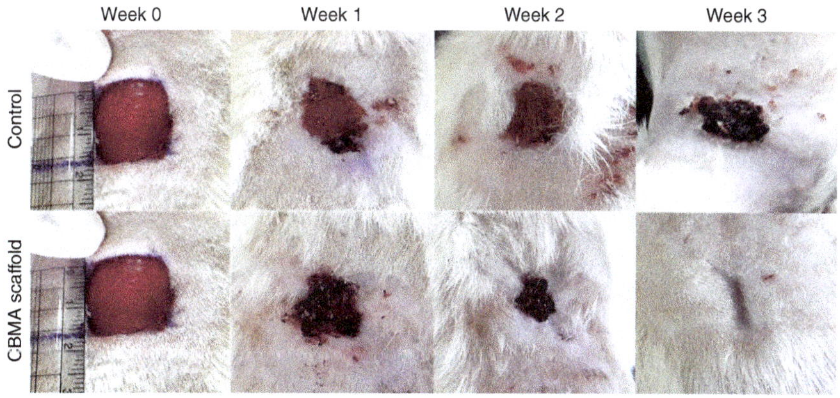

Figure 9.3 Photographs of the *in vivo* wound healing study. Source: Unnithan, A. R., et al. (2016), [11], Figure 06, Pg 07 / with permission of from ELSEVIER.

the clinics. Because the Ag cytotoxic effect is observed when silver concentration is above 58 μg/l, these PSBMA–AgNPs nanocomposite hydrogels are noncytotoxic. Their antibacterial activity was tested toward *Escherichia coli*, *Staphylococcus aureus*, and *Pseudomonas aeruginosa*, and the results showed that the hydrogels inhibited the bacterial growth and also were able to kill bacteria [12]. The wound healing efficiency of the PSBMA–AgNPs hydrogels was tested *in vivo* and its performance was compared to neat PSBMA hydrogels, using bare wounds as a control. The wound size reduction after 15 days was 59%, 80% ,and 98%, respectively, for control, PSBMA, and PSBMA–AgNPs hydrogels. Moreover, it was also reported that no sign of inflammation was observed for the wounds healed with PSBMA–AgNPs hydrogels. The quality of the granulation tissue, vascularization, big rete pegs, and keratinocyte restoration in wounds treated with PSBMA–AgNPs were also significantly improved when compared to other groups. Thus, PSBMA–AgNPs hydrogels showed several benefits, namely (i) noncytotoxicity and biocompatibility, (ii) strong antibiofouling properties, (iii) antibacterial performance via Ag release, and (iv) maintenance of moist wound environment while also allowing for a gaseous exchange [12].

Zhu et al. applied poly(carboxybetaine acrylamide) (PCBAA, Figure 9.2d) and PSBMA hydrogels as wound dressings and compared the *in vivo* performance with poly(2-hydroxyethyl methacrylate) (PHEMA) hydrogels and the commercial product DuoDerm for treating third degree burn – a common and highly challenging skin wound [13]. DuoDerm is a hydrocolloid wound dressing made of sodium carboxymethylcellulose, gelatin, pectin, and adhesive polymers which provides wound exudate absorbency, as well as it keeps a moist gel-like environment that helps promote wound autolytic debridement. The cotton gauze or bandage pads were coated with the PZI hydrogels and thus made them easy for handling and application. Both PZI-coated wound dressings healed better and faster as compared with the controls: on day 14, no wounds were observed in the PZI-treated wounds, whereas obvious skin lesions were still visible in the DuoDerm and PHEMA group. On day 21, wounds treated with PZI hydrogels were completely closed and covered with new epithelium, in contrast to the control groups. Moreover, the regenerated epithelial tissue treated with zwitterionic PCBAA hydrogel was more regular and smoother than PSBMA hydrogel. Thus, the zwitterionic hydrogels, especially PCBAA, significantly enhanced the recovery from burn wounds compared with the commercial dressing DuoDerm and non-zwitterionic PHEMA hydrogels. The authors suggested that the high water content and negligible cell interactions, which characterize zwitterionic hydrogels, create an optimal aqueous environment that facilitates the healing process. In addition, the high water content may promote autolytic debridement, stimulate collagen fiber deposition, and accelerate wound closure. With the highest water content, zwitterionic PCBAA hydrogels performed best.

The excellent performance of PCBAA hydrogels as burn wound dressing was complemented in a following study by imparting antibacterial functionality via AgNPs [14]. AgNPs and the PCBAA hydrogel were formed simultaneously via one-step *in situ* photopolymerization (Figure 9.4). The amount of formed

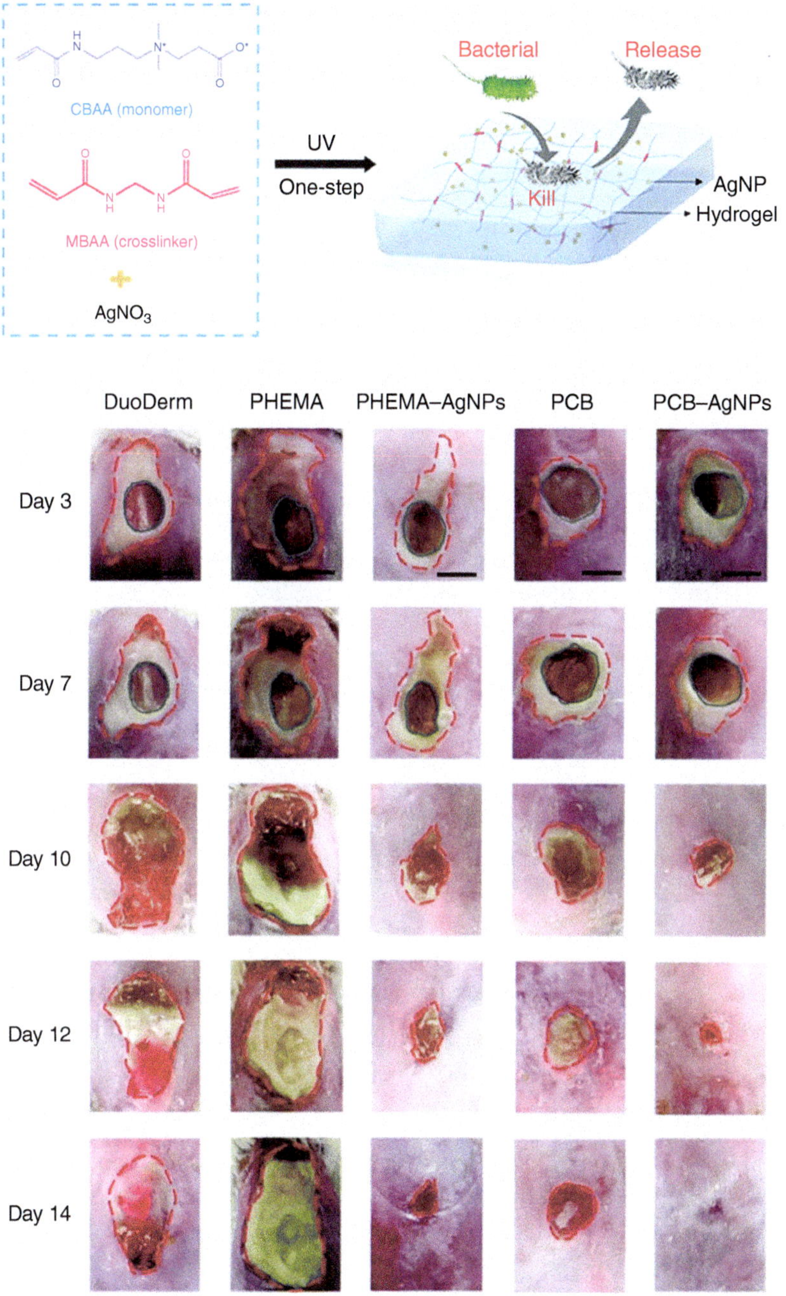

Figure 9.4 One-step synthetic route of zwitterionic PCBAA–AgNPs hydrogel and its effect on wound healing. Source: Zhu, Y., et al. (2017), [14], Figure 07, Pg 07 / with permission of Royal Society of Chemistry.

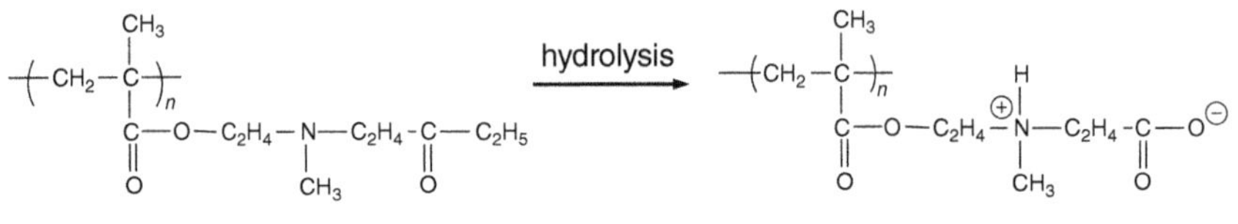

Figure 9.5 High resistance to protein adsorption and mammalian cell attachment is obtained through slow and controlled hydrolysis of carboxybetaine ester analog. Source: Ji et al. [15]/with permission from Royal Society of Chemistry.

AgNPs was followed by the color change of the hydrogels and controlled via the concentration of the $AgNO_3$ solution. The incorporation of AgNPs did not affect either the antifouling property of the hydrogels or its cytotoxicity. The cells viability in PCBAA–AgNPs hydrogels were >80%, i.e. close to that in neat PCBAA hydrogels. PCBAA–AgNPs exhibited the lowest adhesion of both *E. coli* and *S. aureus* strains, which was attributed to the synergistic effects of the antifouling property of PCBAA hydrogel and the antibacterial activity of AgNPs. A murine skin wound infection model was further used to evaluate the therapeutic effect of the PCBAA–AgNPs dressing against *S. aureus* infection. On day 14, the PCBAA–AgNPs closed the wound completely. Due to the lack of antibacterial ability, PHEMA and DuoDerm dressings did not kill *S. aureus* bacteria thus leading to deterioration and wound-size increase. Moreover, the results showed that PCBAA–AgNPs dressing enabled faster wound closure than the PHEMA–AgNPs, which was explained by the unique high water content and strong resistance to bacteria attachment of PZI hydrogels.

Ji et al. [15] have copolymerized carboxybetaine ester analog methacrylate (CB-ester) and poly(ethylene glycol) methacrylate (PEGMA) and used hexamethylene diisocyanate to cross-link them. The PCB hydrogel was obtained after hydrolysis (Figure 9.5) but did not show any antibacterial activity.

To impart antimicrobial functionality of PCB hydrogels, they were loaded with aspirin that is known for its *in vitro* inhibitory effect on the growth of both Gram-negative and Gram-positive bacteria [15]. The PCB hydrogel slowly released the drug and inhibited the microorganism growth exerting at the same time very low cytotoxicity.

9.3.2 Polysulfobetaines

Lalani and Liu [16] were the first to report the PSBMA (Figure 9.2c) application as nonadherent, superabsorbent, and antimicrobial wound dressings. Fibrous membranes were developed via "polymerization – electrospinning – photo-crosslinking" of PSBMA. The cross-linking after the electrospinning was needed to prevent PSBMA dissolution in water. The obtained membranes have a porous structure with randomly oriented nonwoven smooth fibers with an average diameter of 1110.4 ± 145.8 nm (Figure 9.6). They were stable in water and exhibited a water absorption (~353% w/w) that is much higher than the adsorption of the PSBMA hydrogel (81%). The membranes were resistant to protein adsorption and to cell

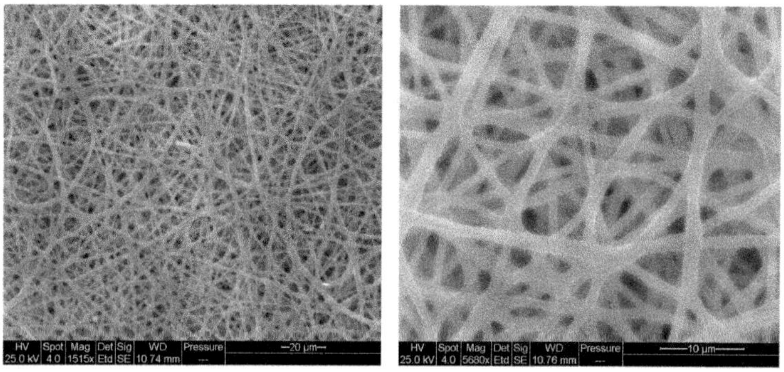

(a) (b)

Figure 9.6 Scanning electron microscopy (SEM) of PSBMA electrospun membranes. Source: Lalani, R., et al. (2012), [16], Figure 03, Pg 04 / with permission American Chemical Society.

attachment. They reduced the bacterial adhesion of the Gram-negative *P. aeruginosa* and the Gram-positive *Staphylococcus epidermidis* when compared with electrospun polycaprolactone (PCL) and tissue-cultured polystyrene (TCPS) [16]. These properties of PSBMA electrospun membranes ensure no-pain dressing change and prevention of wound infection.

Another beneficial characteristic of the developed PSBMA mats as wound dressing material is their ability to absorb high volumes of fluid from highly exudating wounds while keeping the wound hydrated due to the salt philicity of PZI: the wound exudate is a salt solution and the wound dressings based on polyelectrolytes, e.g. alginic acid, are not able to effectively absorb the exudate as they shrink in contact with LMS solutions. The PSBMA mats were also impregnated with Ag^+, and the microbicidal efficacy of the thus obtained PSBMA–Ag mat was demonstrated against both *S. epidermidis* and *P. aeruginosa*. In summary, the electrospun PSBMA mats are nonadherent, superabsorbent, and antimicrobial (when impregnated with Ag^+) wound dressings, which effectively manage wound exudate, support wound healing by maintaining moist wound environment, avoid patients' pain *in situ*, avoid the formation of new wounds upon dressing removal, and allow gas exchange. All these properties are beneficial for efficient wound healing.

Li et al. [17] proposed the application of zwitterionic shape memory polymers for wound dressings: sulfobetaine methacrylate (SBMA) can be copolymerized with 2,3-dihydroxypropyl methacrylate (DHMA) in the presence of boric acid as a cross-linking agent (Figure 9.7a). The shape recovery can be triggered either by heating the samples above T_g or through immersing the samples in water or placing them at humid environment to lower T_g below room temperature (Figure 9.7b). The materials with shape recovery are useful for wound management as they can be expanded temporary to fit easily at the right place of the wound site and then shape recovery-induced contraction is activated either by temperature or by moisture and the polymer seals the wound site (Figure 9.7b).

In practice, the shape memory wound dressing is activated by the wound exudate due to the salt philicity of PSBMA. In this way, besides strong contact and excellent

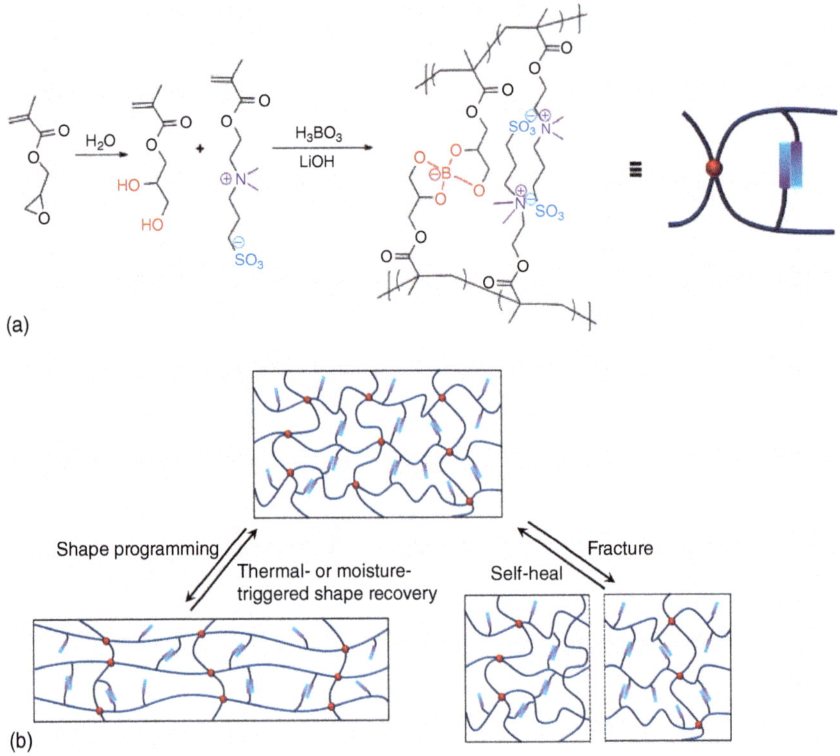

Figure 9.7 Schematic presentation of (a) the synthesis and molecular structure of poly(SBMA-co-DHMA) and (b) shape memory and self-healing processes of the prepared zwitterionic shape memory polymer. Source: Li et al. [17]/with permission from John Wiley & Sons.

anti-adhesion between the regenerated tissue and the dressing, the shape memory dressing can also keep a fresh environment at the wound site to promote wound healing and avoid infection. Poly(SBMA-*co*-DHMA) also possess self-healing ability provided by the presence of two dynamic cross-linking interactions in the system, namely boron ester bonds and electrostatic interactions of PSBMA (Figure 9.7b). Longer self-healing time and higher humidity enhance the self-healing process, and the mechanical properties of the self-healed samples are closed to the starting material.

Wu et al. [18] synthesized PSBMA hydrogels cross-linked with poly(ethylene glycol) dimethacrylate (PEGDMA) and applied them to full-thickness cutaneous wounds in mice. For sake of comparison, the authors prepared pure PEG and SBMA–PEG hydrogels with different SBMA–PEG ratio. All hydrogels were biocompatible and contained more than 90% water in their equilibrium state and demonstrated low protein adsorption (<10%) and excellent antifouling ability as compared to TCPS. When applied as wound dressings, the fastest closure of the full-thickness cutaneous wounds in mice was achieved with the neat PSBMA: on day 20, complete re-epithelialization was observed for PSBMA-treated wounds, whereas only partial re-epithelialization was achieved for PEG-treated wounds. The collagen deposition, another important indicator for wound healing, was significantly more pronounced for PSBMA-treated wounds as compared to the other groups. Moreover, collagen fibers in the PSBMA-treated group were thicker, better organized and aligned, with similar morphology to normal dermal skin, suggesting that PSBMA hydrogel application would avoid scar formation. The PSBMA hydrogel also showed two times higher cell proliferation on day 7, and these proliferating cells are expected to further secret a variety of growth factors to promote the further full-thickness wound healing.

Neovascularization and angiogenesis are crucial events in wound healing, especially for the closure of chronic wounds. The PSBMA hydrogel presented much more vasculatures and more and larger newly formed blood vessels than the PEG hydrogel. These data indicate that the presence of PSBMA promotes the recruitment of endothelial cells to the wound area and enhances the vessel growth for wound healing. At the same time, during the wound healing process, PSBMA hydrogels decreased the pro-inflammatory factors (tumor necrosis factor alpha [TNF-a], interleukin 1β [IL-1b], and inducible nitric oxide synthase [iNOS]). Thus, the healing effects, re-epithelialization ratio, extracellular matrix remodeling, angiogenesis, and macrophage responses during wound healing processes indicate that PSBMA hydrogels promote full-thickness excisional acute wound regeneration in mice by enhancing angiogenesis, decreasing inflammation response, and modulating macrophage polarization.

The effect of mechanical properties of PSBMA hydrogels on their performance as wound dressing was also studied [19]. Different amounts of the cross-linking agent PEGDMA was used to obtain PSBMA hydrogels with different elastic modulus and based on the obtained values, the PSBMA hydrogels were divided into two groups soft (elastic modulus of about 10 kPa) and stiff (modulus of about 50 kPa) materials. The change in the mechanical properties did not influence the ability of PSBMA to reduce the adsorbed protein. Furthermore, all PSBMA hydrogels exhibited neglectable cell attachment. When applied as wound dressing onto full thickness wounds in mice, all PSBMA hydrogels showed enhanced wound regeneration and no obvious sign of inflammation or infection near the wound area. The soft hydrogels showed faster wound regeneration than the stiff hydrogels: after 20 days treatment, both soft PSBMA hydrogels enabled complete wound healing without scar formation, while the stiff hydrogels-treated wounds still had residual wound area. The softer PSBMA hydrogels significantly accelerated skin wound healing via improved granulation tissue formation and epithelial tissue regeneration, as compared to the stiff hydrogels. Moreover, the soft hydrogel-treated wounds had more densely packed collagen fibers with parallel arraignment as compared to the stiff hydrogel-treated wounds where loosely packed collagen fibers running in irregular arrangements were observed.

9.4 PZI as Dressings for Chronic Wounds Management

Wounds usually cause pain and bleeding and often are healed with scar formation, but these are relatively small and soft complications. The most serious condition is the wound infection that results into wound chronification. Bacterial contaminations occur during dressing change or via non-sterile and contaminated dressings, tools for wound treatment, etc. Upon adhesion, the bacteria can form biofilm, which requires orders of magnitude higher antibiotics dosages to be treated as compared to the free diffusing bacteria. From the formed biofilm, bacteria can infiltrate deeper into tissues through the wound, enter the blood circulation or migrate into organs, causing life-threatening complications, such as septicemia, amputation, or even death [14]. Thus, the problem with bacteria adhesion to wound and to wound dressing is crucial for preventing chronification of the wound.

In chronic wounds, the normal process of healing is disrupted at one or more phases, namely hemostasis, inflammation, proliferation, and remodeling [20]. Most often, chronic wounds are arrested into the inflammatory or proliferative phases. The chronic wounds have some peculiarities as compared to the acute ones, namely: [21].

- *elevated matrix metalloproteinases (MMPs) activity* which results into extracellular matrix, fibronectin, and growth factors degradation thus impairing the wound healing;
- *elevated myeloperoxidase (MPO) activity* which catalyzes the formation of reactive oxygen species; the latter's prolonged presence in the wound results into tissue necrosis and permanent tissue damage
- *increased pH of the wound* from the pH of intact skin ~4–6 to 7.15–8.93; alkalinity has an adverse effect on the wound tissue by depriving the wound of oxygen and providing a favorable environment for bacterial growth
- *excessive exudate production*: high levels of exudate trapped under the dressing make the skin more prone to damage and may cause skin stripping (excoriation) leaking out onto the periwound skin.
- the moist environment of chronic wounds is *highly susceptible to bacterial infections* and bacterial biofilms complicate further and delay the wound healing.

Thus, dressings that are used for chronic wound treatment must meet different requirements and have more functionalities as compared to acute wounds dressings.

9.4.1 Dressings for Chronic Wounds Management Based on Polycarboxybetaines

Zhu et al. [22] were the first to report the application of PCB as dressings for chronic wounds healing. They have developed PCB hydrogel wound dressings with an optical sensor to simultaneously monitor the pH and glucose level in diabetic wounds (Figure 9.8). Because the wound exudate composition changes during the wound healing process, the metabolites concentration and pH variation can be used to follow the wound status. Hyperglycemia can cause rigidification of cell membrane and

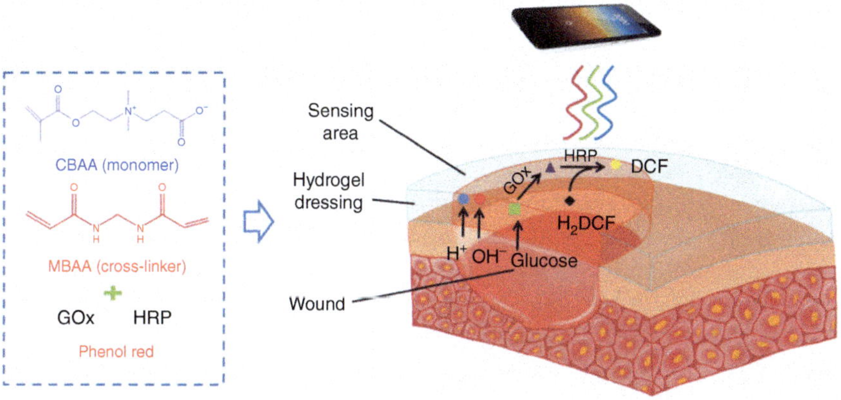

Figure 9.8 Scheme of the multifunctional PCB hydrogel dressing for detection of pH and glucose concentration in wound exudate. Source: Zhu et al. [22]/with permission of John Wiley & Sons.

thus of the blood vessel itself, thus, reducing the blood flow to wound impeding the healing process due to the lack of oxygen and nutrients supply. Hyperglycemia also disturbs the physiologic functions of epidermal keratinocytes that can delay healing of diabetic wounds.

The pH of the skin as well as of acute wounds is acidic (~4–6) and it promotes the neutrophils activity and prevent bacterial colonization [23]. Upon chronification, the pH becomes alkaline (pH 7–9), making the wound prone to bacterial infections. Thus, pH should be monitored in order to early detect the risk of infection and also to serve as an indicator of the different healing phases, assisting effectively the wound management. The *in situ* monitoring of pH and glucose concentration via sensors is usually hampered by the protein adsorption, which takes place immediately when the sensor is introduced.

The PCB hydrogel matrix known for its antibiofoluling performance was upgraded by the incorporation of pH indicator and two glucose-sensing enzymes, namely glucose oxidase (GOx) and horseradish peroxidase (HRP). These hydrogels showed satisfactory cyto-compatibility and a low hemolysis effect (<0.3%). The enzymes encapsulation improved their activity and stability in artificial wound exudate (AWE): free HRP retained only ≈20% while PCB–HRP maintained ≈55% of their initial catalytic activity. It was found that the immobilization had negligible effect on reaction rate of GOx when used in PBS solution but in AWE, PCB–GOx performed much better. The authors explained the enhanced enzymatic activity with the ability of PCB zwitterionic moieties to strongly bind water molecules via ionic solvation and thus to not interfere with the hydrophobic active sites of enzymes. Similar effect was also reported for other enzymes, e.g. acid phosphatase [24].

pH was detected via using a pH-sensitive nontoxic dye (phenol red) which changes its color in the pH range from 4 to 8, the same range at which acute wound becomes a chronic one. On the other hand, it was reported that with wound healing process an alkaline chronic wound gradually progressed to be neutral, and then to an acidic state [25]. The pH was determined by the change of the dressing color (yellow to red with the increase of pH values), while the variation in glucose concentrations was followed under UV light. The design of the PCB hydrogel allowed for using a smartphone to read the detected glucose and pH variation of diabetic mice wound *in vivo*. The healing effect of PCB hydrogels was evaluated and compared to DuoDerm dressings using diabetes mice model. In both control and diabetic groups of mice, the wounds treated with PCB hydrogel healed better than the treated with DuoDerm. The epidermis was nearly intact in PCB-Control and DuoDerm-Control groups, while the epithelial layer of DuoDerm-Diabetes was still incomplete. PCB-Diabetes group showed better recovery and more compact epithelial layer compared with the diabetic wounds treated with DuoDerm. The promoted re-epithelialization is explained by the unique properties of PCB hydrogel, including high water content, nonfouling, and excellent biocompatibility.

In our recent study [21], we showed that PCB hydrogels were able to absorb large amounts of physiological solution (mimicking the wound exudate), expanding at the same time and thus, differ from most of the available at the market wound dressings that shrink upon a contact with the wound exudate. The shrinking causes pain of the patient as well as disrupts the newly formed tissue and in this way impair the proper wound healing. Due to their high swelling ability in salt solutions, the PCB hydrogels were able to absorb the collagenase and MPO, without inhibiting entirely their activity. These enzymes are part of the normal wound healing process and are necessary for the complete wound closure. The high uptake capacity of PCB hydrogels makes them appropriate for controlling the overexpression of these deleterious enzymes in chronic wounds. Moreover, PCB hydrogels did not allow the biofilm formation from *S. aureus,* which is one of the most prevalent bacterial species identified in chronic wounds. The PCB hydrogels are noncytotoxic and biocompatible: no reaction or slight to moderate reaction was observed after their implantation *in vivo* in rats for two months. Additionally, the PCB hydrogels possessed all beneficial characteristics of hydrogel wound dressings such as transparency, preserving wound moisture, and nonadherence to the wound. All these properties proved the great potential of PCB hydrogels as chronic wound dressings [21].

9.4.2 Polysulfobetaines as Dressings for Chronic Wounds Management

Huang et al. [26] have synthesized zwitterionic poly(sulfobetaine acrylamide) (PSBAA)–hectorite nanoclay nanocomposite hydrogels and applied them as chronic wounds dressings. They used the nanocomposite approach to improve the mechanical properties of the hydrogels. For sake of comparison, PSBMA–nanoclay hydrogels were also synthesized. The acrylamide-based PSB hydrogels exhibited stronger mechanical properties than acrylate-based PSB hydrogels. The mechanical properties of PSBAA nanocomposites were comparable with the mechanical properties of PHEMA hydrogels, but the former showed much higher water absorbing ability thus surpassing the PHEMA performance as biomaterial. The different mechanical performance is due to the acrylamide group that can be simultaneously both hydrogen donor and acceptor, while the acrylate group could be only hydrogen acceptor. Thus, the formation of extensive hydrogen bonds network which bridges and strengthens inter- and intramolecular chains is the reason for the better mechanical properties of PSBAA as compared to PSBMA. Consequently, PSBAA was able to absorb larger amount of PBS than PSBMA, indicating the larger capacity of PSBAA to uptake wound exudate. PSBAA nanocomposites exhibited better resistance than PSBMA at the same amount of nanoclay, because PSBAA backbone serves as hydrogen donor to bridge intramolecular chains, thus attracting more water molecules in surroundings.

PSBAA and its nanocomposite hydrogels were also proved to be noncytotoxic and to repel the adsorption of *P. aeruginosa* and *S. epidermidis*. The efficacy of PSBAA/15 (15% nanoclay) was evaluated on full-thickness wounds in normal and diabetic rats and compared to gauze and AQUACEL® wound dressings. AQUACEL is a common clinical hydrofiber wound dressing made from sodium carboxymethylcellulose with high water content and low fouling properties. The samples were placed on the wounds of normal rats and after two days were removed. The PSBAA/15 hydrogel was removed easiest as it did not adhere to the newly formed tissues. In contrast, gauze and AQUACEL dressings adhered to the wounds, which made their removal difficult and painful. The closures of normal and diabetic wounds with PSBAA/15 occurred on day 10 and 12, respectively, which was the fastest closure among all tested dressings. Moreover, zwitterionic nanocomposite hydrogels of PSBAA/15 allowed fast re-epithelialization and collagen deposition, which was again be attributed to the high hydration, low damage of the new tissues during dressing replacement, and low adsorption of proteins such as growth factors, fibrin, and certain protease from exudate.

The PCBAA–clay nanocomposites were functionalized with silver to impart bactericidal functionality [27]. The AgNPs incorporation into zwitterionic nanocomposite hydrogels decreased the tensile strength and compressive modulus by up to 40% and 60%, respectively, compared with PSBAA/15 hydrogels. The effect of AgNPs on mechanical property of hydrogels was ascribed to the fact that AgNPs synthesized on clay interfered the polymer–clay interactions, weakening in this way the physical entanglement and electrostatic interaction. Nevertheless, when compared to the tensile strength of commercial dressing, Kaltostat (~0.9 MPa), which is an alginate dressing indicated as a primary dressing for moderately to highly exuding chronic and acute wounds, PSBAA/Ag15 hydrogel displayed better mechanical properties. The Ag release profile depends on clay amount: PSBAA/Ag5 released Ag^+ 3.4 times faster than PSBAA/Ag15, which is due to the tortured path of silver in polymer/clay network and the recapture of Ag^+ by the negatively charged nanoclay. Therefore, the release rate of Ag^+ in PSBAA–AgNPs hydrogel can be modulated by the amount of the nanoclay, reducing the effect of Ag^+ on regenerative cells.

PSBAA–AgNPs clay nanocomposites exerted protein adsorption resistance and were noncytotoxic. As Ag^+ is a well-known broad-spectrum antimicrobial agent, it was expected that PSBAA/Ag15 will show activity against *P. aeruginosa* and *S. epidermidis*. While no significant zones of inhibition were observed around the

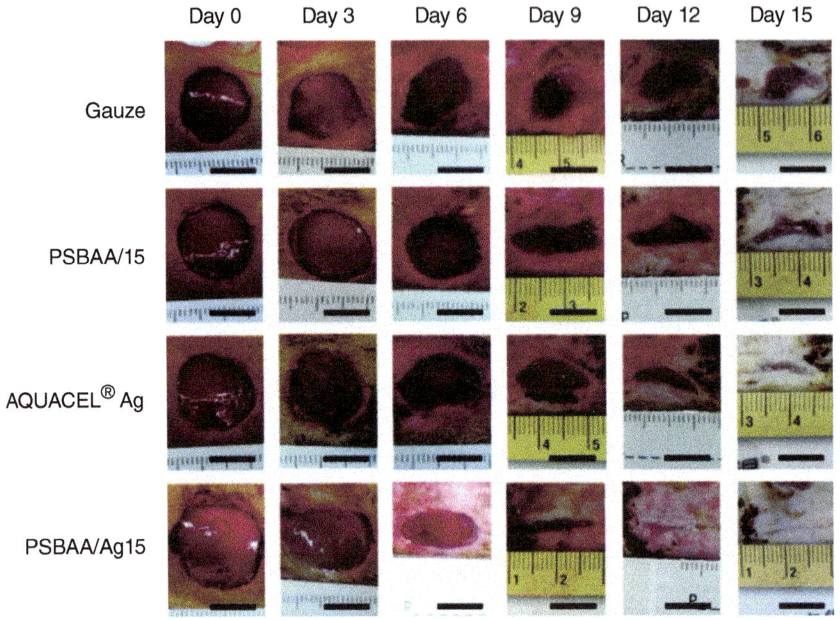

Figure 9.9 Appearance of wounds and wound healing percentage in diabetic rats with bacterial infection using different wound dressings. Source: Huang, K.-T., et al. (2017), [27], Figure 08a, Pg 08 / with permission of Royal Society of Chemistry.

PSBAA/0, PSBAA/15, and pHEMA hydrogels, PSBAA/Ag15 suppressed the growth of these bacteria indicating the effectiveness of the silver.

The authors evaluated the recovery efficacy of PSBAA/Ag15 hydrogels for full-thickness wounds on diabetic rats. In addition, the wounds were applied with *S. epidermidis* to mimic chronic infected wounds diabetic patients. The progress of wound closure was notably improved with PSBAA/Ag15 from day 6 onward compared to gauze and AQUACEL Ag (Figure 9.9). The rapid closure of wounds with PSBAA/Ag15 dressings clearly demonstrates their healing effectiveness for infected wounds on diabetic rats. Complete closure of infected wounds with the PSBAA/Ag15 treatment occurred on day 15. Furthermore, histological examination confirmed the full re-epithelialization and total formation of new connective tissue on the infected wounds after treatment with PSBAA/Ag15. Consequently, the excellent germicidal activity and nonsticky properties of the zwitterionic nanocomposite hydrogels make it excellent material for application in chronic wound healing.

Sener et al. [28] synthesized zwitterionic cryogels (gels formed below freezing temperatures) comprised of CBMA or SBMA, and 2-hydroxyethyl methacrylate (HEMA), without chemical cross-linkers. The cryogels were designed for topical applications and were aimed for injectable, self-healable dressings that provide sustained release of therapeutic molecules. The gels properties were tuned by changing monomer type and ratio as well as the polymerization temperature (room temperature or −20 °C for the cryogels). The zwitterionic–PHEMA gels were mechanically stable after stretching or compression – they could be stretched more

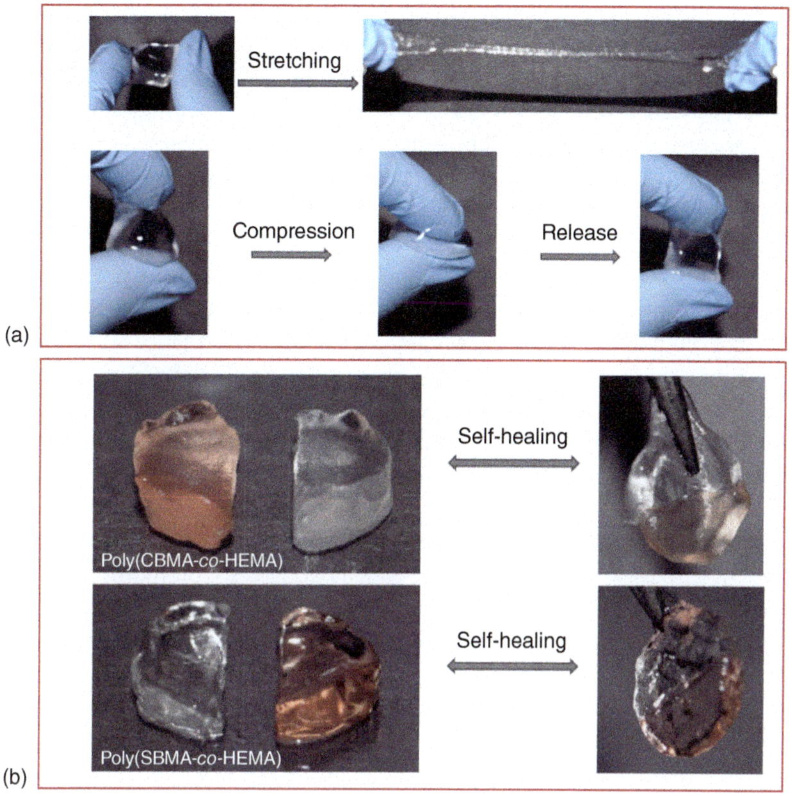

Figure 9.10 Images of PSBMA–PHEMA cryogel showing (a) its durability against stretching and compression and (b) the self-healing ability of zwitterionic–PHEMA cryogels. Source: G. Sener, et al. (2017), [28], Figure 03, Pg 30 / with permission of from ELSEVIER.

than 5× their initial size without breaking and highly compressed without any significant deformation (Figure 9.10a).

Moreover, the gels showed self-healing ability (Figure 9.10b) and some of them were injectable in a controllable manner. PHEMA gels were neither self-healing nor injectable, so these beneficial properties were imparted by the zwitterionic moieties. Rheological tests demonstrated improved mechanical properties for the gels polymerized at cryoconditions compared to the ones prepared at room temperature. These changes were explained by the cryoconcentration effect: monomer concentrations are locally enhanced due to the phase separation of the monomer and water phases during freezing. Thus, a denser polymer network is obtained as compared to gels prepared at room temperature. Moreover, the higher molecular weight polymers obtained at cryoconditions because the slower polymerization rate also enhances the mechanical properties of the hydrogels.

These materials improved the healing of diabetic wounds by allowing topical delivery of small molecule therapeutics including cerium oxide nanoparticles (CNP)-miR146a. The *in vivo* testing of the wound healing effect showed that mice treated with control zwitterionic gel had complete closure at day 20, while when wounds were treated with zwitterionic gel loaded with CNP-miR146a they have healed completely at day 14. This result is attributed to the controlled release of CNP-miR146a which reaches approximately 75% at day 10.

We have performed a study on the potential of PSBMA hydrogels as wound dressings for chronic wounds [2]. PSBMA hydrogels exhibit similar performance to the one described for PCB hydrogels above, namely they were able to absorb large amounts of physiological solution, expanding at the same time and were able to absorb collagenase and MPO from solutions, thus mitigating the deleterious action of these enzymes in chronic wounds. No significant difference in the performance of PSBMA as compared to poly(carboxybetaine methacrylate) (PCBMA) was detected, and both hydrogels demonstrated excellent performance as potential chronic wounds dressings materials. We have further functionalized the PSBMA and PCB hydrogels by imparting debridement activity [29]. Wound debridement is crucial for proper wound care, especially of chronic wounds as it promotes fast and efficient wound healing through removal of necrotic tissue. The latter not only impairs new healthy tissue formation but also increases the odor and the wound exudate, allowing bacteria and other harmful foreign invaders to spread and infect the wound. Hydrogel wound dressings are usually applied for promoting autolytic wound debridement, but this is slow and not a very efficient process. On the other hand, enzymatic products for wound debridement are either ointments or gels and they are easily washed out when used for treating highly exuding wounds. Our study was the first attempt to combine enzymatic debridement functionality with the high swelling ability of polyzwitterionic networks and to produce an innovative dressing with debridement functionality for the healing of highly exuding chronic wounds. To this purpose, PSBMA and PCBMA hydrogels were loaded with the protease subtilisin DY for imparting debridement functionality. The swelling ability and mechanical properties of PZI hydrogels depend on their different propensities to physical network formation. PCBMA hydrogels demonstrated better capacity for wound exudate absorption as well as for exerting higher enzymatic debridement activity. Both PZI hydrogels are noncytotoxic which confirms their appropriateness for direct contact with injured tissues. Thus, the newly developed PZI hydrogels demonstrate the potential to be used as new dressing materials with enzymatic debridement functionality for highly exuding wounds.

9.5 Conclusions

So far, the PZI hydrogels and related materials (nanocomposites, nanofiber membranes, networks, and copolymers) showed excellent performance as wound dressing materials. This excellent performance is defined by the inherent high hydration and protein absorbance resistance that PZI materials possess and that lies also behind their excellent blood and biocompatibility. Following the above described first steps in the field, we are expecting that zwitterionic polymers will bring exceptional developments in the field of biomaterials in the coming decade.

References

1 Georgiev, G., Kamenska, E., Vassileva, E. et al. (2006). Self-assembly, antipolyelectrolyte effect, and nonbiofouling properties of polyzwitterions. *Biomacromolecules* 7: 1329–1334.

2 Ruseva, K., Ivanova, K., Todorova, K. et al. (2019). Poly(sulfobetaine methacrylate)/poly(ethylene glycol) hydrogels for chronic wounds management. *Eur. Polym. J.* 117: 391–401.

3 Chang, Y., Liao, S.-C., Higuchi, A. et al. (2008). A highly stable nonbiofouling surface with well-packed grafted zwitterionic polysulfobetaine for plasma protein repulsion. *Langmuir* 24 (10): 5453–5458. https://doi.org/10.1021/la800228.

4 Wu, J., Lin, W., Wang, Z. et al. (2012). Investigation of the hydration of nonfouling material poly(sulfobetaine methacrylate) by low-field nuclear magnetic resonance. *Langmuir* 28: 7436–7441. https://doi.org/10.1021/la300394c.

5 Y. Zhang, Y. Liu, B. Ren, et al., Fundamentals and applications of zwitterionic antifouling polymers *J. Phys. D: Appl. Phys.*, 52 (40) 2019. https://doi.org/10.1088/1361-6463/ab2cbc.

6 Li, L., Chen, S., Zheng, J. et al. (2005). Protein adsorption on oligo(ethylene glycol)-terminated alkanethiolate self-assembled monolayers: the molecular basis for nonfouling behavior. *J. Phys. Chem. B* 109: 2934–2941.

7 Posnett, J., Gottrup, F., Lundgren, H., and Saal, G. (2009). The resource impact of wounds on health-care providers in Europe. *J. Wound Care* 18 (4): 154–161.

8 Lindholm, C. and Searle, R. (2016). Wound management for the 21st century: combining effectiveness and efficiency. *Int. Wound J.* 13 (Suppl. S2): 5–15.

9 Fujishita, S., Inaba, C., Tada, S. et al. (2008). Effect of zwitterionic polymers on wound healing. *Biol. Pharm. Bull.* 31 (12): 2309–2315.

10 Kitano, H., Tada, S., Mori, T. et al. (2005). Correlation between the structure of water in the vicinity of carboxybetaine polymers and their blood-compatibility. *Langmuir* 21: 11932–11940.

11 Unnithan, A., Nejad, A., Sasikala, A. et al. (2016). Electrospun zwitterionic nanofibers with in situ decelerated epithelialization property for non-adherent and easy removable wound dressing application. *Chem. Eng. J.* 287: 640–648. https://doi.org/10.1016/j.cej.2015.11.086.

12 Nejad, A.G., Park, C.H., and Kim, C.S. (2016). In situ synthesis of antimicrobial silver nanoparticles within antifouling zwitterionic hydrogels by catecholic redox chemistry for wound healing application. *Biomacromolecules* 17: 1213–1223. https://doi.org/10.1021/acs.biomac.6b00039.

13 Zhu, Y., Zhang, J., Yang, J. et al. (2016). Zwitterionic hydrogels promote skin wound healing. *J. Mater. Chem. B* https://doi.org/10.1039/C6TB00540C.

14 Zhu, Y., Zhang, J., Song, J. et al. (2017). One-step synthesis of an antibacterial and pro-healing wound dressing that can treat wound infections. *J. Mater. Chem. B* 5: 8451–8458.

15 Ji, F., Lin, W., Wang, Z. et al. (2013). Development of nonstick and drug-loaded wound dressing based on the hydrolytic hydrophobic poly(carboxybetaine) ester analogue. *ACS Appl. Mater. Interfaces* 5: 10489–10494. https://doi.org/10.1021/am403657t.

16 Lalani, R. and Liu, L. (2012). Electrospun zwitterionic poly(sulfobetaine methacrylate) for nonadherent, superabsorbent, and antimicrobial wound dressing applications. *Biomacromolecules* 13: 1853–1863. https://doi.org/10.1021/bm300345e.

17 Li, G., Wang, Y., Wang, S. et al. (2018). A thermo- and moisture-responsive zwitterionic shape memory polymer for novel self-healable wound dressing applications. *Macromol. Mater. Eng.* 1800603. https://doi.org/10.1002/mame.201800603.

18 Wu, J., Xiao, Z., Chen, A. et al. (2018). Sulfated zwitterionic poly(sulfobetaine methacrylate) hydrogels promote complete skin regeneration. *Acta Biomater.* 71: 293–305. https://doi.org/10.1016/j.actbio.2018.02.034.

19 He, H., Xiao, Z., Zhou, Y. et al. (2019). Zwitterionic poly(sulfobetaine methacrylate) hydrogels with optimal mechanical properties for improving wound healing in vivo. *J. Mater. Chem. B* 7: 1697–1707. https://doi.org/10.1039/C8TB02590H.

20 Enoch, S. and Price, P. (2004). Cellular, molecular and biochemical differences in the pathophysiology of healing between acute wounds, chronic wounds and wounds in the aged. *World Wide Wounds* http://www.worldwidewounds.com/2004/august/Enoch/Pathophysiology-Of-Healing.html.

21 Ruseva, K., Ivanova, K., Todorova, K. et al. (2020). Antibiofilm poly(carboxybetaine methacrylate) hydrogels for chronic wounds dressings. *Eur. Polym. J.* 132: 109673.

22 Zhu, Y., Zhang, J., Song, J. et al. (2019). A multifunctional pro-healing zwitterionic hydrogel for simultaneous optical monitoring of pH and glucose in diabetic wound treatment. *Adv. Funct. Mater.* 1905493. https://doi.org/10.1002/adfm.201905493.

23 Hampton, M.B., Kettle, A.J., and Winterbourn, C.C. (1998). Inside the neutrophil phagosome: oxidants, myeloperoxidase, and bacterial killing. *Blood* 92: 3007.

24 Atanasov, V., Vassileva, E., Kamenova, I. et al. (2006). Double hydrophilic block zwitterionic copolymer as an acid phosphatase folding helper. *Ann. Univ. Sofia Chem.* 98, 99: 327.

25 Schneider, L.A., Korber, A., Grabbe, S., and Dissemond, J. (2007). Influence of pH on wound-healing: a new perspective for wound-therapy? *Arch. Dermatol. Res.* 298: 413.

26 Huang, K.-T., Fanga, Y.-L., Hsieh, P.-S. et al. (2016). Zwitterionic nanocomposite hydrogels as effective wound dressing. *J. Mater. Chem. B* 4: 4206–4215. https://doi.org/10.1039/C6TB00302H.

27 Huang, K.-T., Fang, Y.-L., Hsieh, P.-S. et al. (2017). Non-sticky and antimicrobial zwitterionic nanocomposite dressings for infected chronic wounds. *Biomater. Sci.* 5 (6): 1072–1081. https://doi.org/10.1039/c7bm00039a.

28 Sener, G., Hilton, S.A., Osmond, M.J. et al. (2020). Injectable self-healable zwitterionic cryogels with sustained microRNA – cerium oxide nanoparticle release promote accelerated wound healing. *Acta Biomater.* 101: 262–272.

29 Ruseva, K., Nedkov, P., Alexandrova, R. et al. (2019). Polyzwitterionic hydrogels as wound dressings with enzymatic debridement functionality for highly exuding wounds. *Polym. Int.* 68 (9): 1626–1635. https://doi.org/10.1002/pi.5867.

10

Hyaluronan-Based Hydrogels as Modulators of Cellular Behavior

Sara Amorim[1,2], *Rui L. Reis*[1,2], *and Ricardo A. Pires*[1,2]

[1] *University of Minho, Headquarters of the European Institute of Excellence on Tissue Engineering and Regenerative Medicine, I3Bs – Research Institute on Biomaterials, Biodegradables and Biomimetics, 3B's Research Group, AvePark, Parque de Ciência e Tecnologia, Zona Industrial da Gandra, Barco, 4805-017 Guimarães, Portugal*

[2] *ICVS/3B's - PT Government Associate Laboratory, Braga/Guimarães, Portugal*

10.1 Introduction

The extracellular matrix (ECM) is composed of different bioactive molecules, such as proteins and glycosaminoglycans (GAGs). While the bioactivity of proteins has been well studied throughout the years, the biological relevance of the different GAGs is not yet assessed in such detail. However, it is known that GAGs are involved in biologically relevant events such as activation of growth factors and cytokines, maintenance of protein bioactive conformation for long periods of time (acting as storage depots), acting as coreceptors or mediators of cell–matrix and cell–cell communication, among many others. The interaction of GAGs with different ECM proteins is complex and, in some cases, not completely understood. Importantly, sulfated GAGs, such as heparin, heparan sulfate, chondroitin sulfate, or dermatan sulfate, can be chemically conjugated to proteins to form proteoglycans and/or glycoproteins. However, the only nonsulfated GAG, i.e. hyaluronan (HA), does not bind irreversible to matrix-occurring proteins [1, 2]. In fact, HA is directly extruded by the cells' hyaluronan synthases (HAS1–3) to the pericellular space and ECM, where it assembles into supramolecular forms with other ECM components, allowing its recognition by specific cell surface receptors [3–5]. HA has a simple, linear structure, and negative charge due to the glucuronic acid (GlcA). GlcA is linked to the *N*-acetyl glucosamine (GlcNAc) through ß-glycosidic bonds, forming a disaccharide unit that is repeated to form the polysaccharide structure of different length. In fact, the bioactivity of HA is linked to its molecular weight (M_w), contributing to the biofunctionality and homeostasis of the ECM and of the tissue's parenchyma [6]. The biological alterations of the ECM composition due to variations on the amount and size of HA are associated with different pathological states, e.g. cancer, fibrosis, osteoarthritis, and among others. This association is at the basis of using HA in the development of *in vitro* models.

Multifunctional Hydrogels for Biomedical Applications, First Edition.
Edited by Ricardo A. Pires, Iva Pashkuleva, and Rui L. Reis.

HA-based biomaterials can be tuned to recapitulate different HA biofunctions – as a biochemical stimulus, its interaction(s) with cell surface receptors, its cellular internalization, and its role as a mechanical support that confers resistance to external physical impact. In this chapter, we gather the latest developments on HA-based biomaterials to modulate cellular behaviors such as (i) biochemical guidance of stem cells' (SCs) differentiation and (ii) mechanotransduction through the manipulation of the viscoelastic properties of the HA-based hydrogel. In addition, the most recent reports that indicate an association between the dysregulated synthesis/degradation of HA and cancer cells [7, 8] is also included with particular emphasis on HA-based systems targeting HA-mediated cancer cells' behavior.

10.2 Biological Relevance of Hyaluronan

10.2.1 Hyaluronan in Biological Tissues and Fluids

HA is one of the main constituents of biological tissues contributing to their physical and biochemical homeostasis. Its function depends on its concentration and M_w. As an example, the capacity of HA of high M_w (HM_w) to adsorb high amounts of water and swell to large volumes contributes to the increased density and viscosity of some biological fluids, being essential to the rheological properties of synovial joint fluid [9]. In fact, the lack of HM_w HA, caused by its degradation into shorter chains, compromises the lubrication and mechanical support of the joints, which is associated with the appearance of osteoarthritis [10]. HA content in synovial fluids is essential to reduce the friction of articular cartilage thus avoiding the mechanical wear during movement [11]. Based on this HA biofunction, HA-based viscosupplementation has been proposed as a therapy towards improvement of the joints lubrification and biomechanics, while reducing pain [12]. HA is also considered crucial to maintain the hydration of the skin, due to its high capacity to retain water, being an essential component of the ECM of skin cells [13]. The presence of HA in other tissues and organs such as blood vessels [14], umbilical cord [15], vitreous body of the eye [16] contributes not only to their hydration but also to act as a mechanical support.

10.2.2 Hyaluronan as a Signaling Molecule

Whereas the function of the HA of HM_w is usually related with its ability to act as a mechanical support of connective tissues, HA of lower M_w (LM_w) is reported to be involved in the activation of different biochemical signaling pathways, e.g. through the interaction with CD44 and Troll-like receptors (TLRs) inducing the release of proinflammatory cytokines triggering the NF-κB signaling cascade [17, 18]. The distort balance of HA of different M_w within the ECM is linked to different pathological states. As an example, the overexpression of HAS3 and, consequently, the overproduction of HA of LM_w (1×10^5–2×10^5 Da), leads to the accumulation of short chains of HA which is associated with carcinogenesis and cancer aggressiveness [19]. The biorecognition of HA is mediated by specific HA receptors, such as the hyaladherins

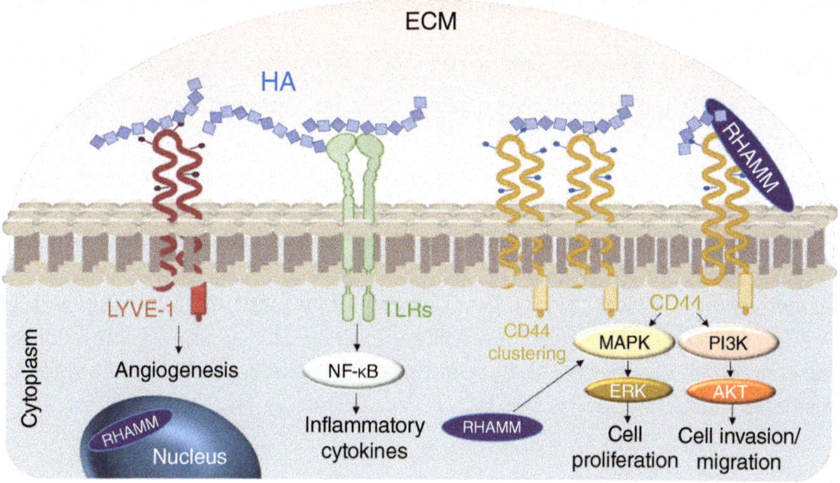

Figure 10.1 HA interactions with different cell surface receptors and the activation of subsequent signaling cascades that lead to cell migration or proliferation, as well as angiogenic or inflammatory outcomes. Source: Amorim et al. [25]/with the permission from Elsevier.

CD44 and receptor for HA-mediated motility (RHAMM). CD44 is a transmembrane glycoprotein and is one of the most studied and well-known receptors for HA [20]. The interaction between HA and CD44 triggers different cellular behaviors, such as proliferation and migration [21], as well as inducing M_w-specific responses, i.e. anti- or proinflammatory [22] and cancer cells' activity or latency [4]. The presence of several HA-binding motifs in the terminal amino acid sequence of the CD44 protein allows its coupling through numerous hydrogen bonding interactions with the –COOH groups present in the HA chemical structure, i.e. glucuronic acid, that can be from the same or different chains of HA [4, 23]. It is known that HA oligomers up to 6-mer can bind in a monovalent manner to the CD44 receptor [24], whereas native HM_w HA is able to induce the formation of receptor complexes through CD44 clustering [4], triggering different signaling cascades (Figure 10.1).

The signal transduction of HA also occurs through the RHAMM, also known as CD168, which is upregulated in different cancers [26]. In contrast to CD44, RHAMM is a cytoplasmic and nuclear protein associated to centrosomes, microtubules, and the mitotic spindle [27, 28]. The intracellular colocalization of short HA's fragments (i.e. 10–30 kDa) with RHAMM at the nuclei suggests their role on nuclei separation and cell division. In addition, HA is able to promote the RHAMM-mediated activation of the mitogen-activated protein kinase (MAPK) pathway inducing ERK1/2, FAK, and Src signaling cascades [29]. RHAMM lacks the link module domain and its interaction with HA is through a BX7B motif present in its carboxylic terminus [23]. Extracellular RHAMM is usually anchored to different proteins, namely, receptor tyrosine kinase (RTK's) and CD44, potentiating the interactions HA-RHAMM. The complexes generated by the combination of CD44/RHAMM-HA can modulate cellular migration and proliferation, through the regulation of ERK and AKT pathways, associated with the malignant phenotype of cancer cells [28].

The presence of HA in biological fluids, specifically in the lymph, leads to its uptake through the LYmphatic Vessel Endothelial hyaluronan receptor 1 (LYVE-1) activating lymphatic endothelial proliferation [30]. Moreover, the expression of the transmembrane protein HyAluronan Receptor for Endocytosis (HARE) in the sinusoidal endothelial cells of the liver and lymph nodes is responsible for the systemic clearance of HA; however, it is also able to modulate the biological outcomes in an HA M_w-dependant manner (ranging from small to medium HA chain sizes, 40–400 kDa) [31]. In fact, the mid-range small HA to mid-range high HA M_w (40–400 kDa) have been observed to stimulate HARE- and NF-κB-mediated gene expression, whereas the HA presenting an M_w ranging out of these values are considered inert [32].

10.3 Hyaluronan-Based Systems for Biomedical Applications

10.3.1 Hydrogels for Tissue Engineering

The above-mentioned bioactivity of HA inspired the development of different HA-based hydrogels for tissue engineering. Despite HA ability to absorb water and generate highly viscous fluids, this GAG does not have the capacity to gel on its own under physiological conditions. However, the HA's linear and simple chemical structure allows its modification at three different functional groups (primary alcohol, carboxylic acid, and amine functionalities) enabling its gelation and crosslinking. This strategy has been used to generate hydrogels that mimic the presence of HA in the ECM and its role in the modulation of cellular behavior [33]. In addition, the reduced content of HA in the matrix of tissues affected by different pathologies, such as osteoarthritis or skin aging, motivated the development of injectable HA-based hydrogels for treatment/repair of the damaged tissues.

10.3.1.1 Differentiation of Stem Cells

The capacity of SCs to differentiate into different lineages has been exploited in the context of tissue engineering and regenerative medicine [34]. The interaction between HA and its receptors anchored on the surface of SCs (e.g. CD44, RHAMM, TLR4, HARE, or LYVE-1) can trigger the activation of intracellular signaling cascades that may lead to their differentiation into the chondrogenic, osteogenic, or adipogenic lineages [35, 36]. In addition, the presence of HA in the cellular microenvironment is also known to modulate the ability of SCs to adhere and self-renew [37]. These characteristics are the basis of the interest in the development of HA-based hydrogels to mimic the microenvironment of SCs, providing both mechanical and biochemical cues for their differentiation. As previously mentioned, native HA alone is not able to gel under physiological conditions. Methacrylation of HA (Me-HA) at the carboxylic acid group from the glucuronic acid residues is the most common strategy to generate a polymer that is crosslinkable under UV radiation. The controlled exposure to the UV light can be used to tune the mechanical properties of these hydrogels making them suitable to mimic tissues of different stiffnesses [38]. As an example, HA-based hydrogels with a low stiffness (~500 Pa) promote the differentiation of human-induced pluripotent stem cells (hiPSCs) into neural progenitor cells (NPSs) [39]. The stemness markers (e.g. NANOG and SOX2) of human dental pulp stem cells (DPSCs) are upregulated when encapsulated in soft hydrogels (stiffness of ~680 Pa) generated using 2-aminoethyl methacrylate (AEMA)-modified HA, showing that the cellular behavior is modulated not only by the mechanical properties but also by biochemical factors [40]. The encapsulation of mesenchymal stem cells (MSCs) into Me-HA-based hydrogels promoted their chondrogenic differentiation, while inert poly(ethylene glycol) (PEG) hydrogels, with matching elastic modulus, did not produce the same outcome. The authors hypothesize that the interaction between HA and CD44 (expressed by MSCs) is at the basis of this observation [41].

HA-based hydrogels can also be used in the development of composite matrices that combine HA with different materials such as polymers, ceramics, naturally occurring ECM components (Figure 10.2). These combinations allow to tune: the mechanical properties and stability of the hydrogels [42]; their cell adhesive properties [43]; and to generate more accurate mimics the ECM's composition [44–46]. As an example, enzymatically cross-linked tyramine conjugated HA (HA-TA) has been proposed in combination with platelet lysates (PLs) for the chondrogenic differentiation of human MSCs. It was observed an increased deposition of ECM, forming a dense matrix of collagen type II and proteoglycans, that prompted cartilage regeneration through chondrogenic differentiation of MSCs [47]. The combination of Me-HA with MMP degradable peptide sequences induces the differentiation of MSCs through the upregulation of chondrogenic markers [48]. Likewise, the presence of peptides that mimic *N*-cadherin, a transmembrane protein and key player on cell–cell communication, in the formulation of Me-HA-based hydrogels promoted early chondrogenic differentiation of MSCs through the production of cartilage matrix [49], as well as their osteogenic differentiation when in presence of Me-HA functionalized with RGD peptide [50]. On the other hand, the blending of nonmodified HA with decellularized ECM derived from small intestinal submucosa induced the secretion of growth factors (i.e. IL-8, VEGF, and HGF) associated to the differentiation of human adipose-derived SCs toward superficial lamina propria fibroblasts [51]. The assembly of HA with silk fibroin and its impact in cellular proliferation has been also reported. The hydrogels of HA-silk fibroin/gelatin-chondroitin sulfate showed to enhance the MSCs' proliferation [52] and their ability to differentiate toward chondrocytes [53], when compared to the bare silk fibroin scaffolds. Moreover, increasing the content of HA on the silk fibroin-HA hydrogels promoted the expression of chondrogenic-specific genes, such as Col2a, Agg, and Sox9, showing the potential of these hydrogels to induce the chondrogenic differentiation of human umbilical cord-derived MSCs [54]. Finally, it has been also shown that silk fibroin interpenetrated network containing HA

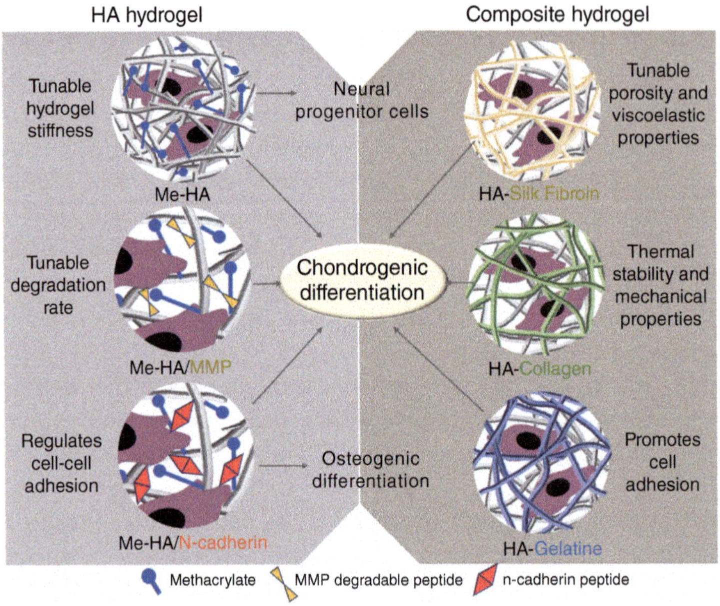

Figure 10.2 Promotion of the differentiation of stem cells by: hydrogels composed of HA as the main component of the 3D matrix; or HA blended with other biomaterials, forming a composite hydrogel.

is able to induce the differentiation of human bone marrow-derived MSC toward chondrogenesis for regeneration of the nucleus pulposus [55].

Collagen (Col) is one of the main constituents of the ECM, and its bioactivity has been widely exploited in the development of hydrogels for biomedical applications. The presence of Col in HA-based hydrogels enhanced the thermal stability and mechanical properties of the gels [56]. The conjugation of a Col mimetic peptide onto the maleimide-modified HA backbone crosslinked with MMP-sensitive peptide (known to be a regulator of the differentiation of bone MSCs and a key player on cartilage formation) has been shown to enhance the chondrogenic differentiation of bone marrow MSCs [57]. Moreover, it is also possible to promote the chondrogenic phenotype using hydrogels that combine Alginate, HA, and Col, as well as self-crosslinked hydrogels based on the combination of Col and HA-modified with *N*-hydroxyl sulfosuccinimide (with a degree of substitution of 32%) [58]. In fact, Col-free Alginate-HA hydrogels have been also shown to promote the differentiation of periodontal ligament SCs into chondrocytes [59]. The lack of adhesive properties on HA-based hydrogels are overcome by combining HA with gelatin (Gel) which has amino acids sequences that promote cellular adhesion (e.g. RGD). In this context, the HA-Gel hydrogels present an improved adhesion, proliferation, and differentiation of human MSCs toward the chondrogenic lineage [60], as well as the promotion of myotube formation and C2C12 differentiation into myoblasts [61]. Overall, HA alone, or in combination with other biomaterials, can generate hydrogels that can guide the differentiation of SCs into the chondrogenic lineage, serving as a basis for cartilage repair.

10.3.1.2 Space Filling Hydrogels

The well-known viscoelastic properties of HM_W HA (i.e. >500 kDa) make it an essential component for the lubrication of articular cartilage, for the absorption of the energy of impact, as well as for the reduction of wear generated by friction in the joints. There is a direct correlation between increased degradation of HA and age, as well as increased production of reactive oxygen species [62]. Intra-articular injection of HA-based hydrogels has been proposed to overcome this problem, to reduce the pain and promote tissue regeneration by guiding cellular behavior. The use of HA-based dermal fillers for cosmetic purposes has been also explored, where their injection into the dermis act as space fillers, reducing wrinkles and improving the moisture of skin [62, 63].

The use of injectable *in situ* forming hydrogels are preferable to the preformed ones, as they are easier to encapsulate therapeutic agents, and its administration requires a minimal invasive injection, rather than a surgical incision. Moreover, the use of injectable hydrogels increases the effectiveness of the delivery of bioactive molecules and of the filling of *in situ* defects, while reducing the convalescence period and the risk of infection [64, 65]. These advantages led to a strong emphasis on the development of injectable HA-based hydrogels for regenerative medicine. However, a major challenge is still to be overcome: the control of the degradation rate of HA [66]. It has been proposed the modification of HA to tune its rheological properties, making it suitable for *in situ* gelation while presenting a controlled degradation rate. As an example, biorthogonal Diels–Alder click crosslinking reaction was used to conjugate HA with bone morphogenetic protein-2 (BMP-2) mimetic peptide generating hydrogels for bone tissue engineering [67]. In this case, the cross-reaction between tetrazine (Tet) and trans-cyclooctene (TCO) both immobilized in the HA structure allows the fast HA crosslinking under physiological conditions. Another reported strategy is the combination of tyrosine-modified HA and human-like Col that is crosslinked by 1,4-butanedioldiglycidyl ether, generating hydrogels that can be used as soft tissue fillers [68]. Crosslinking can also be achieved by UV radiation using tyramine-substituted HA (HAT) in the presence of riboflavin photosensitizer, generating hydrogels with tunable mechanical properties and good biocompatibility, being a promising material to fill defects in articular cartilage [69]. Interestingly, HAT hydrogels can be also enzymatically crosslinked using horseradish peroxidase (HRP) and galactose oxidase [70]. In fact, injectable enzymatically crosslinked HAT hydrogels containing epigallocatechin-3-gallate (EGCG, a scavenger of radical oxygen species and anti-inflammatory agent) can promote cartilage regeneration with controlled inflammation [71]. Schiff's base reactions has been also tested to crosslink hydrogels composed by a combination of HA monoaldehyde and carbohydrazide-modified Gel. This system did not compromise biocompatibility and show the formation of a dense angiogenic network [66].

The ability to control the rheological properties of Me-HA makes it suitable not only for the differentiation of SCs (as previously described) but also for intra-articular viscosupplementation or to act as a dermal filler [72–74].

10.3.2 3D Cancer Models

HA is overexpressed in the ECM of cancer cells where it is a key player in tumor invasion and metastasis [75]. In fact, HA as one of the main components of the ECM and is known to modulate cellular behavior through its direct interaction with cell surface receptors (e.g. CD44 and RHAMM) or indirectly by modulating the mechanical/physical properties of the ECM, e.g. stiffness and porosity.

Based on its different bioactivities, HA-based systems that mimic either the intratumoral hypoxic environment, which is associated to tumor proliferation and vascularization [7, 76, 77], or the 3D tumor microenvironment to study the behavior of cancer cells have been developed. In brain cancers, abnormal levels of HA are associated with cancer cell proliferation, invasion, chemotherapeutic resistance, and cancer relapse [78, 79]. In this case, 3D systems can provide insights in the role of HA present in the tumor microenvironment, particularly in its ability to modulate brain cancer invasion. In fact, a combination of HA and Gel has been proposed to mimic the brain ECM including a combination of healthy glial cells and glioblastoma (GBM) cancer cells to study its invasive characteristics [78]. HA is abundant in the healthy brain; however, there is a low amount of fibrillar proteins. In contrast, brain tumors are usually rich in Col, laminin, and fibronectin that are responsible for the fibrotic nature and high stiffness of the cancerous tissue [80, 81]. The combination of HA with different proteins has been proposed to better mimic the cancer microenvironment. In addition, the lack of adhesive sites in the HA backbone requires its combination with cell adhesive molecules, e.g. Gel or RGD peptide, to promote integrin-based cellular attachment [82, 83]. As previously mentioned, it is necessary for the chemical modification of the HA's structure to allow crosslinking, while improving the stability of the hydrogel over time. Thiol-functionalized HA was used to enable crosslinking with PEG through Michael-type addition [84]. The combination of HA-PEG with the incorporation of RGD peptide [85], as well as Me-HA with Gel methacrylamide (GelMA) [86], was used to study the impact of erlotinib treatment, a molecule that inhibits the activity of epidermal growth factor receptor (EGFR) in GBM tumor. Moreover, the results showed that the overexpression of the CD44 receptor is correlated with the chemoresistance to erlotinib activity. In fact, this CD44-linked resistance is transversal to a series of different tumors, being recognized as a cancer SC marker [87]. In this context, it is commonly proposed the targeting of CD44 in the development of cancer therapies. As an example, HA hydrogels with different crosslinking densities interact selectively only with CD44+ breast cancer cells through preferential adhesion [88]. The gelation rate and crosslinking density of HA-phenol based hydrogels can be tuned by the concentration of HRP and hydrogen peroxide (H_2O_2), modulating their capacity to enrich the hydrogel with cancer SCs. In addition, the invasive character of MCF-7 breast cancer cells was recapitulated in HA-based hydrogels generated by (i) the combination of oxidized HA with an aldehyde (AHA) and hydrazide-modified HA for glycidyl methacrylate (GHHA) [89] and (ii) a double network of poly(Nϵ-acryloyl L-lysine) (pLysAAm) and HA (synthesized through a two-step photo-polymerization process) [90]. In general, these hydrogels generated a promising *in vitro* 3D microenvironment model from the MCF-7 cancer cells.

In addition to mimicking the 3D tumor microenvironment, HA-based hydrogels have been developed for the screening of anticancer drugs. As an example, HA-based models designed to be crosslinked with MMP cleavable peptide (and modified with multiphoton labile nitrodibenzofuran, NDBF) have been proposed to monitor the response of MDA-MB-231 and MDA-MB-468 breast cancer cells to cetuximab, a drug that binds and inhibits the activity of EGFR – a growth factor associated with the aggressive phenotypes of breast cancers [91]. Moreover, an *in situ* cross-linkable hydrogel composed by an amino derivative of HA and vinylsulfone functionalized β-cyclodextrins (sensitive to Michael reaction-mediated crosslinking at 37 °C) was developed for the release of doxorubicin. The released doxorubicin induced the recession of colorectal carcinoma tissue [92]. HA-based hydrogels for localized chemo-photothermal therapy against breast cancers have been also developed [93]. Dopamine conjugated HA (using *N*-(3-dimethylaminopropyl)-*N*′-ethylcarbodiimide hydrochloride, EDC, and *N*-hydroxysuccinimide, NHS) crosslinked using sodium selenite (Se) as a coordinating agent has been also proposed for the same application. This system takes advantage of the known Se anticancer properties and its combination with Indocyanine green (ICG) confers photothermal therapeutic characteristics to the hydrogels. To increase their stability, Shi et al. [94] proposed the formation of *in situ* dynamic hydrogels based on a combination of covalent conjugation and the self-healing capacity of HA through the interactions of imine and hydrazine. Cross-linking agents can elicit intrinsic toxicity in the hydrogels, however, using 4-(4,6-dimethoxy-1,3,5-triazin-2-yl)-4-methyl-morpholinium chloride (DMTMM) instead of EDC/NHS chemistry to graft phenylboronic acid (PBA) to HA reduce the cytotoxicity of the HA-based hydrogels. In fact, they showed to be cytocompatible with MDA-MB-231 breast cancer cells, as well as hiPSCs-derived NPC cell line (UTY1) and exhibiting anti-oxidative protection toward NPC when in contact with H_2O_2 and in the presence of doxorubicin.

The blending of HA with other biocompatible materials has been used to develop systems to study the behavior of cancer cells, namely the impact of the HA's M_w on cancer progression. Under this approach, Alginate (Alg) has been one of the most used components due to its easy handling and ability to physical or chemical crosslinking in the presence and absence of HA [95, 96]. The covalent crosslinking of oxidized Alg with HA-generated hydrogels that were tested with breast cancer cells, i.e. 4T-1 and SKBR3. These gels recapitulated the aggressiveness and invasive character of the cancer cells when in contact with HA of low M_w (i.e. 35 kDa) [97]. Furthermore, the blending of Alg and HA without prior chemical modification was also used to study the invasive behavior of a gastric cancer cell line, MKN45, in the presence of bone marrow MSCs that mimicked the tumor microenvironment. This study showed that HA of low M_w (i.e. 6.4 kDa) promote the invasive character of the cancer cells [98]. Finally, to mimic the fibrillar structure of the ECM, hydrogels composed by Col and HA (crosslinked using EDC) were used to mimic the tumor microenvironment and study the proliferation and invasion of melanoma cancer cells [99]. Once more, the HA of low M_w showed to promote the adhesion and invasive behavior of BRO cell line, when compared to soluble HA, where only increased proliferation was observed.

10.4 Conclusion and Future Remarks

The important role of HA in different tissues and organs is well established. This knowledge has been used in the development of therapies using bioactive HA making them important components to be considered when developing tissue engineering and regenerative medicine approaches. The perturbation of the homeostasis of HA in soft tissues (and in its ECM) is associated to different pathologies, which increases the interest of mimicking its presentation in the biological environments. The versatility of HA, in particular the ability to chemical modify it at its –COOH and –OH groups, allows researchers to fine tune their mechanical properties, bioactivity and stability of the HA-based hydrogels. They have been used to study the behavior of different cell types (healthy and cancer ones) in an *in vitro* biomimetic environment, or to drive the differentiation of SCs. It has been proposed systems that exploit the thermoresponsiveness, self-healing, and pH-sensitivity of HA-based hydrogels. They have been used to generate injectable *in situ* gelation systems or *in vitro* models throughout the years and developments that are expected to continue in the coming years.

Acknowledgments

We acknowledge the financial support from the Portuguese Foundation for Science and Technology (FCT) under the CancerCage project (PTDC/NAN-MAT/28468/2017) and M-ERA-NET under the INCIPIT project (M-ERA-NET2/0001/2016) and the European Commission (EC) Horizon 2020 programme, under grant agreement numbers 668983–FORECAST.

References

1 Soares da Costa, D., Reis, R.L., and Pashkuleva, I. (2017). Sulfation of glycosa minoglycans and its implications in human health and disorders. *Annu. Rev. Biomed. Eng.* 19: 1–26.
2 Richter, R.P., Baranova, N.S., Day, A.J. et al. (2018). Glycosaminoglycans in extracellular matrix organisation: are concepts from soft matter physics key to understanding the formation of perineuronal nets? *Curr. Opin. Struct. Biol.* 50: 65–74.
3 Stern, R., Asari, A.A., and Sugahara, K.N. (2006). Hyaluronan fragments: an information-rich system. *Eur. J. Cell Biol.* 85 (8): 699–715.
4 Yang, C.X., Cao, M.L., Liu, H. et al. (2012). The high and low molecular weight forms of hyaluronan have distinct effects on CD44 clustering. *J. Biol. Chem.* 287 (51): 43094–43107.

5 Day, A.J. and Sheehan, J.K. (2001). Hyaluronan: polysaccharide chaos to protein organisation. *Curr. Opin. Struct. Biol.* 11 (5): 617–622.

6 Tavianatou A.G., Caon I., Franchi M. et al. (2019). Hyaluronan: molecular size-dependent signaling and biological functions in inflammation and cancer. *FEBS J.* 286 (15): 2883–2908.

7 Chanmee, T., Ontong, P., and Itano, N. (2016). Hyaluronan: a modulator of the tumor microenvironment. *Cancer Lett.* 375 (1): 20–30.

8 Turley, E.A., Wood, D.K., and McCarthy, J.B. (2016). Carcinoma cell hyaluronan as a "portable" cancerized prometastatic microenvironment. *Cancer Res.* 76 (9): 2507–2512.

9 Zhang, Z. and Christopher, G.F. (2015). The nonlinear viscoelasticity of hyaluronic acid and its role in joint lubrication. *Soft Matter* 11 (13): 2596–2603.

10 Faust, H.J., Sommerfeld, S.D., Rathod, S. et al. (2018). A hyaluronic acid binding peptide-polymer system for treating osteoarthritis. *Biomaterials* 183: 93–101.

11 Tamer, T.M. (2013). Hyaluronan and synovial joint: function, distribution and healing. *Interdiscip. Toxicol.* 6 (3): 111–125.

12 Gaumet, M., Badoud, I., and Ammann, P. (2018). Effect of hyaluronic acid-based viscosupplementation on cartilage material properties. *Osteoarthritis Cartilage* 26: S136.

13 Papakonstantinou, E., Roth, M., and Karakiulakis, G. (2012). Hyaluronic acid: a key molecule in skin aging. *Dermatoendocrinol.* 4 (3): 253–258.

14 Sadowitz, B. et al. (2012). The role of hyaluronic acid in atherosclerosis and intimal hyperplasia. *J. Surg. Res.* 173 (2): e63–e72.

15 Cowman, M.K., Lee, H.G., Schwertfeger, K.L. et al. (2015). The content and size of hyaluronan in biological fluids and tissues. *Front. Immunol.* 6: 261.

16 Tram, N.K. and Swindle-Reilly, K.E. (2018). Rheological properties and age-related changes of the human vitreous humor. *Front. Bioeng. Biotechnol.* 6: 199.

17 Sainio, A. and Jarvelainen, H. (2020). Extracellular matrix-cell interactions: focus on therapeutic applications. *Cell. Signalling* 66: 109487.

18 Scuruchi, M., D'Ascola, A., Avenoso, A. et al. (2016). 6-Mer hyaluronan oligosaccharides modulate neuroinflammation and α-synuclein expression in neuron-like SH-SY5Y cells. *J. Cell. Biochem.* 117 (12): 2835–2843.

19 Kultti, A., Zhao, C., Singha, N.C. et al. (2014). Accumulation of extracellular hyaluronan by hyaluronan synthase 3 promotes tumor growth and modulates the pancreatic cancer microenvironment. *Biomed. Res. Int.* 2014: 817613.

20 Vuorio, J., Vattulainen, I., and Martinez-Seara, H. (2017). Atomistic fingerprint of hyaluronan-CD44 binding. *PLoS Comput. Biol.* 13 (7): e1005663.

21 Murakami, T., Otsuki, S., Okamoto, Y. et al. (2019). Hyaluronic acid promotes proliferation and migration of human meniscus cells via a CD44-dependent mechanism. *Connect Tissue Res.* 60 (2): 117–127.

22 Gao, Y., Sun, Y., Yang, H. et al. (2019). A low molecular weight hyaluronic acid derivative accelerates excisional wound healing by modulating pro-inflammation, promoting epithelialization and neovascularization, and remodeling collagen. *Int. J. Mol. Sci.* 20 (15).

23 Misra, S., Hascall, V.C., Markwald, R.R. et al. (2015). Interactions between hyaluronan and its receptors (CD44, RHAMM) regulate the activities of inflammation and cancer. *Front. Immunol.* 6: 201.

24 Cyphert, J.M., Trempus, C.S., and Garantziotis, S. (2015). Size matters: molecular weight specificity of hyaluronan effects in cell biology. *Int. J. Cell Biol.* 2015: 563818.

25 Amorim, S. et al. (2021). Extracellular matrix mimics using hyaluronan-based biomaterials. *Trends Biotechnol.* 39 (1): 90–104.

26 Wang, D., Narula, N., Azzopardi, S. et al. (2016). Expression of the receptor for hyaluronic acid mediated motility (RHAMM) is associated with poor prognosis and metastasis in non-small cell lung carcinoma. *Oncotarget* 7 (26): 39957–39969.

27 Tolg, C., McCarthy, J.B., Yazdani, A. et al. (2014). Hyaluronan and RHAMM in wound repair and the "cancerization" of stromal tissues. *Biomed. Res. Int.* 2014: 103923.

28 Hamilton, S.R., Fard, S.F., Paiwand, F.F. et al. (2007). The hyaluronan receptors CD44 and Rhamm (CD168) form complexes with ERK1,2 that sustain high basal motility in breast cancer cells. *J. Biol. Chem.* 282 (22): 16667–16680.

29 Skandalis, S.S., Karalis, T., and Heldin, P. (2020). Intracellular hyaluronan: importance for cellular functions. *Semin. Cancer Biol.* 62: 20–30.

30 Jackson, D.G. (2019). Hyaluronan in the lymphatics: the key role of the hyaluronan receptor LYVE-1 in leucocyte trafficking. *Matrix Biol.* 78, 79: 219–235.

31 Pandey, M.S. and Weigel, P.H. (2014). Hyaluronic acid receptor for endocytosis (HARE)-mediated endocytosis of hyaluronan, heparin, dermatan sulfate, and acetylated low density lipoprotein (AcLDL), but not chondroitin sulfate types A, C, D, or E, activates NF-κB-regulated gene expression. *J. Biol. Chem.* 289 (3): 1756–1767.

32 Pandey, M.S., Baggenstoss, B.A., Washburn, J. et al. (2013). The hyaluronan receptor for endocytosis (HARE) activates NF-κB-mediated gene expression in response to 40–400-kDa, but not smaller or larger, hyaluronans. *J. Biol. Chem.* 288 (20): 14068–14079.

33 Wolf, K.J. and Kumar, S. (2019). Hyaluronic acid: incorporating the bio into the material. *ACS Biomater. Sci. Eng.* 5 (8): 3753–3765.

34 Tewary, M., Shakiba, N., and Zandstra, P.W. (2018). Stem cell bioengineering: building from stem cell biology. *Nat. Rev. Genet.* 19 (10): 595–614.

35 Solis, M.A., Chen, Y.H., Wong, T.Y. et al. (2012). Hyaluronan regulates cell behavior: a potential niche matrix for stem cells. *Biochem. Res. Int.* 2012: 346972.

36 Pre, E.D., Conti, G., and Sbarbati, A. (2016). Hyaluronic acid (HA) scaffolds and multipotent stromal cells (MSCs) in regenerative medicine. *Stem Cell Rev. Rep.* 12 (6): 664–681.

37 Gerecht, S., Burdick, J.A., Ferreira, L.S. et al. (2007). Hyaluronic acid hydrogel for controlled self-renewal and differentiation of human embryonic stem cells. *Proc. Natl. Acad. Sci. U. S. A.* 104 (27): 11298–11303.

38 Ondeck, M.G. and Engler, A.J. (2016). Mechanical characterization of a dynamic and tunable methacrylated hyaluronic acid hydrogel. *J. Biomech. Eng.* 138 (2): 021003.

39 Wu, S., Xu, R., Duan, B. et al. (2017). Three-dimensional hyaluronic acid hydrogel-based models for in vitro human iPSC-derived NPC culture and differentiation. *J. Mater. Chem. B* 5 (21): 3870–3878.

40 Niloy, K.K., Gulfam, M., Compton, K. B. et al. (2019). Methacrylated hyaluronic acid–based hydrogels maintain stemness in human dental pulp stem cells. *Regener. Eng. Transl. Med.* 6: 262–272.

41 Chung, C. and Burdick, J.A. (2009). Influence of three-dimensional hyaluronic acid microenvironments on mesenchymal stem cell chondrogenesis. *Tissue Eng. Part A* 15 (2): 243–254.

42 Amorim, S., Reis, R.L., and Pires, R.A. (2020). Biomatrices that mimic the cancer extracellular environment. In: *Biomaterials for 3D Tumor Modeling* (ed. S.C. Kundu and R.L. Reis), 91–106. Elsevier.

43 Gallagher, L.B., Dolan, E.B., O'Sullivan, J. et al. (2020). Pre-culture of mesenchymal stem cells within RGD-modified hyaluronic acid hydrogel improves their resilience to ischaemic conditions. *Acta Biomater.* 107: 78–90.

44 Lou, J., Stowers, R., Nam, S. et al. (2018). Stress relaxing hyaluronic acid-collagen hydrogels promote cell spreading, fiber remodeling, and focal adhesion formation in 3D cell culture. *Biomaterials* 154: 213–222.

45 Addington, C.P., Dharmawaj, S., Heffernan, J.M. et al. (2017). Hyaluronic acid-laminin hydrogels increase neural stem cell transplant retention and migratory response to SDF-1α. *Matrix Biol.* 60, 61: 206–216.

46 Seidlits, S.K., Drinnan, C.T., Petersen, R.R. et al. (2011). Fibronectin-hyaluronic acid composite hydrogels for three-dimensional endothelial cell culture. *Acta Biomater.* 7 (6): 2401–2409.

47 Jooybar, E., Abdekhodaie, M.J., Alvi, M. et al. (2019). An injectable platelet lysate-hyaluronic acid hydrogel supports cellular activities and induces chondrogenesis of encapsulated mesenchymal stem cells. *Acta Biomater.* 83: 233–244.

48 Feng, Q., Zhu, M., Wei, K. et al. (2014). Cell-mediated degradation regulates human mesenchymal stem cell chondrogenesis and hypertrophy in MMP-sensitive hyaluronic acid hydrogels. *PLoS One* 9 (6): e99587.

49 Bian, L., Guvendiren, M., Mauck, R.L. et al. (2013). Hydrogels that mimic developmentally relevant matrix and N-cadherin interactions enhance MSC chondrogenesis. *Proc. Natl. Acad. Sci. U. S. A.* 110 (25): 10117–10122.

50 Zhu, M., Lin, S., Sun, Y. et al. (2016). Hydrogels functionalized with N-cadherin mimetic peptide enhance osteogenesis of hMSCs by emulating the osteogenic niche. *Biomaterials* 77: 44–52.

51 Huang, D., Wang, R., and Yang, S. (2016). Cogels of hyaluronic acid and acellular matrix for cultivation of adipose-derived stem cells: potential application for vocal fold tissue engineering. *Biomed. Res. Int.* 2016: 6584054.

52 Sawatjuia, N., Damrongrungruang, T., Leeanansaksiri, W. et al. (2014). Fabrication and characterization of silk fibroin-gelatin/chondroitin sulfate/hyaluronic acid scaffold for biomedical applications. *Mater. Lett.* 126: 207–210.

53 Sawatjui, N., Damrongrungruang, T., Leeanansaksiri, W. et al. (2015). Silk fibroin/gelatin-chondroitin sulfate-hyaluronic acid effectively enhances in vitro chondrogenesis of bone marrow mesenchymal stem cells. *Mater. Sci. Eng. C Mater. Biol. Appl.* 52: 90–96.

54 Jaipaew, J., Wangkulangkul, P., Meesane, J. et al. (2016). Mimicked cartilage scaffolds of silk fibroin/hyaluronic acid with stem cells for osteoarthritis surgery: morphological, mechanical, and physical clues. *Mater. Sci. Eng. C Mater. Biol. Appl.* 64: 173–182.

55 Chung, T.-W., Chen, W.-P., Tai, P.-W. et al. (2020). Roles of silk fibroin on characteristics of hyaluronic acid/silk fibroin hydrogels for tissue engineering of nucleus pulposus. *Materials* 13 (12).

56 Mahapatra, C., Jin, G.Z., and Kim, H.W. (2016). Alginate-hyaluronic acid-collagen composite hydrogel favorable for the culture of chondrocytes and their phenotype maintenance. *Tissue Eng. Regen. Med.* 13 (5): 538–546.

57 Ren, Y., Zhang, H., Qin, W. et al. (2020). A collagen mimetic peptide-modified hyaluronic acid hydrogel system with enzymatically mediated degradation for mesenchymal stem cell differentiation. *Mater. Sci. Eng. C Mater. Biol. Appl.* 108: 110276.

58 Gao, Y., Liu, Q., Kong, W. et al. (2020). Activated hyaluronic acid/collagen composite hydrogel with tunable physical properties and improved biological properties. *Int. J. Biol. Macromol.* 164: 2186–2196.

59 Ansari, S., Diniz, I.M., Chen, C. et al. (2017). Alginate/hyaluronic acid hydrogel delivery system characteristics regulate the differentiation of periodontal ligament stem cells toward chondrogenic lineage. *J. Mater. Sci. Mater. Med.* 28 (10): 162.

60 Moulisová, V., Poveda-Reyes, S., Sanmartín-Masiá, E. et al. (2017). Hybrid protein-glycosaminoglycan hydrogels promote chondrogenic stem cell differentiation. *ACS Omega* 2 (11): 7609–7620.

61 Poveda-Reyes, S., Moulisova, V., Sanmartín-Masiá, E. et al. (2016). Gelatin-hyaluronic acid hydrogels with tuned stiffness to counterbalance cellular forces and promote cell differentiation. *Macromol. Biosci.* 16 (9): 1311–1324.

62 Fakhari, A. and Berkland, C. (2013). Applications and emerging trends of hyaluronic acid in tissue engineering, as a dermal filler and in osteoarthritis treatment. *Acta Biomater.* 9 (7): 7081–7092.

63 La Gatta, A., Salzillo, R., Catalano, C. et al. (2019). Hyaluronan-based hydrogels as dermal fillers: the biophysical properties that translate into a "volumetric" effect. *PLoS One* 14 (6): e0218287.

64 Wang, L., Dong, S., Liu, Y. et al. (2020). Fabrication of injectable, porous hyaluronic acid hydrogel based on an in-situ bubble-forming hydrogel entrapment process. *Polymers* 12 (5): 1138.

65 Park, K.M. and Park, K.D. (2017). Injectable hydrogels: properties and applications. In: *Encyclopedia of Polymer Science and Technology* (ed. H.F. Mark), 1–16. Wiley.

66 Hozumi, T., Kageyama, T., Ohta, S. et al. (2018). Injectable hydrogel with slow degradability composed of gelatin and hyaluronic acid cross-linked by Schiff's base formation. *Biomacromolecules* 19 (2): 288–297.

67 Park, S.H., Park, J.Y., Ji, Y.B. et al. (2020). An injectable click-crosslinked hyaluronic acid hydrogel modified with a BMP-2 mimetic peptide as a bone tissue engineering scaffold. *Acta Biomater.* 117: 108–120.

68 Liu, Y. and Fan, D. (2019). Novel hyaluronic acid-tyrosine/collagen-based injectable hydrogels as soft filler for tissue engineering. *Int. J. Biol. Macromol.* 141: 700–712.

69 Donnelly, P.E., Chen, T., Finch, A. et al. (2017). Photocrosslinked tyramine-substituted hyaluronate hydrogels with tunable mechanical properties improve immediate tissue-hydrogel interfacial strength in articular cartilage. *J. Biomater. Sci. Polym. Ed.* 28 (6): 582–600.

70 Wang, L., Jinrui, L., Zhang, D. et al. (2020). Dual-enzymatically crosslinked and injectable hyaluronic acid hydrogels for potential application in tissue engineering. *RSC Adv.* 10 (5): 2870–2876.

71 Jin, Y., Koh, R.H., Kim, S.-H. et al. (2020). Injectable anti-inflammatory hyaluronic acid hydrogel for osteoarthritic cartilage repair. *Mater. Sci. Eng. C Mater. Biol. Appl.* 115: 111096.

72 Highley, C.B., Prestwich, G.D., and Burdick, J.A. (2016). Recent advances in hyaluronic acid hydrogels for biomedical applications. *Curr. Opin. Biotechnol.* 40: 35–40.

73 Tsanaktsidou, E., Kammona, O., and Kiparissides, C. (2019). On the synthesis and characterization of biofunctional hyaluronic acid based injectable hydrogels for the repair of cartilage lesions. *Eur. Polym. J.* 114: 47–56.

74 Cheng, L., Ji, K., Shih, T.Y. et al. (2017). Injectable shape-memorizing three-dimensional hyaluronic acid cryogels for skin sculpting and soft tissue reconstruction. *Tissue Eng. Part A* 23 (5–6): 243–251.

75 Liu, M., Tolg, C., and Turley, E. (2019). Dissecting the dual nature of hyaluronan in the tumor microenvironment. *Front. Immunol.* 10: 947.

76 Wang, Y., Mirza, S., Wu, S. et al. (2018). 3D hydrogel breast cancer models for studying the effects of hypoxia on epithelial to mesenchymal transition. *Oncotarget* 9 (63): 32191–32203.

77 Bonnesœur, S., Morin-Grognet, S., Thoumire, O. et al. (2020). Hyaluronan-based hydrogels as versatile tumor-like models: tunable ECM and stiffness with genipin-crosslinking. *J. Biomed. Mater. Res. A* 108 (5): 1256–1268.

78 Ma, L., Li, Y., Wu, Y. et al. (2020). 3D bioprinted hyaluronic acid-based cell-laden scaffold for brain microenvironment simulation. *Bio-Des. Manuf.* 3 (3): 164–174.

79 Xiao, W., Sohrabi, A., and Seidlits, S.K. (2017). Integrating the glioblastoma microenvironment into engineered experimental models. *Future Sci. OA* 3 (3): FSO189.

80 Pedron, S., Becka, E., and Harley, B.A. (2015). Spatially gradated hydrogel platform as a 3D engineered tumor microenvironment. *Adv. Mater.* 27 (9): 1567–1572.

81 Cha, J., Kang, S.G., and Kim, P. (2016). Strategies of mesenchymal invasion of patient-derived brain tumors: microenvironmental adaptation. *Sci. Rep.* 6 (1): 24912.

82 Nakod, P.S., Kim, Y., and Rao, S.S. (2020). Three-dimensional biomimetic hyaluronic acid hydrogels to investigate glioblastoma stem cell behaviors. *Biotechnol. Bioeng.* 117 (2): 511–522.

83 Chen, J.E., Pedron, S., and Harley, B.A.C. (2017). The combined influence of hydrogel stiffness and matrix-bound hyaluronic acid content on glioblastoma invasion. *Macromol. Biosci.* 17 (8): 1700018.

84 Xiao, W., Ehsanipour, A., Sohrabi, A. et al. (2018). Hyaluronic-acid based hydrogels for 3-dimensional culture of patient-derived glioblastoma cells. *J. Vis. Exp.* 138: 58176.

85 Xiao, W., Zhang, R., Sohrabi, A. et al. (2018). Brain-mimetic 3D culture platforms allow investigation of cooperative effects of extracellular matrix features on therapeutic resistance in glioblastoma. *Cancer Res.* 78 (5): 1358–1370.

86 Pedron, S., Wolter, G.L., Chen, J.E. et al. (2019). Hyaluronic acid-functionalized gelatin hydrogels reveal extracellular matrix signals temper the efficacy of erlotinib against patient-derived glioblastoma specimens. *Biomaterials* 219: 119371.

87 Morath, I., Hartmann, T.N., and Orian-Rousseau, V. (2016). *CD44: more than a mere stem cell marker. Int. J. Biochem. Cell Biol.* 81 (Pt A): 166–173.

88 Tan, S., Yamashita, A., Gao, S.J. et al. (2019). *Hyaluronic acid hydrogels with defined crosslink density for the efficient enrichment of breast cancer stem cells. Acta Biomater.* 94: 320–329.

89 Suo, A., Xu, W., Wang, Y. et al. (2019). *Dual-degradable and injectable hyaluronic acid hydrogel mimicking extracellular matrix for 3D culture of breast cancer MCF-7 cells. Carbohydr. Polym.* 211: 336–348.

90 Xu, W., Qian, J., Zhang, Y. et al. (2016). *A double-network poly(Nϵ-acryloyl L-lysine)/hyaluronic acid hydrogel as a mimic of the breast tumor microenvironment. Acta Biomater.* 33: 131–141.

91 Fisher, S.A., Tam, R.Y., Fokina, A. et al. (2018). *Photo-immobilized EGF chemical gradients differentially impact breast cancer cell invasion and drug response in defined 3D hydrogels. Biomaterials* 178: 751–766.

92 Fiorica, C., Palumbo, F.S., Pitarresi, G. et al. (2020). A hyaluronic acid/cyclodextrin based injectable hydrogel for local doxorubicin delivery to solid tumors. *Int. J. Pharm.* 589: 119879.

93 Yang, M., Lee, S.Y., Kim, S. et al. (2020). Selenium and dopamine-crosslinked hyaluronic acid hydrogel for chemophotothermal cancer therapy. *J. Controlled Release* 324: 750–764.

94 Shi, W., Hass, B., Kuss, M.A. et al. (2020). Fabrication of versatile dynamic hyaluronic acid-based hydrogels. *Carbohydr. Polym.* 233: 115803.

95 Bidarra, S.J. and Barrias, C.C. (2019). 3D culture of mesenchymal stem cells in alginate hydrogels. *Methods Mol. Biol.* 2002: 165–180.

96 Neves, M.I., Araújo, M., Moroni, L. et al. (2020). Glycosaminoglycan-inspired biomaterials for the development of bioactive hydrogel networks. *Molecules* 25 (4): 978.

97 Zhao, Y.F., Qiao, S.P., Shi, S.L. et al. (2017). Modulating three-dimensional microenvironment with hyaluronan of different molecular weights alters breast cancer cell invasion behavior. *ACS Appl. Mater. Interfaces* 9 (11): 9327–9338.

98 Amorim, S., Soares da Costa, D., Pashkuleva, I. et al. (2021). 3D hydrogel mimics of the tumor microenvironment: the interplay among hyaluronic acid, stem cells and cancer cells. *Biomater. Sci.* 9 (1): 252–260.

99 Sapudom, J., Ullm, F., Martin, S. et al. (2017). Molecular weight specific impact of soluble and immobilized hyaluronan on CD44 expressing melanoma cells in 3D collagen matrices. *Acta Biomater.* 50: 259–270.

11

Hydrogel Fibers Produced via Microfluidics

Kongchang Wei, Claudio Toncelli, René M. Rossi, and Luciano F. Boesel

Empa, Swiss Federal Laboratories for Materials Science and Technology, Laboratory for Biomimetic Membranes and Textiles, Lerchenfeldstrasse 5, St. Gallen 9014, Switzerland

11.1 Introduction to Microfluidics and Microfluidic Wet Spinning

11.1.1 Fundamentals of Microfluidics

Microfluidics has become a popular tool to manipulate a small volume of fluids with high precision by integrating, automatizing, and parallelizing complex processes within miniaturized components [1]. Examples of its applications are found in the sorting of biological entities [2], as with cells, bacteria, and other corpuscular entities, point of care detection and diagnostics [3], and *in vitro* simulation and modeling of biological processes including the so-called organ-on-chip [4], and control of sophisticated chemical reactions [5], to name but a few. Microfluidics uses the laminar flow conditions dictated by the reduced section of the channels used (i.e. 0–1000 μm) to achieve laminar flow separation and mixing only by diffusion forces. Indeed, the velocity of an incompressible fluid is described by the Navier–Stokes equation:

$$\rho\frac{\partial v}{\partial t} + \rho(u \cdot \nabla)u = -\nabla p + \eta\nabla^2 u + \rho g \tag{11.1}$$

where u (m/s) is the fluid velocity field, ρ (kg/m^3) is the density, η (m^2/s) is the kinematic viscosity, and ρg (g/cm^2/s^2) is the contribution related to an external acceleration field, whether due to gravity or electrostatic forces. This formula, *per se* complicated and difficult to solve, is notably simplified when considering the behavior of fluids within narrow channel geometries. The Reynolds number (*Re*) is a dimensionless number defined as the ratio between the inertial forces and viscous forces:

$$Re = \frac{\rho u d}{\mu} \tag{11.2}$$

where d (m) is the channel diameter and μ (Pa·s) is the dynamic viscosity of the fluid. When $Re \ll 1$, Eq. (11.1) becomes the following differential equation:

$$0 = -\nabla p + \eta\nabla^2 u + \rho g \tag{11.3}$$

Multifunctional Hydrogels for Biomedical Applications, First Edition.
Edited by Ricardo A. Pires, Iva Pashkuleva, and Rui L. Reis.

The solution to this equation yields a parabolic velocity profile where, in the case of cylindrical channel geometry, the velocity is maximal at the center of the channel and tends to zero as it approaches the channel walls. Hence, the Reynolds number determines whether the fluid is in its laminar or turbulent flow condition, with values <2300 considered as laminar.

One of the advantages of having liquids operate in laminar flow conditions is the possibility of limiting mixing at the liquid interfaces dictated only by Fick's diffusion laws. This concept is particularly useful for the development of the microfluidic wet spinning (MWS) technology discussed in the next Section 11.1.2. A detailed review of flow dynamics in microfluidic channels can be found elsewhere [6, 7].

11.1.2 Application of Microfluidics to Fiber Production: Microfluidic Wet Spinning

When the separation of laminar flows within a microfluidic channel occurs in the presence of a polymer solution and a nonsolvent solution, it is possible to provoke *in situ* fiber coagulation directly. If the spinning dope is coaxially aligned as the core flow with a sheath flow constituted by the coagulating solution, then fiber solidification occurs at the liquid–liquid interface. On the other hand, conventional wet spinning of fibers provokes the coagulation of fibers by spinning a polymer solution directly into a large liquid coagulation bath [8]. Thus, wet spinning has a relatively limited choice of coagulating solutions, which are mostly water in order to limit costs. Instead, the relatively small volume of fluids operating with MWS opens a larger choice of coagulating solvents, therefore expanding the range of materials that can be processed via this technique.

The sheath flow solution has the function of reducing the friction with the channel wall during fiber coagulation and/or inducing phase separation and fiber solidification [9]. Hence, microfluidic laminar flow separation between sheath and core fluids permits fine control of the fiber coagulation directly inside the microfluidic reactor [10].

By manipulating the shape of the microchannels where the spinning dope solution is flowing, in principle any fiber shape can be obtained, including grooved [11], flat [12], core–shell [13], hollow [14], Janus [15], helical [16, 17], heterogeneous, and knotted (Figure 11.1) [19, 20]. Among anisotropic fibers, semilunar [21], double anchor [22], triangular [23], kidney bean [23], trilobed-wheel, maple leaf, six-angled star, T-shaped, U-shaped, and H-shaped constructs have already been produced [24].

Additionally, while conventional wet spinning provokes fiber coagulation only through a phase inversion process, other methods are available in MWS to fix the fiber structure in place according to the dictated flow conditions and channel geometries, namely photopolymerization [25], ionic cross-linking [26], chemical cross-linking [27], and solvent evaporation [28]. These features considerably expand the range of materials that can be processed into functional fibers (Figure 11.2).

The ratio between core and sheath fluids as well as their absolute values can also influence another important parameter during microfluidic fiber processing,

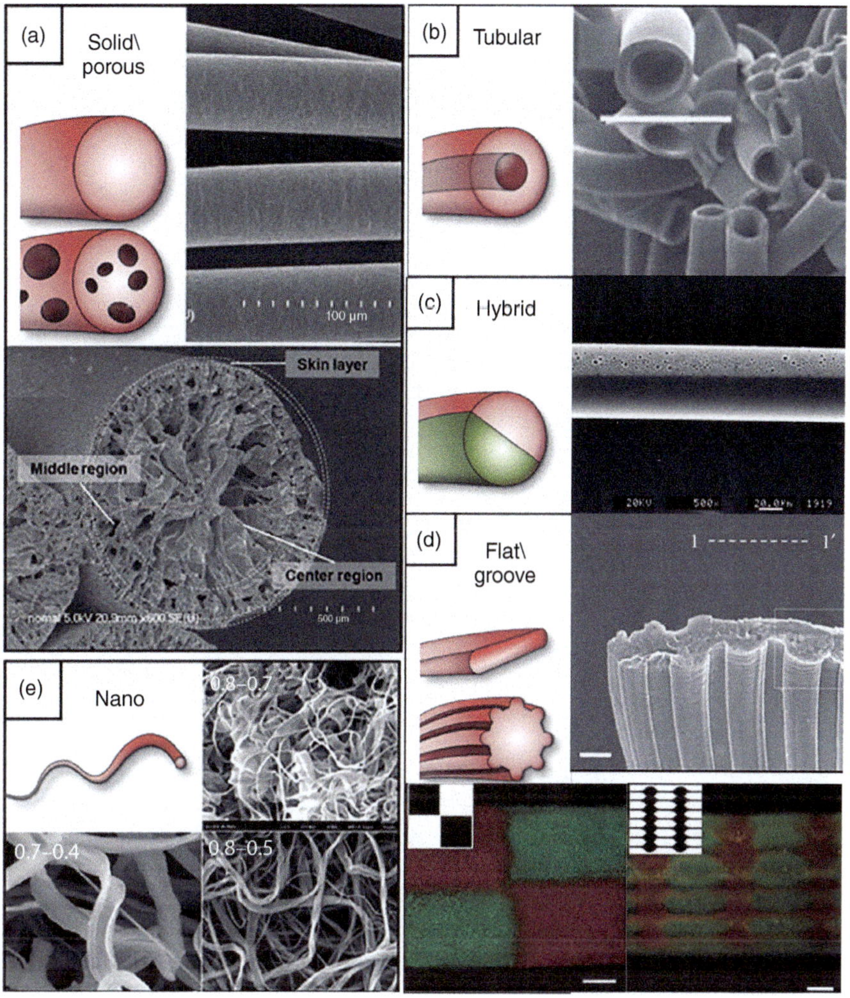

Figure 11.1 Examples of various fiber morphologies attainable with the use of microfluidic wet spinning. (a) Solid and porous fibers. (b) Tubular or core-shell fibers. (c) Hybrid/Janus fibers. (d) Flat and grooved fibers. (e) Nanoscaled fibers. Source: Jun et al. [18], Figure 04, Pg 11/with permission of from the Royal Society of Chemistry.

namely hydrodynamic focusing. Coaxial sheath flows exert a radial hydrodynamic pressure on the core flow during the fiber solidification mechanism as illustrated in Figure 11.2. This pressure affects the final fiber diameter and porosity as well as the alignment of the macromolecular chains, in turn influencing the extent and size of the crystalline domains as well as the tensile strength, Young's modulus, and elongation at break [29].

Besides the above-mentioned fiber geometries that can be achieved by varying the design of the microfluidic spinneret, manipulation of the sheath flow can lead to other interesting features such as the segmented bamboo-like fibers depictured in a previous study [30]. Additionally, multi-material fibers and liquid-filled fibers

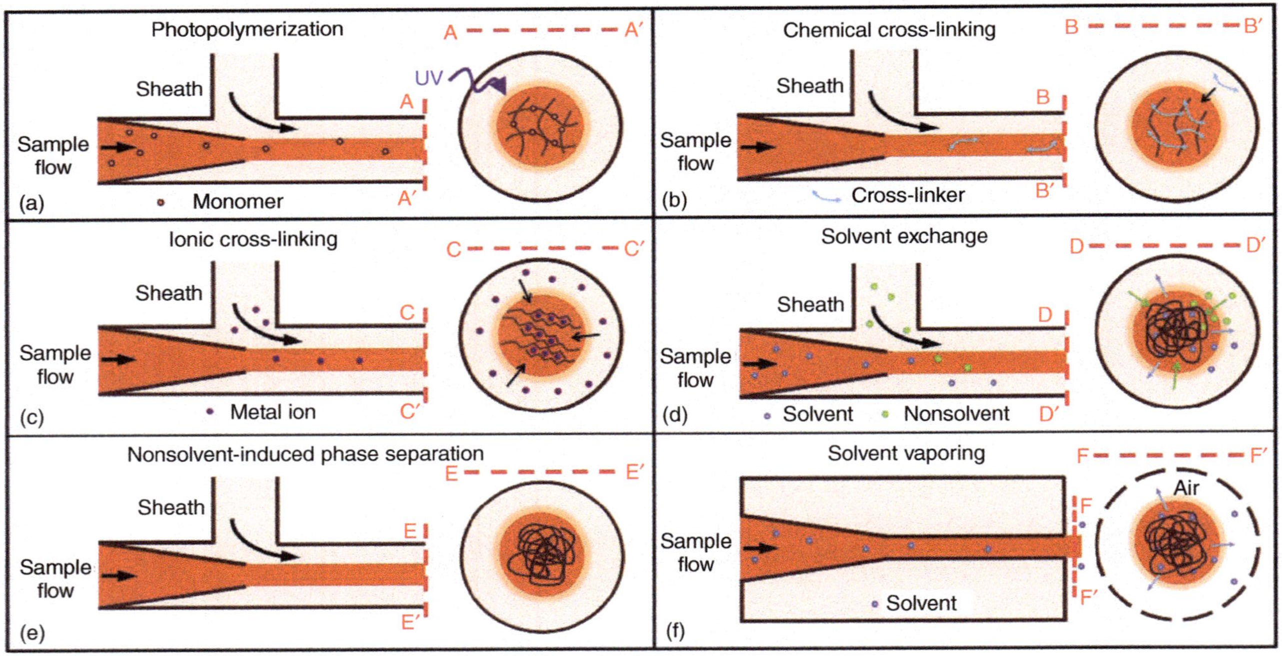

Figure 11.2 Different fiber coagulation strategies used to produce functional fiber by MWS. (a) Photoinitiated polymerization or crosslinking. (b) Chemical crosslinking. (c) Ionic crosslinking. (d) Solvent exchange. (e) Nonsolvent induced phase separation. (f) Solvent evaporation. Source: Du et al. [9]/with permission from Wiley-VCH.

can be produced by adding an extra set of sheath flow to the microfluidic design shown in Figure 11.2 or by introducing two different spinning dopes in the core and sheath flows and then using a coagulation bath for the precipitation of both polymers [31].

While it is theoretically possible to introduce a disparate number of materials as the coaxial layers within the same fiber, a limitation occurs regarding the possibility of fabricating a chip with an increasing number of coaxial sheath flows (see Section 11.2 for a more detailed discussion on the topic). Not only can the fiber network itself be precisely assembled within the microfluidic reactor, but also nanocapsules, nanoparticles, and other functional nano-objects can be selectively introduced in predetermined regions of the fiber by opportunely introducing them in the microfluidic spinneret prior to fiber coagulation [32].

11.2 Fabrication of Chips for Microfluidic Wet Spinning

To produce different geometries and hybrid structures via MWS, specific development of chips should tackle the different fiber coagulation kinetics by accommodating a versatile design of the microchannel with tunable residence times. Additionally, the chip should resist hydrodynamic pressures high enough to let high viscosity polymer solutions flow within microsized channels, display good transparency to visualize the fiber solidification process and therewith tackle any clogging issues, and permit easy integration of valves and fittings to connect with the external pumping system. Most importantly, the channel walls should show high shape fidelity to the target morphology and ensure that a homogeneous hydrodynamic pressure is exerted by the sheath flow on the core flow to induce the so-called hydrodynamic focusing. This feature is particularly important since by using three-dimension (3D) hydrodynamic focusing, we can vary the morphology (including the extent and size of the crystalline domains), the fiber size and also the porosity [29]. In order to produce multi-material fibers, several sheath flows need to be aligned with the core flow, and thus it would be highly desirable to develop a chip where sheath flows could be coaxially coupled on request as in a modular system. A microfluidic chip encompassing all these features has yet to be produced, so in practice a compromise needs to be found according to the type of application.

An overview of the chip fabrication methods is given in Table 11.1. Soft lithography of poly(dimethyl siloxane) (PDMS) is considered to be the most popular technique for prototyping and standard microfluidic chip fabrication [51]. The reasons are multifold: PDMS is easy to mold, optically transparent, oxygen-permeable, cheap, biocompatible, highly flexible and can easily conform and adapt to soft surfaces for wearable applications [52]. Features are mostly developed by casting PDMS on ultraviolet (UV) masks fabricated by standard photoresists used in the semiconductor industry followed by plasma bonding to another PDMS slab or to a different compatible material (e.g. quartz, glass, silicon) to fabricate the desired closed channel features [12, 29, 30].

Table 11.1 Overview of the chip fabrication methods used for microfluidic wet spinning of fibers.

Substrate	Fabrication method	Channel geometry	Fiber geometry	References
PDMS	Soft lithography	Square	C/NC[a)]	[12, 29, 30, 33–35]
PDMS	Soft lithography and application of negative pressure on PDMS membrane	Round	C/NC[a)]	[36–40]
PDMS + stainless steel needles	Gluing coaxial tubings	Round	C	[41, 42]
PDMS + stainless steel needles	Templating PDMS with stainless steel needles	Round	C[a)]	[43]
Concentric glass capillary within PDMS (or epoxy thermoset)	Assembly of glass capillaries during PDMS (or epoxy thermoset) cross-linking	Round	C[a)]	[44]
Concentric glass capillary within PMMA	PMMA micromilling and capillary insertion	Round	C[a)]	[25, 45]
PMMA	CO_2-laser engraving	Square	NC[a)]	[46, 47]
PMMA	Microcarving	Square	NC[a)]	[48]
Photo-polymerizing resin	Polyjet 3D printing	Round	C[a)]	[49]
Photo-patternable resin	Nanoscribe 3D printing	Round	C[a)]	[50]

Abbreviations: C, circular; NC, noncircular.

a) Multi-material fabrication

While PDMS soft lithography has been proven to be very effective at laboratory scale, several hurdles exist in bringing this technology to mass production, since cleanroom environments with sophisticated instruments are typically necessary and the entire fabrication process is relatively time-consuming. Furthermore, this method yields conventionally square channels, which do not permit homogeneous 3D hydrodynamic focusing. A useful method to produce a circular channel with a modified soft lithography processing has been developed by Lee's group (Figure 11.3a) [36–40]. Initially, a standard PDMS is fabricated with square channel geometry and a thin PDMS membrane is fixed on the top of the PDMS mold. Upon application of negative pressure, the PDMS membrane forms a concave hemicylindrical channel. This deformed membrane geometry is then replicated using SU-8 followed by UV curing. The SU-8 mold is then used to fabricate the hemicylindrical channels with PDMS, and then two identical slabs are aligned and bonded by plasma. Although this method has been shown to produce perfectly circular channels, it is even more time-consuming than standard PDMS soft lithography considering the challenge of achieving perfect slab alignment and its tedious and time-consuming fabrication procedure consisting of multiple soft lithography steps. On the other hand, it has been shown that microfiber patterning can be easily transferred with this technology [11].

A simpler construct is described by the group of Chen [41, 42], in which a hollow PDMS tube is used for the sheath fluid and a stainless steel needle is coaxially inserted in the tube and fixed at its edge by acrylic glue. It is important to notice that this chip does not allow any modularity and can, therefore, be used only to fabricate mono-material fibers. Recently, a templating method with PDMS using selected arrays of hypodermic needles as templates within a silicone elastomer matrix was developed by our group (Figure 11.3c) [43]. Interestingly, this method has demonstrated the possibility of fabricating microfluidic chips depicting two series of coaxial sheath fluids along with the main core flow, which can be translated to the fabrication of core–shell fibers.

Another standard material for microfluidics is glass, thanks to its biocompatibility, chemical inertness, high optical transparency, and good mechanical properties to withstand high hydraulic pressures inside microfluidic channels [51]. The fabrication of glass microfluidic chips, consisting mainly of powder blasting and hydrofluoric acid etching, uses either high-speed powder erosion or chemicals to carve the desired features in the chip, whose patterned surfaces are then bonded to another glass slab to seal the channel. On the other hand, high temperatures are generally needed during bonding, jeopardizing the cost efficiency and scalability of the process.

A pioneering method for the development of a coaxial microfluidic chip for wet spinning was developed in 2004 by W. Jeong et al. by combining the use of glass micropipettes with a premolded PDMS substrate (Figure 11.3b) [44]. Most of the literature research on MWS uses this standard chip fabrication procedure [16, 20, 26, 53–64], although in later cases PDMS, which is too flexible to support the inherently fragile glass capillaries, has been replaced by more mechanically stable two-component epoxy glue. A variation of this method that uses a blunt

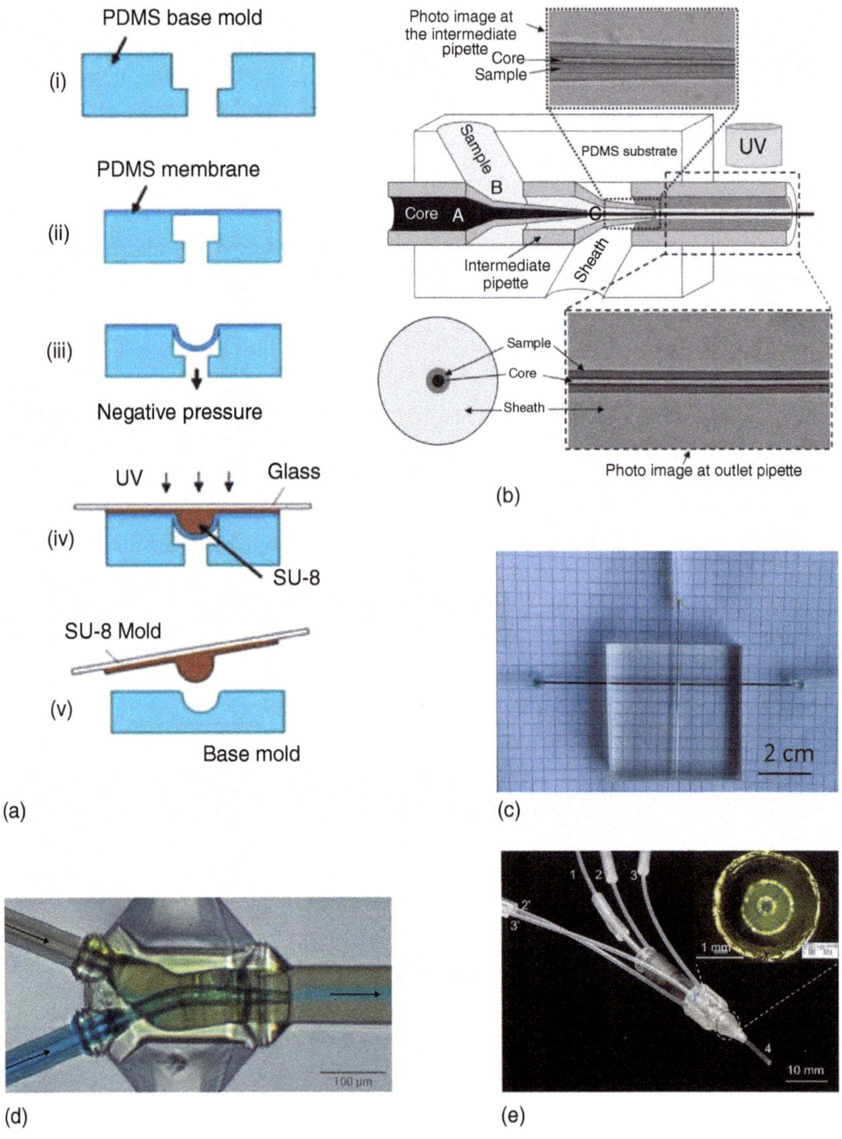

Figure 11.3 Overview of some fabrication methods for microfluidic spinnerets: (a) development of round channels by PDMS soft lithography. Source: Kang et al. [36]/with permission of Royal Society of Chemistry. (b) Fabrication of coaxial microfluidic chip by glass capillary assembly. (c) Production of a microfluidic chip by a templating method in PDMS with arrays of coaxially aligned stainless steel needles. Source: Gursoy et al. [43], Figure 01, Pg 03/MDPI/CC BY 4.0. (d) Development of 3D-printed microfluidic spinneret from Nanoscribe©. Source: Lölsberg J, et al. [50], Figure 05, Pg 05/with permission of from the Royal Society of Chemistry. (e) Fabrication of coaxial microfluidic spinneret by inserting stainless steel needles within 3D-printed chip. Source: Hu et al. [49], Figure 02, Pg 03/with permission of from Elsevier.

stainless steel tube coaxially inserted within a glass capillary has recently been presented [19, 65]. Alternatively, poly(methyl methacrylate) (PMMA), thanks to its high optical transparency, has also been used as the matrix to embed aligned glass capillaries for chip fabrication. In this case, the channels in the PMMA matrix are fabricated by micromilling technologies [25, 45]. However, it needs to be taken into account that the length and size of the drilling bits are limited, restricting their adaptability for different chip lengths.

Despite being a relatively simple method of fabricating microfluidic chips for wet spinning with a glass capillary that is resistant to high temperature and pressure as well as suitable for etching in different organic solutions, the assembly and alignment of the capillaries rely heavily on experience and manual operation, which limits the possibilities for widespread use of this method in manufacturing facilities [66].

Other methods that do not require any intermediate bonding step, as with open microfluidics [67], represent a solution for microfluidics in point-of-care diagnostic and consumable applications thanks to their easier simplicity in fabrication but cannot be used for fiber fabrication since the fluids flow in a passive manner with the use of capillarity. Similar considerations are also valid for paper-based and thread-based microfluidics [3, 68].

Subtractive manufacturing methods, namely CO_2 laser engraving [46] and microcarving [48], are also widely used to obtain microfluidic chips in PMMA in a layer-by-layer fashion and then further assembled by a screwing system or by epoxy glue. A homemade method of utilizing plastic disposable pipette tips for the development of coaxial flow has been shown by C. Chen et al. [69], where two pipette tips have been coaxially aligned and kept in place by gluing them together. While the method is simple, problems with reproducibility might arise due to the low homogeneity in flow alignment between the subsequent pipette tips.

Thermoplastic polymers, such as PMMA, are increasingly seen by the microfluidic community as an appealing alternative to reduce the fabrication time and cost of microfluidic chips, with processing techniques like microinjection molding and hot embossing, which have been used for the development of micro- and nanofluidic devices [70]. However, despite being high-throughput techniques, these processing methods still suffer from high prototyping cost due to tedious and cost-inefficient mold fabrication.

In this regard, additive manufacturing has also had a large impact on microfluidics, although the field is still considered to be in its infancy. Many advantages can be clearly pointed out when considering 3D printing with respect to the more standard soft lithography: when considering prototyping, 3D printing is economically convenient and is regarded as environmentally friendly since minimal waste is generated [71]. Additionally, 3D printing can be easily integrated with all the positive features of digital design, such as predicting the printing feasibility as well as modeling device performance and final cost [72]. In this section, we will limit our discussion to photopolymer inkjet printing (i.e. polyjet) and direct laser writing, since these are the only 3D printing methods used in the literature to build up microfluidic spinnerets. A deeper discussion of the advantages and disadvantages of different

3D printing technologies for the fabrication of microfluidic chips, namely selective laser sintering, fusion deposition modeling, 3D printing, laminated object manufacturing, and stereolithography printing, can be found in specific reviews [71–77]. Polyjet technology was first used in a study by M. Hu et al. to produce microfluidic chips for wet spinning of fibers like the one depicted in Figure 11.3e [49]. Polyjet technology deposits drops of photopolymer that solidify when exposed to UV light on the build tray. After removal of the support, the chip can be retrieved.

The spinneret body and the connection funnel of a triple-orifice spinneret were designed using Solidworks and fabricated with this technology. However, due to the orifices' thin wall and the stringent requirement for them to be concentric, they could not be 3D-printed, and thus two concentric blunt stainless steel needles were utilized for this purpose. Although it displays very high resolution (down to 10 μm), this method still does not yield completely smooth channels for MWS and may lead to microflow instabilities along with the flow pattern.

On the other hand, direct laser writing has proven to be a very precise technique for manufacturing with resolution down to hundreds of nanometers. Although direct laser writing is traditionally considered among the additive manufacturing techniques, it is actually a subtractive manufacturing technique since a solid mixture of materials is further cross-linked by either one- or two-photon polymerization with the non-cross-linked area untouched by the laser cleaned away in a subsequent washing step. One example of a microfluidic spinneret produced with this technology has been reported by J. Lölsberg et al. [50], who presented a microfluidic spinneret design for the fabrication of single-digit micrometer fibers by using a nozzle outlet of 12 μm (Figure 11.3d). While the use of this technique will certainly lead to an astonishing versatility in fiber fabrication in the next years, including extension of the produced fiber geometries, the equipment is still cost-prohibitive for industrial fabrication and standard high-throughput production of microfluidic chips.

11.3 Biomedical Applications of Hydrogel Fibers Produced via Microfluidics

Bulk hydrogels are emerging biomaterials with ECM-mimicking properties [78–80]. Hydrogel fibers produced by MWS have been investigated in many biomedical applications, including cell culturing and tissue engineering, fibrous biomedical devices, and drug delivery and controlled release, among others [10, 81, 82]. In Table 11.2, a summary of the selection of materials for different applications is given together with the fiber morphologies. Alginate is the most used material, due to its good biocompatibility and biodegradability, mild gelation condition, and high gelation rate [136]. Instead of using alginate alone (Table 11.2, Alg), non-gelling additives are useful to reinforce the alginate hydrogel fibers or to improve the bioactivity such as cell–material interactions (Table 11.2, Alg + Additives). By blending alginate with other gelling materials, additional functions and properties can be introduced (Table 11.2, Alg + Other gelling materials). Albeit rarely, chemically modified alginates can be also (Table 11.2, Alg Derivatives) used with or without other gelling materials. Only a few alginate-free materials have been used for the production of hydrogel fibers via MWS (Table 11.2, Alg-free materials).

11.3.1 Tissue Engineering

Microfluidic spun hydrogel fibers can encapsulate cells directly, making them particularly attractive for tissue engineering and cell transplantation applications [10, 18, 82, 86, 137]. Many efforts have been dedicated to the fabrication of cell-laden hydrogel fibers by MWS for engineering of various tissues. These fibers are generally fabricated *in vitro* to mimic the intrinsic morphologies and functions of human tissues, such as muscle fibers, blood vessels, liver microstructures, pancreatic islets, and neural networks. Taking advantage of microfluidics, the structures of cell-laden hydrogel fibers can be tailored to give many different forms, ranging from simple solid fibers to hollow fibers with straight or helix channels, core–shell fibers with cells encapsulated in a core layer or shell layer, knotted microfibers with cell-encapsulated knots, and so on. More importantly, in addition to simple encapsulation of single-cell type, MWS also enables the facile fabrication of heterogeneous constructs with spatially well-defined distribution of multiple cell types [9]. Microfluidic spun cell-laden hydrogel fibers were first used as microscale single-fiber scaffolds for cell encapsulation and tissue engineering and then evolved to become living building units for assembling macroscale artificial tissues and organs with high complexity.

11.3.1.1 Single-Fiber Scaffolds

As single-fiber scaffolds, microfluidic spun hydrogel fibers have been used not only for encapsulation and culturing of a single cell type but also for spatially controlled encapsulation and co-culturing of multiple cell types. Particularly, the emerging trends in using hydrogel fibers as co-culturing scaffolds have advanced the field of tissue engineering [9].

Mono-culturing System The works in MWS of cell-laden hydrogel fibers very often involve only a single cell type [44, 88]. For example, meter-long cell-laden hydrogel fibers exhibiting specific tissue morphologies and functions were prepared with a microfluidic chip composed of double-coaxial channels (Figure 11.4). Living cells were suspended in the core fluid containing extracellular matrix (ECM) proteins, which were subsequently encapsulated by alginate-based hydrogel shell during the MWS process. The hydrogel shell prevented the ECM proteins from diffusing away from the cells, thus promoting cell proliferation and functions within the produced hydrogel fibers. Finally, the alginate shell was degraded by alginate lyase, yielding a purely biological microfiber. Multiple cell types, including fibroblasts, endothelial cells, neurons, and myocytes, were used to establish mono-culturing systems with such microfluidic spun hydrogel fibers, showing their great potential for reconstructing fiber-shaped functional tissues that can mimic muscle fibers, blood vessels, and nerve networks. The *in vivo* transplantation of 20-cm-long primary islet cell fibers into the subrenal capsular space of a diabetic mouse demonstrated that

Table 11.2 A summary of gelling materials for different biomedical applications of microfluidic wet spun hydrogel fibers.

Material	Solidification method	Application	Morphology	References
Alg[a)]	Ionic cross-linking	Cell culturing for tissue engineering/regeneration	Cylindrical solid fibers	[83–87]
			Cylindrical hollow fibers	[61, 88–92]
			Cylindrical fibers with grooves	[93]
			Cylindrical hollow fibers with multilayered walls	[94, 95]
			Cylindrical fibers with multiple channels/cores	[63, 96]
			Cylindrical fibers with spatiotemporally coded complexity	[38]
			Flat fibers with grooves	[12]
			Sandwich-type fibers	[33, 97, 98]
			Spindle, hemispherical, and petal-knotted microfibers	[19]
			Planar sheets with mosaic patterns	[99, 100]
		Sensors and actuators	Cylindrical solid fibers	[35, 44]
			Cylindrical hollow fibers	[44]
			Solid, string-of-beads, and Janus topographies	[41]
			Helical cylindrical fibers	[17, 101, 102]
		Drug delivery/cancer research/microbiology	Cylindrical solid fibers	[34, 47, 103]
Alg + additives (ionic cross-linking)				
	(With chitosan as additive)	Cell culturing for tissue engineering	Cylindrical solid fibers	[60]
		Drug delivery	Cylindrical solid fibers	[104]
	(With VdECMs[b)] as additive)	Cell culturing for tissue engineering	Cylindrical hollow fibers	[105, 106]

	(With PVA[c)] as additive)	Cell culturing for tissue engineering	Cylindrical hollow fibers	[107]
	(With PNIPAM[d)] and graphene oxide as additives)	Actuators	Cylindrical bilayered solid fibers	[108]
	(With PEDOT: PSS[e)] as additive)	Flexible electronics	Cylindrical core–shell solid fibers	[109]
Alg + other gelling materials				
Alg + p(NIPAM-AA)[f)]	Ionic cross-linking	Actuators	Cylindrical solid and hollow fibers	[110]
Alg + GelMA[g)]	Ionic cross-linking + UV polymerization	Cell culturing for tissue engineering	Cylindrical solid fibers	[111–114]
			Cylindrical hollow fibers	[114]
Alg + GelMA + PEGOA[h)]			Cylindrical hollow fibers	[115]
Alg + GelMA + PEGTA[i)]			Cylindrical hollow fibers	[116]
Alg + GelMA + CS-AEMA[j)] + HAMA[k)]			Cylindrical solid fibers	[117]
Alg + PEGDA[l)]		Actuators	Helical fibers with Janus, triplex, and core–shell cross-sectional structures	[118]
		Wound dressing/healing materials	Cylindrical solid fibers	[119]
Alg + PEG-Fibrinogen		Cell culturing for tissue engineering	Cylindrical solid fibers	[120]
Alg + PAAm[m)]		Sensor	Cylindrical solid fibers	[121]
		Actuators	Cylindrical solid fibers	[56]
		Optogenetic manipulation	Cylindrical solid fibers	[122]
		Actuators	Helical cylindrical fibers	[17]
	Ionic cross-linking + free radical polymerization	Actuators	Cylindrical core–shell solid fibers	[123]

(*continued*)

Table 11.2 (Continued)

Material	Solidification method	Application	Morphology	References
Alg derivatives (with or without other gelling materials)				
Alg-Ph[n)]	Enzymatic cross-linking	Cell culturing for tissue engineering	Cylindrical solid fibers	[124]
Alg-Ph + gelatin-Ph[o)]				[125]
AlgMe[p)]	Ionic cross-linking and UV polymerization		Cylindrical hollow fibers with bi-layered walls	[126]
AlgOx[q)] + gelatin	Ionic cross-linking and amine–aldehyde chemical reaction		Cylindrical solid fibers as channel templates	[127]
Alg-free materials				
PEGDA	UV polymerization	Sensors	Mosaicked microfibers with rectangular cross section	[128]
GelMA		Cell culturing for tissue engineering	Cylindrical solid fibers with grooves	[11, 129]
GelMA-PEGDA		Microfluidic 3D bioprinting	Multi-material microstructures	[130]
MeHA[r)]/GelMA/NorHA[s)]/PEGDA		Microfluidic 3D bioprinting	Cylindrical solid, hollow, and intermittent fibers	[131]
PEGDA + 4-HBA[t)] + AA[u)]		Sensors	Barcoded strips	[132]
Chitosan	Ionic cross-linking	Cell culturing for tissue engineering	Cylindrical solid fibers	[133]

Bacterial cellulose	Ethanol-induced coagulation	Drug delivery	Cylindrical core–shell solid fibers	[134]
HA-EDA-C18[v)]	Coagulation induced by different ionic strengths	Drug delivery	Cylindrical solid fibers	[135]

a) Alg: alginate.
b) VdECMs: vascular tissue-specific decellularized extracellular matrices.
c) PVA: poly(vinyl alcohol).
d) PNIPAM: poly(*N*-isopropylacrylamide).
e) PEDOT: PSS: poly(3,4-ethylenedioxythiophene): poly (4-styrenesulfonate).
f) p(NIPAM-AA): poly(*N*-isopropylacrylamide-*co*-acrylic acid).
g) GelMA: methacrylamide-modified gelatin.
h) PEGOA: 8-arm poly(ethylene glycol) (PEG) acrylate with tripentaerythritol core.
i) PEGTA: 4-arm poly(ethylene glycol)-tetra-acrylate.
j) CS-AEMA: chondroitin sulfate amino ethyl methacrylate.
k) HAMA: hyaluronic acid methacrylate.
l) PEGDA: poly(ethylene glycol) diacrylate.
m) PAAm: polyacrylamide.
n) Alg-Ph: phenolic hydroxyl alginate.
o) Gelatin-Ph: phenolic hydroxyl gelatin.
p) AlgMe: methacrylated alginate.
q) AlgOx: oxidized alginate.
r) MeHA: methacrylated hyaluronic acid.
s) NorHA: norbornene-functionalized hyaluronic acid.
t) 4-HBA: 4-hydroxybutyl acrylate.
u) AA: acrylic acid.
v) HA-EDA-C18: hyaluronic acid amphiphilic derivative.

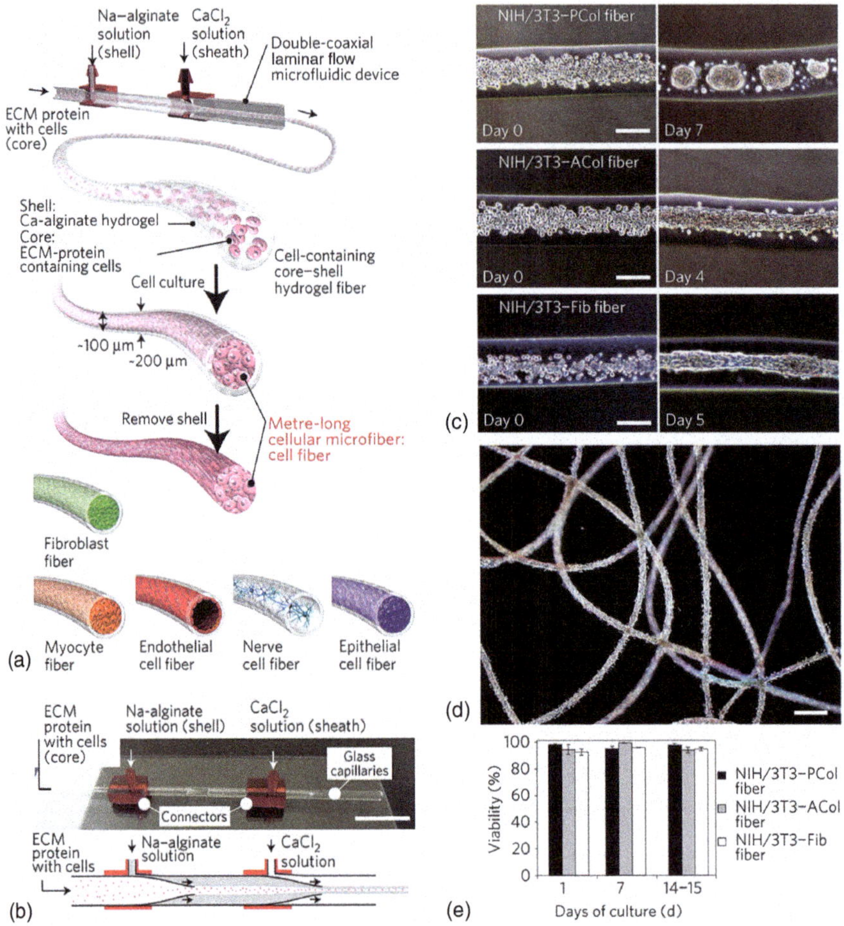

Figure 11.4 (a) A cell-containing ECM-protein/Ca-alginate core–shell hydrogel microfiber is continuously generated in a double-coaxial microfluidic device. The cells in the gelated ECM protein migrate and form a fiber-shaped cellular construct with cell-to-cell contacts. The Ca–alginate shell can be selectively removed with an enzymatic reaction. Various types of cells can be applied to the cell fibers. (b) An image (top) and an explanatory illustration (bottom) of the double-coaxial laminar flow microfluidic device. The device was composed of pulled glass capillaries and connectors. A double-coaxial laminar flow consisting of a pre-gel solution of ECM proteins with cells (core), a pre-gel solution of Na-alginate (shell), and a $CaCl_2$ solution (sheath) was generated in the device, and a cell-containing ECM-protein/Ca-alginate core–shell hydrogel microfiber was continuously formed. (c) Sequential images of the behaviors of NIH/3T3 cells in the different types of ECM protein. NIH/3T3 cells in ACol and Fib formed cell fibers. In contrast, NIH/3T3 cells in PCol (pepsin-solubilized type-I collagen) did not form cell fibers. (d) An image of the NIH/3T3–ACol (acid-solubilized type-I collagen) fiber on day 4. (e) Viability of the cells in NIH/3T3 fibers. The results are shown as the mean ± s.d. of three independent fibers. Scale bars: 1 mm (b); 100 μm (c); and 500 μm (d). Source: Onoe et al. [61], Figure 01, Pg 02/Permission from Springer Nature.

insulin secretion from the living fiber could be regulated by the surrounding glucose concentration [61]. Hydrogel-fiber-based mono-culturing systems have also found applications in liver-like tissue engineering [19, 60], blood vessels [105], neurons [33, 89, 90], and cartilage [85].

For some tissue engineering applications, cells could also be seeded on the fiber scaffolds after microfluidic spinning fabrication instead of being encapsulated during spinning. For example, neural cells were seeded on microgrooved fibers produced by microfluidic spinning. Alignment of the seeded cells on the microgrooved fiber surface was observed, which is of great importance for the formation of neural pathways. It may have important potential in tissue regeneration for peripheral nerve or spinal cord injuries [12, 38, 93]. Artificial muscle tissues have also been engineered by culturing myoblasts on the surface of grooved methacrylated gelatin (GelMA) hydrogel fibers. The alignments of myoblasts as well as the myotube formations are augmented by topographical cues on the fiber surface [11, 129].

Co-culturing System One of the key challenges in tissue engineering is heterotypic placement and co-culturing of distinct cell types in the microstructure of tissue engineering scaffolds [138], which could be addressed by the unique capability of MWS in spatiotemporally manipulating the dimension, composition, and morphology of complex hydrogel fibers [38, 63, 99, 139]. Therefore, MWS meets the demand for complex constructs involving co-culturing of multiple cell types [115, 130]. Such complex cell-laden hydrogel fibers are useful for the development of artificial microtissues mimicking blood vessels, the liver, neuron networks, muscles, among others.

Early examples of using microfluidic spun cell-laden hydrogel fibers in a co-culturing system were demonstrated by embedding hydrogel fibers in bulk hydrogel matrix [84, 91, 124, 127] or seeding a second cell type on the preformed cell-laden hydrogel fibers [125]. However, heterotypic placement and co-culturing of distinct cell types within the hydrogel microfibers have not yet been demonstrated in these examples. Recently, hydrogel fibers with concentric layers of different cell types were fabricated by using multi-flow microfluidic spinning, proving that complex heterogeneous hierarchical architectures that have strong potential in tissue engineering applications can be realized by one-step MWS biofabrication [63, 95, 106, 115, 124]. This concept has been intensively demonstrated in microvessel tissue engineering, where co-culturing of endothelium cells (ECs) and smooth muscle cells (SMCs) is found to be of crucial importance for the development of blood vessels [63, 95, 106, 115]. For example, Gao et al. reported the development of biomimetic tissue-engineered blood vessels that include an endothelium layer surrounded by a smooth muscle layer by using a triple-coaxial microfluidic spinning technology (Figure 11.5) [106]. Other co-culturing examples of microfluidic spun hydrogel fibers also include tissue engineering of liver-like constructs [97, 100].

11.3.1.2 Assembled Fiber Scaffolds

Hydrogel fibers can be used as functional building units for assembling macroscopic scaffolds [9]. The novel concept of cell-laden textiles was based on the ability of

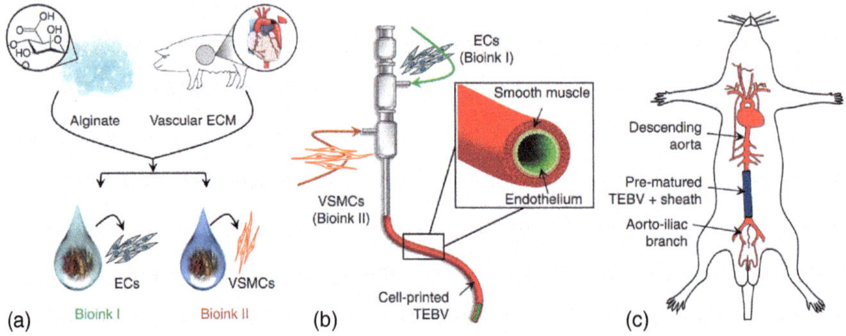

Figure 11.5 (a) The formulation of vascular tissue-specific bioinks to promote the cellular activities of endothelial cells (ECs) and vascular smooth muscle cells (VSMCs). (b) Triple-coaxial cell printing of biomimetic tissue-engineered blood vessels (TEBVs). (c) *In vivo* evaluation of prematured TEBVs through an interpositional abdominal aorta graft in a rat model. Source: Gao G et al. [106]/ with permission from AIP Publishing.

microfluidic spinning in producing hierarchically cell-laden hydrogel fibers. This has led to the emerging field of tissue/organ weaving and the next-generation tissue-engineered products for regenerative medicine applications. Such a tissue/organ weaving concept has been demonstrated by assembling microfluidic spun hydrogel fibers into macroscopic constructs either by hand or by machine [63, 82, 140].

Microfluidic Tissue/Organ Weaving By applying the textile weaving technique, hydrogel fibers can be assembled into macroscale scaffolds for the development of artificial tissues/organs. Liberski et al. presented the concept of "organ weaving" for the first time. Living threads consisting of cell-laden alginate hydrogel fibers were woven by a hand-weaving process [94]. In a typical example, Tamayol et al. reported the microfluidic fabrication of hydrogel fibers containing NIH-3T3 fibroblasts, HepG2s, or human umbilical vein endothelial cells (HUVECs). These hybrid hydrogel fibers with different cell types could be assembled by weaving, braiding, or direct writing into a 3D liver model, where the cells remained active over 16 days of culturing and the level of albumin in the media increased continuously [111]. Onoe et al. demonstrated that such living cell-laden textiles could be produced by machine instead of hand-weaving. They developed a microfluidic weaving machine working in culture medium, which can be coupled with the microfluidic spinning device to assemble higher-order cellular constructs. Compared to those woven by hand, such cellular constructs feature organized spatial patterns and well-controlled and reproducible production [61]. This integration of modern microfluidic spinning technology with traditional textile industry is considered highly promising in the bottom–up regeneration of complex, large tissue defects, thus benefiting a variety of applications in tissue engineering and biomedical research, as is also demonstrated in recent researches [98, 126].

Microfluidic 3D Bioprinting More recently, microfluidic 3D bioprinting, which integrates MWS with 3D bioprinting, is rapidly emerging for the construction of complex tissue-engineered constructs [130]. Such a combination features the advantage of precise control over both microstructures and macrostructures of the produced cell-laden constructs, where the microstructures of the hydrogel fiber building units are controlled by the MWS, while the macrostructures of 3D cell-laden constructs are defined by the 3D bioprinting technique. Consequently, this microfluidic-based 3D bioprinting technology provides a powerful and versatile approach for creating biomimetic heterogeneous tissue models, which may advance the fields of regenerative medicine and drug discovery [141]. Firstly, such hydrogel constructs fabricated with microfluidic 3D bioprinting have been used as general fibrous tissue engineering scaffolds, which permit high diffusion capability of molecules and enable better viability of encapsulated cells than nonfibrous scaffold even in massive cell culture [86, 133]. Special interest has been shown in fabricating vascularized artificial tissue constructs with microfluidic 3D bioprinting to address one of the most challenging issues in tissue engineering, namely the vascularization of artificial tissues with clinically relevant dimensions [112, 116]. Specific tissues have been targeted by the microfluidic 3D bioprinting approach, including cartilage [117], cardiac muscles [113], skeletal muscles [120, 129], and blood vessels [92, 142]. A typical example of microfluidic 3D bioprinting was presented recently by Zhang et al. Microfluidic spinning was used to produce endothelialized hydrogel fibers, which could be precisely assembled into a macroscale anisotropic architecture by 3D bioprinting (Figure 11.6). Cardiomyocytes were seeded on the resultant constructs to induce the formation of myocardium and to generate aligned myocardium capable of spontaneous and synchronous contraction. An endothelialized-myocardium-on-a-chip platform was then developed after being cultivated in a microfluidic perfusion bioreactor. This platform shows great potential for cardiovascular toxicity evaluation and could be developed for constructing endothelialized human myocardium [113].

11.3.2 Sensors and Actuators

Microfluidic spun hydrogel fibers have shown great promise in fabricating advanced biomedical devices, as they could combine the excellent biocompatibility of hydrogels with the large surface-to-volume ratio of fibers. This combination of properties makes them particularly attractive for biomedical devices such biosensors, actuators, and flexible bioelectronics [9, 143].

11.3.2.1 Sensors

Compared with conventional bulk hydrogels, microfiber-shaped hydrogel sensors have additional characteristics such as excellent flexibility and rapid responsivity [9]. As the very first example of continuous microfibers produced by a concentric-flow microfluidic device, hydrogel fibers were used to demonstrate

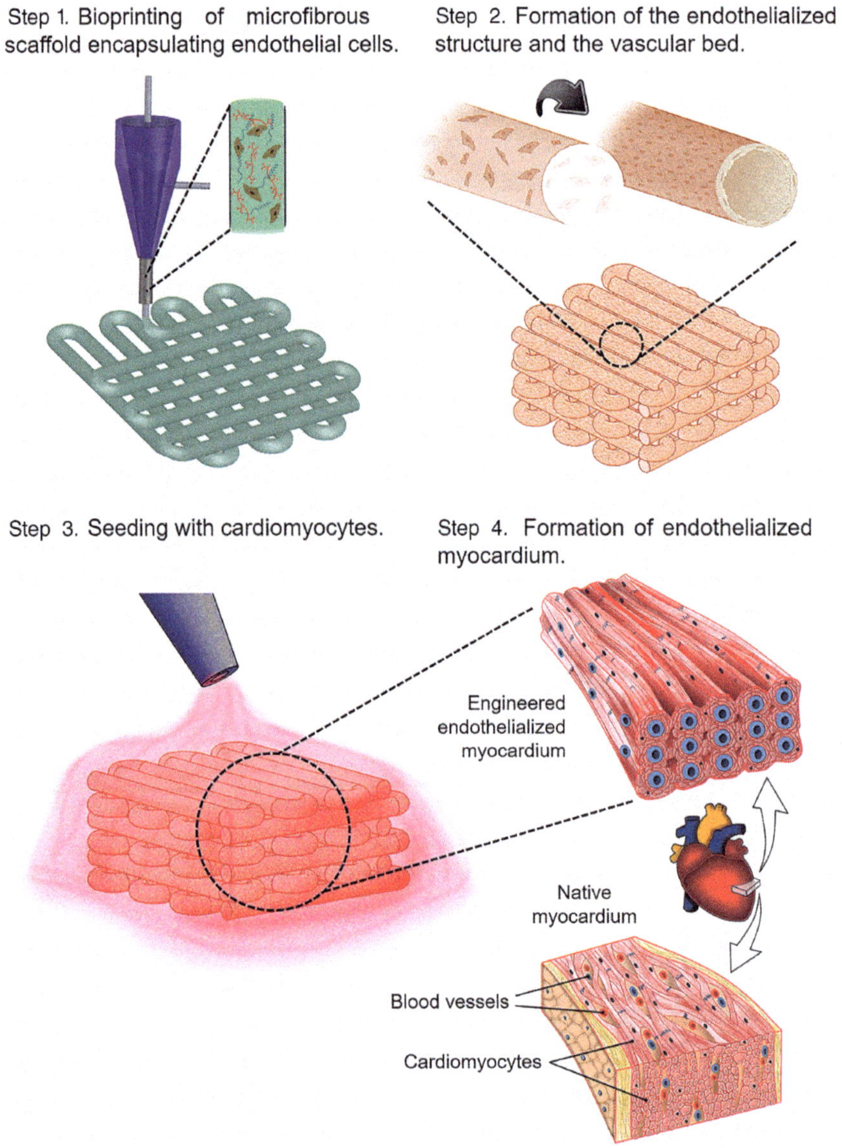

Figure 11.6 Schematics showing the procedure of fabricating endothelialized myocardium using the 3D bioprinting strategy. Step 1: bioprinting of a microfibrous scaffold using a composite bioink encapsulating endothelial cells. Step 2: formation of the vascular bed through migration of HUVECs to the peripheries of the microfibers. Step 3: seeding of cardiomyocytes into the interstitial space of the endothelialized scaffold. Step 4: formation of engineered endothelialized myocardium structurally resembling the native myocardium. Source: Zhang et al. [113]/with permission from Elsevier.

biosensing applications [44]. Since then, two main types of biosensors have been produced with hydrogel fibers, namely fluorescence-based optical sensors and deformation-based strain sensors.

Optical Sensors The first microfluidic spun hydrogel fibers were demonstrated as fluorescence-based optical sensors, in which hydrogel fibers entrapping two enzymes (glucose oxidase [GOx] and horseradish peroxide [HRP]) were produced by a concentric-flow microfluidic device. In the presence of glucose, Amplex Red induced fluorescence within the hydrogel fibers, which were used for glucose sensing [44]. While the basic principle remains similar to this pioneering example, many attempts have been dedicated to achieving multiple biosensing by hydrogel fibers. A typical example is presented by Kim et al., where enzyme-immobilized barcoded strips for multiple bioanalysis were produced by MWS with a microfluidic device called microstrip fabrication apparatus (MFA). Two pairs of coenzymes, namely HRP/GOx and HRP/lactate oxidase (LOx), were loaded into the barcoded microstrips. Simultaneous detection of glucose and lactate was realized [132]. A more recent example presented by Cho et al. also realized multiplex biomolecular analysis, where human and rabbit immunoglobulins G (IgG) were incorporated in poly(ethylene glycol) diacrylate (PEGDA) hydrogel fibers during MWS. Fluorescein isothiocyanate (FITC)-human anti-IgG and tetramethylrhodamine (TRITC)-rabbit anti-IgG in a mixed analyte solution were detected simultaneously [128].

Other than biomolecules, hydrogel fibers are also useful as optical sensors for monitoring bio-relevant environmental changes [41]. For example, the pH value of a wound is closely correlated with a broad range of biological processes, including protease activity, angiogenesis, and bacterial infection. It can be used as an important indication of the physiological condition of skin wounds [144]. Hydrogel fibers, being flexible, can conformably contact skin for long-term monitoring of epidermal wound pH, thus providing real-time monitoring of the wound healing process. Tamayol et al. reported encapsulation of pH-responsive dyes in mesoporous polyester beads which were loaded in hydrogel fibers during MWS. These hydrogel fibers were assembled on a transparent medical tape to form a pH-responsive wound dressing. Such a hydrogel-fiber-based wound dressing allows real-time pH measurement by using a smartphone camera for onsite readout [35].

Strain Sensors Hydrogel fibers composed of stimuli-responsive materials are of great interest due to their capability to change shape in response to a wide range of external stimuli (pH, temperature, magnetic field, electric field, etc.). Specifically, shrinking or swelling in response to changes in corresponding external stimuli, such as temperature or pH, is the most common strain sensing mechanism of such "smart" hydrogel fibers. The reversibility of such volume changes is of particular interest for hydrogel fiber sensors, since it can allow repeated usage. For example, Peng et al. reported MWS of electro-responsive hydrogel fibers composed of graphene oxide (GO), polyacrylamide, and alginate. Such hydrogel fibers can undergo macroscopic bending upon electro-stimulation, making them promising materials for electro-sensing in biological systems [56]. Wei et al. reported the microfluidic spinning of tough and conductive hydrogel fiber networks, which can

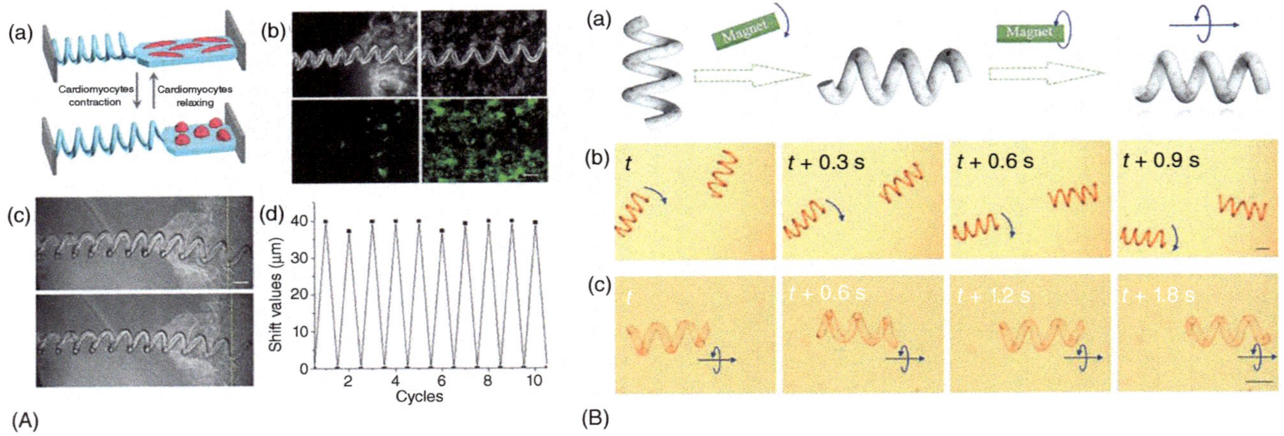

Figure 11.7 Application of helical microfibers as mechanical sensors (A) or microactuators (B). (A-a) Schematic illustration of a microfiber–film complex used as a mechanical sensor for cardiomyocytes. (A-b) Cross-sectional confocal laser scanning microscopy (CLSM) images of the helical microfiber and cardiomyocytes on GelMA film. The scale bar is 150 μm. (A-c) Microscopy images of the helical microfiber corresponding to the beating activity of the cardiomyocytes. The scale bar is 150 μm. (A-d) Records of the changes in 10 helical pitches according to the beating cycles of the cardiomyocytes [17]. (B-a) Illustration of the helical micromotor responding to the clockwise rotary and 3D rotating magnetic field. (B-b) Movement of the helical micromotors under different direction magnets. (B-c) Corkscrew motion of the helical micromotor in a 3D rotating magnetic field. Scale bars: 250 mm. Source: From Yu et al. [118], Figure 05, Pg 06/with permission of Wiley-VCH.

be used as wearable sensors for detecting human motions [121]. More advanced biosensing applications based on fiber deformation were also demonstrated in systems involving living cells [17]. Yu et al. reported the microfluidic fabrication of alginate helical microfibers that can be employed as mechanical sensors for cardiomyocytes with beating ability (Figure 11.7A). In this system, a helical hydrogel microfiber was tied to an elastic GelMA hydrogel film on which the cardiomyocytes were then seeded. The cardiomyocytes beating on the elastic film were then visualized by helical microfibers undergoing cycles of elongation and contraction [17].

11.3.2.2 Actuators

Micro-scale Actuators Recently, artificial microactuators have attracted considerable attention due to their great promise in material transfer and assembly, drug delivery, and environmental remediation [9]. Hydrogel fiber strain sensors based on stimuli-responsive volume change can also be used as microactuators, which can perform motions by transforming varying types of energy into mechanical movements [56, 101]. Among them, helical hydrogel fibers, or hydrogel microsprings, are most intriguing due to their ability to mimic the motility of natural microorganisms [145]. For example, Yoshida and Onoe reported magnetic-responsive hydrogel microsprings produced by microfluidic spinning. The magnetically responsive helical microfibers could be stretched by exerting a magnetic field and then recover to their original states upon removal of the magnetic field [101]. Yu et al. also reported micromotors consisting of magnetically actuated helical PEGDA hydrogel microfibers (Figure 11.7B) [118]. Tang et al. described the microfluidic fabrication of a rigid hollow helical alginate/protamine/silica hydrogel microfiber loaded with Fe_3O_4 nanoparticles [102]. The prepared hydrogel microfibers can achieve rotation-based locomotion and provide good mechanical strength for supporting cargo transportation. These highly biocompatible and fuel-free intelligent helical micromotors could be applied in biomedical fields, especially in targeted drug delivery.

In addition, pH, temperature, and light can also be used to stimulate the actuation of hydrogel fibers [108, 110, 118]. For example, Kim et al. reconfigured the barcoded hydrogel microstrips used for multiple bioanalysis by implementing pH-responsive poly(acrylic acid) (PAA) into the polymer network. The resultant hydrogel microstrips with PAA located at predefined sites can swell in a controllable manner, thus allowing programmable microactuation based on pH variation [132]. Yu et al. reported that temperature-responsive helical hydrogel microfibers were produced by copolymerizing temperature-responsive *N*-isopropylacrylamide (NIPAM) monomers into the fibers. The produced hydrogel fibers could perform reversible deformation upon alternating the surrounding temperature [17, 118].

Other than reversible shape change, chemical fuels can also be used to realize microactuation of hydrogel fibers. Yu et al. reported the encapsulation of catalytic platinum (Pt) nanoparticles in a core–shell helical micromotor, which could be propelled by oxygen microbubbles generated by the catalytic reaction between Pt nanoparticles and surrounding hydrogen peroxide [118].

Macroscale Actuators Hydrogel microfibers have also found applications in constructing macroscopic actuators [108, 110, 123]. Nakajima et al. reported the microfluidic fabrication of stimuli-responsive hydrogel fibers composed of poly(*N*-isopropylacrylamide-*co*-acrylic acid) (pNIPAM-AA) and sodium alginate (Na–alginate). These fibers can undergo folding and pumping movements triggered by temperature or pH change. Macroscale 3D structures were assembled by bundling microfibers together, yielding an artificial muscle-like actuator that might be useful for soft robot applications [110]. Liu et al. reported the fabrication of macroscopic hydrogel fiber bundles and hydrogel films from temperature-responsive core–shell hydrogel fibers. The simple device made of hydrogel fibers can act as an artificial "muscle" that can lift up to 180 times the mass of the hydrogel actuator. In addition, when such hydrogel microfibers were embedded in parallel on the top layer of a poly(vinyl alcohol) (PVA) hydrogel, the hybrid hydrogel exhibited fast bending transformation perpendicular to the axis of the microfibers [123].

11.3.3 Controlled Drug Delivery

Microfibers are promising drug delivery biomaterials due to their high surface-to-volume ratio, enabling the release of drugs into the surrounding environment over a large area [9, 146]. MWS has been used for hydrogel fiber production with applications in synergistic encapsulation and controlled release of drugs. Taking advantage of MWS in continuous fiber production and excellent morphological control, a variety of drug-loaded fibers of controllable dimensions and morphologies have been reported. These drug-delivering fibers can be categorized as passive or active drug release systems.

Ahn et al. used isopropyl alcohol (IPA) in the sheath flow of the MWS process to generate alginate microfibers. Compared to conventional alginate hydrogel fibers cross-linked solely by $CaCl_2$, these fibers with IPA-induced polymer aggregation possessed better drug encapsulation ability [34]. In addition to IPA-induced polymer aggregation, Zhang et al. demonstrated that the strengthened degree of cross-linking achieved by incorporation of chitosan could further increase the ampicillin drug-loading capacity and prolong the drug release profile of alginate microfibers [104]. Agnello et al. reported the microfluidic spinning of microfibers from a hyaluronic acid amphiphilic derivative. Such microfibers with ionic-strength-sensitive properties were used for loading and release of dexamethasone as a model drug molecule [135].

While passive control of drug release from microfibers usually relies on the diffusion properties of the drugs, and the porous structure and degradation profile of the fibers, active control of drug release uses external stimuli as triggers to manipulate the diffusion of drugs from the porous fibers and could thus provide better control over the drug release profile in an on-demand manner. For example, Lin et al. reported the fabrication of magnetic iron-oxide-loaded microfibers. The fibers produced can realize magnetic-controlled drug release from alginate microfibers [47]. Jiang et al. prepared composite hollow microfibers with K^+-responsive controlled release behavior [147]. Chen et al. reported electrically responsive drug release

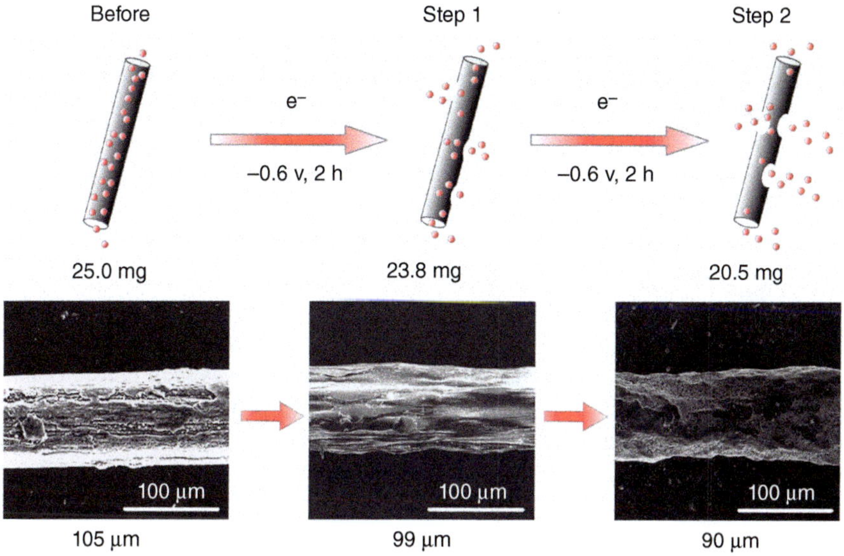

Figure 11.8 Weight and morphology changes of the as-prepared microfiber before and after electrical stimulation. Source: Chen et al. [69], Figure 05, Pg 35/with permission of from Elsevier.

core–shell hybrid microfibers (Figure 11.8) [69, 134]. In this study, multifunctional core–shell hybrid microfibers were synthesized using a combination of coaxial spinning and a subsequent dip-coating process. These hydrogel fibers contain a hydrogel core of bacterial cellulose (BC) and a conductive polymer shell layer of poly(3,4-ethylenedioxythiophene) (PEDOT). A model drug, diclofenac sodium, was loaded in the core layer of the microfibers. The enhanced drug release from the microfibers was realized by external electrical stimulation.

11.3.4 Other Biomedical Applications

Microfluidic spun hydrogel fibers have also been explored in other biomedical applications, including flexible electronics [109], cancer research [47, 148], microbial culturing [103], optogenetic manipulation [122], wound dressing/healing materials [96, 119], drug assays [149], and so on.

11.4 Hydrogel Optical Fibers

Optical fibers (OFs) are standard materials used in telecommunication/data transmission, home illumination, and industrial sensors [150]. Light is guided in an OF by the total internal reflection between core and cladding, for which the refractive index of the core must be higher than that of the cladding. While most of the OFs used commercially are made of silica (glass optical fibers [GOFs]), polymer optical fibers (POFs) are becoming increasingly important. POFs are typically made of a

PMMA core and a fluoropolymer as cladding. This ensures good transmission properties due to both an adequate difference between the refractive indices (RIs) of the core and cladding (1.52 and 1.35, respectively) as well as low light attenuation losses of these two polymers. On the other hand, PMMA is stiff and brittle. While this is not of concern for the standard applications of POFs, it makes them unsuitable for biomedical applications, where contact with body tissues, sharp bending, and high mechanical loading during fabrication of the devices may be found [151]. To address these issues, elastomeric and ductile POFs with thermoplastic siloxanes or cyclic olefin copolymers as the core have been investigated [152–154].

These fibers, however, are not adequate for implants or for light-guiding in inner tissues. Due to their properties (soft, rubbery nature, high water content, and compatibility with cells), hydrogel materials offer more advantages than conventional, hydrophobic waveguides for in-body applications. This research field, however, has only recently been investigated. This section will describe the materials used to produce hydrogel optical fibers (HOFs) as well as the potential applications of these innovative waveguides.

11.4.1 Materials

The field of HOFs derives from the initial studies on hydrogel waveguides, going back to the early 1990s [155]. Hydrogel waveguides have been produced with both natural and synthetic precursors: agarose, alginate, gelatin, cellulose derivatives, PVA, poly(ethylene glycol) (PEG), PEGDA, P(AAm-*co*-EGDA), and polyacrylamide (PAAm) have been reported in the literature [154, 156, 157]. Only in the last decade, however, have the findings for planar waveguides been translated to HOFs: the first core-only (PVA) and core-cladding (PEGDA–Alg) HOFs were reported in 2014 and 2015, respectively [158, 159]. PEGDA is the most investigated synthetic polymer due to its widespread utilization in soft and implantable devices, nontoxicity, and ease of use. Among the natural polymers, alginate, being widely used in biomedical applications and having a simple gelation system with divalent cations, has been the preferred choice [160]. Compared with the variety of hydrogels used for other biomedical applications or with the choice of materials for standard POFs, this list clearly shows potential for an increase in the number of precursor polymers for HOFs in the future. As mentioned in the introduction, a large difference between the core and cladding RIs is crucial to allow the guiding of large amounts of light. Table 11.3 displays the reported fibers with their compositions for core and cladding as well as their respective RIs. For core-only fibers, the cladding will be the environment around the HOF (air, water, tissue, etc.), which leads to changing boundary conditions for reflection and, consequently, light losses. Table 11.3 also shows the reported attenuation for the produced fibers. As a comparison, commercial PMMA presents attenuation lower than 0.02 dB/cm (at 650 nm), while POFs used in textile sensors present attenuation of 0.14–0.50 dB/cm [151, 152]. The high attenuation of HOFs means that light can only be guided for a few tens of centimeters. This is still a strong limitation of HOFs that should be improved by a better choice of materials (with intrinsically lower attenuation) or by a more adequate processing method.

Table 11.3 A summary of material selection and optical properties of hydrogel optical fibers.

Core	n_{core}	Cladding	n_{clad}	Attenuation (dB/cm)	References
Alg/PAAm	1.41	Alg	1.37	0.45 (air), 0.80–1.00 (water)	[161]
P(AAm-*co*-EGDA)	1.46	Alg	1.34	0.32 (air), 0.28 (tissue)	[162]
	n/a		n/a	1–6	[163]
PEGDA	1.46	Alg	1.33	0.32 (air), 0.42 (tissue)	[159]
	1.40		1.33	<1	[164, 165]
	n/a		n/a	0.4	[166]
PEGDA	n/a	None	—	1.2–1.3	[159, 167]
PVA	n/a	None	—	0.6 (air), 0.9 (water)	[158]
Alg/PAAm	1.41	None	—	0.56 (in air)	[161]
Alg/PAAm	1.35	None	—	0.25 (swollen)	[122]

For definitions of abbreviations, see the footnote of Table 11.2.

Although most of the current literature describes molding as the processing choice, all the materials reported in Table 11.3 have already been processed by microfluidics (see Section 11.3 and Table 11.2). It is expected, therefore, that the optical properties of HOFs will profit from the morphology control provided by MWS in future.

One remarkable advantage of HOFs over conventional POFs is the ease of tailoring their properties by changing their chemistry. Attenuation and RI may, for example, be controlled by the precursor concentration in water, the molecular weight (MW) of the precursor, the cross-linking degree, the type of cross-linking mechanism (ionic or covalent), or the use of a co-monomer (Figure 11.9a,b) [159, 163, 168]. In general, optical properties of PEG-based HOFs improve by using higher precursor MW or solution concentrations (Figure 11.9a). The phenomenon has been assigned to the formation of pores, after gelation, which are more abundant and larger for lower concentrations or lower MW, as well as to the phase separation between water-rich and polymer-rich phases [159, 163, 166–168]. Interestingly, the opposite behavior has been observed for alginate-based materials: higher concentration leads to increased attenuation [159, 162, 163]. Accordingly, in HOFs composed of a blend of PAAm and Alg, attenuation decreased with the increase in the content of the synthetic polymer up to a concentration of 40 wt% [122]. Jiang et al. used finite elements modeling to investigate the design parameters and allow the rational design of core-cladding HOFs, specially based on the effects of changes in fiber length or diameter and the RIs of the materials on the attenuation [162]. For HOFs with micrometric dimensions, attenuation increased with a decrease in core diameter below 3.5 μm or a decrease in cladding thickness below 0.25 μm. The effect was stronger for shorter wavelengths and for core-only fibers. The RIs for both natural and synthetic hydrogels increase with the concentration: the lower the concentration, the closer the RI is to that of water (1.33). That means that even core–cladding HOFs would have

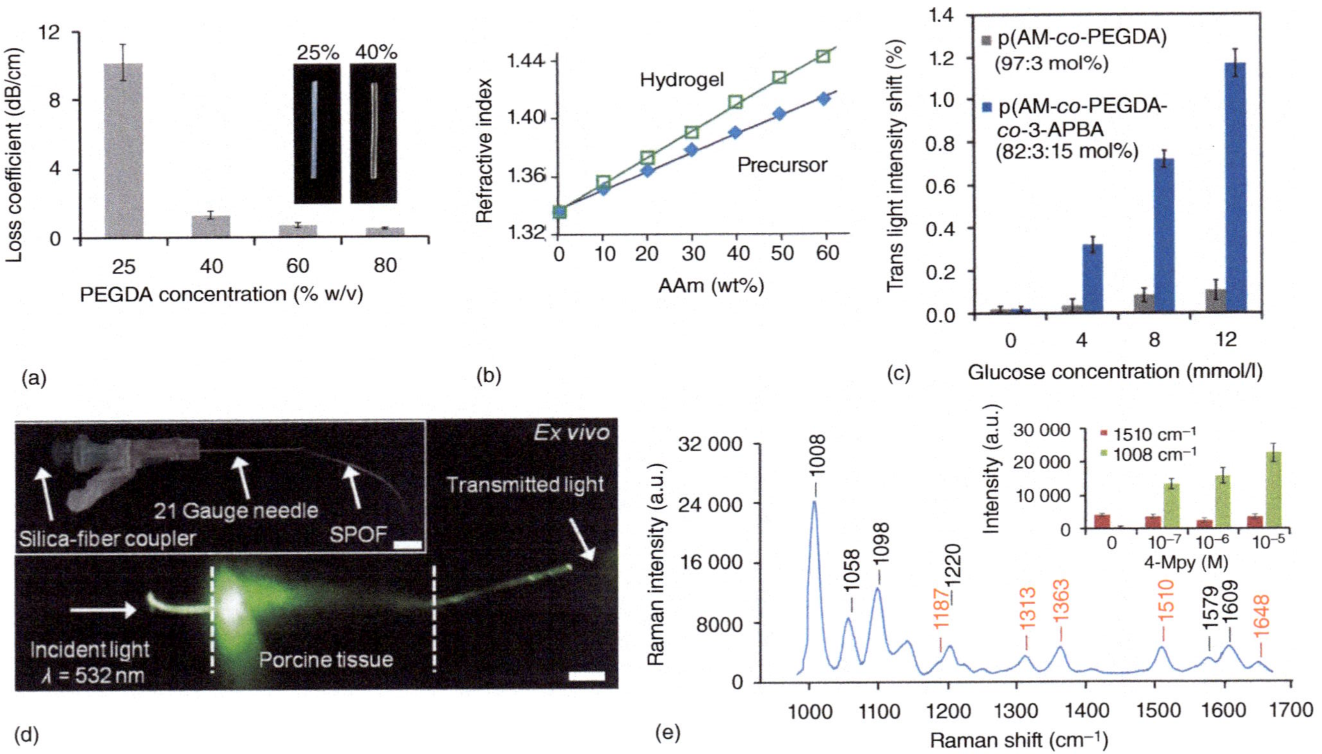

Figure 11.9 (a) Dependence of attenuation of PEGDA HOFs on the concentration of the precursor solution; the inset shows photographs of 2-cm-long HOFs [167]; (b) RI of Alg/PAAm precursors and cross-linked hydrogels as a function of AAm concentration. Source: Guo et al. [161]/with permission of John Wiley & Sons.; (c) detection of glucose (in the range of 0–12 mM) due to the RI shift in poly(AAm-EGDA-APBA) HOFs. Source: Yetisen et al. [163]/with permission of John Wiley & Sons.; (d) light attenuation of an HOF implanted into porcine tissue (scale bar = 3 mm). The inset shows an HOF being injected through a 21-gauge needle (scale bar = 5 mm). Source: Jiang et al. [162], Figure 05, Pg 08/with permission of John Wiley & Sons, Inc.; (e) multiplex SERS detection of two molecules (R6G and 4-Mpy). The inset shows the intensity of two peaks as a function of concentration of 4-Mpy when the R6G was kept constant at 10^{-4} M [167]. Source: (a and e) Reprinted with permission. © The Optical Society. (b and d) © Wiley-VCH Verlag GmbH & Co. KGaA. Reproduced with permission. (c) © 2017 The Authors. Published by WILEY-VCH Verlag GmbH & Co. KGaA, Weinheim.

different transmission properties in air or in contact with tissues, due to swelling of the cladding. Accordingly, Choi et al. observed a 50% increase in the attenuation for PEGDA/Alg fibers after insertion into tissues [159], while Yetisen et al. observed a 10% increase in the attenuation after inserting P(AAm-*co*-EGDA)/Alg fiber into tissue phantoms [163]. Core-only fibers, lacking the protective effect of the cladding, are more sensitive to swelling or interaction with tissues: PEGDA HOFs without cladding had a fourfold increase in attenuation after insertion into tissue [159], while Alg/PAAm fibers without cladding had a threefold increase in attenuation when the outer RI matched that of the core [161].

The versatility in the production of HOFs allows their functionalization for sensing purposes via different methods. Small MW molecules may be diffused into the hydrogel after their fabrication; this physical entrapment, however, may lead to leakage during use [159, 162]. This functionalization method may be interesting when using fluorescent dyes, which are photobleached after a certain time. The dyes could then be simply replaced by washing and doping cycles [159]. The presence of functional groups on hydrogels allows their functionalization via chemical reactions in water, another advantage when compared to conventional POFs, which can only be functionalized in organic solvents [163, 166]. Last, HOFs can also be functionalized by incorporation, during their production, of nanoparticles that are then physically entrapped, but with low diffusion or leakage (due to their size and stiffness). Graphene nanoplatelets, metal nanoparticles [162, 167], and quantum-dots (QDs) [164, 169] have already been incorporated into HOFs or other hydrogel waveguides by this method. The drawback of nanoparticle incorporation is the strong increase in attenuation with the increase in particle size, explained by the Mie and Rayleigh scattering theories for scattering elements higher or lower than the wavelength of incident light, respectively [170]. Guo et al. observed an increase in attenuation with a concentration of 90-nm silver nanoparticles (AgNPs); the attenuation increase peaked at 422 nm, corresponding to the peak absorption of the particles [167]. Microparticles (approx. 3 μm) of metal–organic frameworks (MOFs), due to the much larger size, induced a larger effect [165]. Very small nanoparticles such as QDs with diameters lower than 6 nm can still contribute to Rayleigh scattering. Moreover, their major contribution to attenuation will derive from the strong absorption peaks of QD [164]. This effect is similar to that found when doping HOFs with dyes: Choi et al. found a 50-fold increase in attenuation of HOFs at the wavelength corresponding to the absorption peak of rhodamine when compared to other wavelengths [159]. This effect depends on the concentration and extinction coefficient of the dyes.

The use of hydrophilic polymers with functional groups allows the use of reactions in water to improve interfacial bonding between core and cladding. The presence of voids or even nanoscale roughness that may arise during the fabrication process (due to inadequate interfacial bonding) is an important source of attenuation (interfacial scattering). Guo et al. used 1-ethyl-3-[3-dimethylami- nopropyl]-carbodiimide hydrochloride (EDC)-*N*-hydroxysuccinimide (NHS) reactions in water to covalently couple Alg cladding to a core made of a blend of Alg and PAAm, creating a fiber with a robust interface [161].

11.4.2 Applications

HOFs have been investigated mostly for sensing [159, 161, 163–167], photothermal therapy [159, 162], and optogenetics [122, 158]. The high permeability of hydrogels to hydrophilic substances makes HOFs perfectly suited for biomedical sensors or sensors in aqueous media. Accordingly, HOFs have been investigated for glucose sensing [163, 166], blood oxygenation [159], strain sensors [161], detection of organic molecules [165, 167], and metal ion sensing [164].

Glucose sensing with HOFs was achieved by the covalent immobilization of phenylboronic acid (PBA) derivatives on P(ethylene glycol diacrylate [EGDA]-*co*-AAm) or PEGDA fibers [163, 166]. Yetisen et al. synthesized a copolymer of P(EGDA-*co*-AAm-*co*-3-acrylamido-phenylboronic acid [APBA]), which was subsequently used as the core of an HOF, with Alg as the cladding [163]. Upon exposure to glucose, *cis*-diol groups of the sugar complexed with the anionic boronate species, leading to changes in the osmotic pressure of the hydrogel. A higher concentration of glucose leads to an increase in the fiber diameter and a decrease in the RI, leading to changes in the light propagation inside the fiber, which could be used to detect the glucose concentration (Figure 11.9c). The sensitivity could be fine-tuned not only by changing the percentage of PBA in the terpolymer but also by changing the ratio of the other two co-monomers: 3 mol% of EGDA was found to give the best results. Being a reversible covalent bond, the sensor could be reset by washing the HOFs in acetate buffer and PBS. In a similar approach, Elsherif et al. used a post-functionalization step to decorate PEGDA fiber tips with 3-APBA [166]. Both sensors were used to detect glucose in the millimole range.

Guo et al. developed strain sensors based on core/cladding HOFs that could find applications in wearable sensors or implantable devices [161]. Sensitivity was obtained by doping fluorescent dyes (optical absorbers/scatterers) into the core: application of strain changed the dispersion of the dyes, leading to changes in the attenuation. Sensitivity of 0.062 dB/% strain was achieved. The full power of OF sensors was demonstrated by multiplexing: when doping three dyes with different absorption curves, multiple sensing regions could be implemented on a single fiber.

The facile fabrication of multiple sensing regions has also been explored for chemical sensing. Zhou et al. dissolved two types of QDs in PEGDA to prepare fiber cores with regions responding to different excitation wavelengths [164]. By making the appropriate choice of QD, the HOFs were made sensitive only to Fe^{3+} ions and were only negligibly sensitive to other metal ions (alone or in a complex mixture). Moreover, the use of two QD types (one being insensitive to metals) allowed a precise and robust ratiometric detection of Fe^{3+} (limit of detection [LOD]: 14 nM). Highly sensitive and specific sensors were also designed by preparing PEGDA/Alg HOFs doped with MOF microparticles [165]. A nitroaromatic explosive (picric acid) could be detected at concentrations as low as 5.7 ppm without interference with other nitroaromatic compounds or metal ions.

Besides fluorescence detection, HOFs have also been proposed as a platform for surface-enhanced Raman spectroscopy (SERS), a technique which allows specific, label-free bio- and chemical analysis down to single molecule level [167]. The use of HOFs (as opposed to rigid OFs) could allow the implementation of SERS for *in vivo* real-time monitoring. Guo et al. mixed AgNPs with PEGDA solution, which was used to fabricate core-only fibers. Excitation of the fibers at 785 nm led to highly sensitive detection of rhodamine 6G (R6G, LOD: 100 nM) or 4-mercaptopyridine (4-Mpy, LOD: 10 nM). Here, as in the previous examples, multiplexing could be achieved by analyzing different Raman peaks of the molecules when present in a mixture (Figure 11.9e) [167].

Another application of metal-nanoparticle-doped HOFs is photothermal therapy, where implantable HOFs could help to concentrate the heat generation only in the desired tissue/organ volume (Figure 11.9d). Choi et al. mixed gold nanoparticles (AuNPs, 50-nm diameter) with precursor PEGDA solution before fiber formation [159]. Pumping of laser light at the plasmon-resonance-enhanced absorption peak wavelength (532 nm) resulted in a temperature increase of 16 °C. The HOFs, unlike glass OFs, were also soft enough to be implanted into the intestines of mice for *in vivo* applications. Jiang et al. demonstrated that AuNPs maintained their intrinsic plasmonic properties in the HOFs when compared to freestanding Au colloids [162].

Implantable HOFs could also find applications in optogenetics, where their low stiffness, modulated not only by material choice but also by water absorption, is more compatible with brain tissue (~1 kPa) than the currently used GOFs (~10 GPa) [122, 158]. After four weeks of implantation in mouse brain, neither the ductility nor the optical properties of PAAm/Alg core-only fibers were significantly affected; moreover, optogenetic modulation with HOFs was as effective as in mice implanted with GOFs. On the other hand, the HOF elicited a much lower inflammatory response and much higher neuronal survival than GOFs; the neuronal density remained almost unchanged up to 500-μm distance from the implanted HOF.

11.5 Conclusions

MWS has become, in recent years, a prime technique to produce hydrogel fibers for biomedical applications. That is mainly due to the mild processing conditions, excellent control over the morphology of produced fibers, and possibility of doping or functionalization of the fibers in predetermined regions directly during the production stages. Hydrogel fibers can then be produced with tailored mechanical and biochemical properties. Most importantly, biological components such as cells and proteins can be encapsulated in a spatiotemporally controlled manner via MWS, making MWS a promising 3D-biofabrication technology. For a more widespread use of the technology, the design of modular chips allowing the fabrication of multi-material fibers is required. Although soft lithography has been for decades the predominant technique for the fabrication of microfluidic chips, the development of bench-top stereolithography 3D printers, together with strong research in new photopolymers, will lead to an upcoming revolution in chip fabrication and will slowly help translate MWS into industrial settings. HOFs, being a specialty fiber whose morphology plays a crucial role in performance, are expected to profit strongly in the near future from the control and modularity offered by MWS.

Acknowledgments

Funding for this work was provided by the Swiss National Science Foundation (SNSF) and Innosuisse BRIDGE Discovery funding opportunity (project number 40B2-0_180983).

References

1 Rapp, E.B. (2017). Introduction, Chapter 1. In: *Microfluidics: Modeling, Mechanics and Mathematics* (ed. S. Holt), 3–7. Oxford/Cambridge: Matthew Deans.

2 Shields, C.W., Reyes, C.D., and Lopez, G.P. (2015). Microfluidic cell sorting: a review of the advances in the separation of cells from debulking to rare cell isolation. *Lab Chip* 15 (5): 1230–1249.

3 Li, H. and Steckl, A.J. (2019). Paper microfluidics for point-of-care blood-based analysis and diagnostics. *Anal. Chem.* 91 (1): 352–371.

4 Tian, C., Tu, Q., Liu, W.M., and Wang, J.Y. (2019). Recent advances in microfluidic technologies for organ-on-a-chip. *Trends Anal. Chem.* 117: 146–156.

5 Liu, Y. and Jiang, X. (2017). Why microfluidics? Merits and trends in chemical synthesis. *Lab Chip* 17 (23): 3960–3978.

6 Rapp, B.E. (2017). Fluids, Chapter 9. In: *Microfluidics: Modelling, Mechanics and Mathematics*, 243–263. Oxford/'Cambridge: Matthew Deans.

7 Zhang, J. and Hoshino, K. (2018). Microfluidics and micro total analytical systems, Chapter 3. In: *Molecular Sensors and Nanodevices: Principles, Designs and Applications in Biomedical Engineering*, 2e (ed. S. Holt), 113–179. London/San Diego/Cambridge: Mathew Deans.

8 Paul, D.R. (1968). Diffusion during coagulation step of wet-spinning. *J. Appl. Polym. Sci.* 12 (3): 383–402.

9 Du, X.Y., Li, Q., Wu, G., and Chen, S. (2019). Multifunctional micro/nanoscale fibers based on microfluidic spinning technology. *Adv. Mater.* 31: 1903733.

10 Cheng, J., Jun, Y., Qin, J.H., and Lee, S.H. (2017). Electrospinning versus microfluidic spinning of functional fibers for biomedical applications. *Biomaterials* 114: 121–143.

11 Shi, X.T., Ostrovidov, S., Zhao, Y.H. et al. (2015). Microfluidic spinning of cell-responsive grooved microfibers. *Adv. Funct. Mater.* 25 (15): 2250–2259.

12 Kang, E., Choi, Y.Y., Chae, S.K. et al. (2012). Microfluidic spinning of flat alginate fibers with grooves for cell-aligning scaffolds. *Adv. Mater.* 24 (31): 4271–4277.

13 Meng, J.K., Wu, G., Wu, X.J. et al. (2020). Microfluidic-architected nanoarrays/porous core-shell fibers toward robust micro-energy-storage. *Adv. Sci.* 7 (1): 1901931.

14 Nguyen, T.P.T., Tran, B.M., and Lee, N.Y. (2018). Microfluidic approach for the fabrication of cell-laden hollow fibers for endothelial barrier research. *J. Mater. Chem. B* 6 (38): 6057–6066.

15 Jung, J.H., Choi, C.H., Chung, S. et al. (2009). Microfluidic synthesis of a cell adhesive janus polyurethane microfiber. *Lab Chip* 9 (17): 2596–2602.

16 Yang, H.L. and Guo, M.Y. (2019). Bioinspired polymeric helical and superhelical microfibers via microfluidic spinning. *Macromol. Rapid Commun.* 40 (12): 1900111.

17 Yu, Y.R., Fu, F.F., Shang, L.R. et al. (2017). Bioinspired helical microfibers from microfluidics. *Adv. Mater.* 29 (18): 1605765.

18 Jun, Y., Kang, E., Chae, S., and Lee, S.H. (2014). Microfluidic spinning of micro- and nano-scale fibers for tissue engineering. *Lab Chip* 14 (13): 2145–2160.

19 Xie, R.X., Xu, P.D., Liu, Y.P. et al. (2018). Necklace-like microfibers with variable knots and perfusable channels fabricated by an oil-free microfluidic spinning process. *Adv. Mater.* 30 (14): 1705082.

20 Wu, Z.Q., Wang, J., Zhao, Z. et al. (2018). Microfluidic generation of bioinspired spindle-knotted graphene microfibers for oil absorption. *ChemPhysChem* 19 (16): 1990–1994.

21 Choi, C.H., Yi, H., Hwang, S. et al. (2011). Microfluidic fabrication of complex-shaped microfibers by liquid template-aided multiphase microflow. *Lab Chip* 11 (8): 1477–1483.

22 Boyd, D.A., Shields, A.R., Howell, P.B., and Ligler, F.S. (2013). Design and fabrication of uniquely shaped thiol-ene microfibers using a two-stage hydrodynamic focusing design. *Lab Chip* 13 (15): 3105–3110.

23 Boyd, D.A., Adams, A.A., Daniele, M.A., and Ligler, F.S. (2014). Microfluidic fabrication of polymeric and biohybrid fibers with predesigned size and shape. *J. Vis. Exp.* 83: e50958.

24 Liu, W., Xu, Z.N., Sun, L.X. et al. (2017). Polymerization-induced phase separation fabrication: a versatile microfluidic technique to prepare microfibers with various cross sectional shapes and structures. *Chem. Eng. J.* 315: 25–34.

25 Lan, W.J., Du, Y.J., Guo, X.Q. et al. (2018). Flexible microfluidic fabrication of anisotropic polymer microfibers. *Ind. Eng. Chem. Res.* 57 (1): 212–219.

26 Shin, S., Park, J.Y., Lee, J.Y. et al. (2007). On the fly continuous generation of alginate fibers using a microfluidic device. *Langmuir* 23 (17): 9104–9108.

27 Wu, F., Ju, X.J., He, X.H. et al. (2016). A novel synthetic microfiber with controllable size for cell encapsulation and culture. *J. Mater. Chem. B* 4 (14): 2455–2465.

28 Ma, K.Z., Du, X.Y., Zhang, Y.W., and Chen, S. (2017). In situ fabrication of halide perovskite nanocrystals embedded in polymer composites via microfluidic spinning microreactors. *J. Mater. Chem. C* 5 (36): 9398–9404.

29 Haynl, C., Hofmann, E., Pawar, K. et al. (2016). Microfluidics-produced collagen fibers show extraordinary mechanical properties. *Nano Lett.* 16 (9): 5917–5922.

30 Yu, Y., Wen, H., Ma, J.Y. et al. (2014). Flexible fabrication of biomimetic bamboo-like hybrid microfibers. *Adv. Mater.* 26 (16): 2494–2499.

31 Tang, Z.H., Jia, S.H., Wang, F. et al. (2018). Highly stretchable core-sheath fibers via wet-spinning for wearable strain sensors. *ACS Appl. Mater. Interfaces* 10 (7): 6624–6635.

32 Shang, L.R., Yu, Y.R., Liu, Y.X. et al. (2019). Spinning and applications of bioinspired fiber systems. *ACS Nano* 13 (3): 2749–2772.

33 Yamada, M., Sugaya, S., Naganuma, Y., and Seki, M. (2012). Microfluidic synthesis of chemically and physically anisotropic hydrogel microfibers for guided cell growth and networking. *Soft Matter* 8 (11): 3122–3130.

34 Ahn, S.Y., Mun, C.H., and Lee, S.H. (2015). Microfluidic spinning of fibrous alginate carrier having highly enhanced drug loading capability and delayed release profile. *RSC Adv.* 5 (20): 15172–15181.

35 Tamayol, A., Akbari, M., Zilberman, Y. et al. (2016). Flexible pH-sensing hydrogel fibers for epidermal applications. *Adv. Healthc. Mater.* 5 (6): 711–719.

36 Kang, E., Shin, S.J., Lee, K.H., and Lee, S.H. (2010). Novel PDMS cylindrical channels that generate coaxial flow, and application to fabrication of microfibers and particles. *Lab Chip* 10 (14): 1856–1861.

37 Park, J.Y., Lee, D.H., Lee, E.J., and Lee, S.H. (2009). Study of cellular behaviors on concave and convex microstructures fabricated from elastic PDMS membranes. *Lab Chip* 9 (14): 2043–2049.

38 Kang, E., Jeong, G.S., Choi, Y.Y. et al. (2011). Digitally tunable physicochemical coding of material composition and topography in continuous microfibres. *Nat. Mater.* 10 (11): 877–883.

39 Cheng, J., Park, D., Jun, Y. et al. (2016). Biomimetic spinning of silk fibers and in situ cell encapsulation. *Lab Chip* 16 (14): 2654–2661.

40 Jun, Y., Kim, M.J., Hwang, Y.H. et al. (2013). Microfluidics-generated pancreatic islet microfibers for enhanced immunoprotection. *Biomaterials* 34 (33): 8122–8130.

41 Zhang, Y., Wang, C.F., Chen, L. et al. (2015). Microfluidic-spinning-directed microreactors toward generation of multiple nanocrystals loaded anisotropic fluorescent microfibers. *Adv. Funct. Mater.* 25 (47): 7253–7262.

42 Tong, Y.L., Xu, B., Du, X.F. et al. (2018). Microfluidic-spinning-directed conductive fibers toward flexible micro-supercapacitors. *Macromol. Mater. Eng.* 303 (6): 1700664.

43 Gursoy, A., Iranshahi, K., Wei, K. et al. (2020). Facile fabrication of microfluidic chips for 3D hydrodynamic focusing and wet spinning of polymeric fibers. *Polymers* 12 (3): 633.

44 Jeong, W., Kim, J., Kim, S. et al. (2004). Hydrodynamic microfabrication via "on the fly" photopolymerization of microscale fibers and tubes. *Lab Chip* 4 (6): 576–580.

45 Lan, W.J., Li, S.W., Lu, Y.C. et al. (2009). Controllable preparation of microscale tubes with multiphase co-laminar flow in a double co-axial microdevice. *Lab Chip* 9 (22): 3282–3288.

46 Xu, T., Ding, X.T., Liang, Y. et al. (2016). Direct spinning of fiber supercapacitor. *Nanoscale* 8 (24): 12113–12117.

47 Lin, Y.S., Huang, K.S., Yang, C.H. et al. (2012). Microfluidic synthesis of microfibers for magnetic-responsive controlled drug release and cell culture. *PLoS One* 7 (3): e33184.

48 Hu, X.L., Tian, M.W., Pan, N. et al. (2019). Structure-tunable graphene oxide fibers via microfluidic spinning route for multifunctional textiles. *Carbon* 152: 106–113.

49 Hu, M., Deng, R.S., Schumacher, K.M. et al. (2010). Hydrodynamic spinning of hydrogel fibers. *Biomaterials* 31 (5): 863–869.

50 Lölsberg, J., Linkhorst, J., Cinar, A. et al. (2018). 3D nanofabrication inside rapid prototyped microfluidic channels showcased by wet-spinning of single micrometre fibres. *Lab Chip* 18 (9): 1341–1348.

51 Nielsen, J.B., Hanson, R.L., Almughamsi, H.M. et al. (2020). Microfluidics: innovations in materials and their fabrication and functionalization. *Anal. Chem.* 92 (1): 150–168.

52 McDonald, J.C. and Whitesides, G.M. (2002). Poly(dimethylsiloxane) as a material for fabricating microfluidic devices. *Acc. Chem. Res.* 35 (7): 491–499.

53 Chaurasia, A.S., Jahanzad, F., and Sajjadi, S. (2017). Preparation and characterization of tunable oil-encapsulated alginate microfibers. *Mater. Des.* 128: 64–70.

54 Peng, L., Liu, Y., Gong, J.H. et al. (2017). Continuous fabrication of multi-stimuli responsive graphene oxide composite hydrogel fibres by microfluidics. *RSC Adv.* 7 (31): 19243–19249.

55 Li, D., Jacobsen, M.M., Rim, N.G. et al. (2017). Introducing biomimetic shear and ion gradients to microfluidic spinning improves silk fiber strength. *Biofabrication* 9 (2): 025025.

56 Peng, L., Liu, Y., Huang, J.N. et al. (2018). Microfluidic fabrication of highly stretchable and fast electro-responsive graphene oxide/polyacrylamide/alginate hydrogel fibers. *Eur. Polym. J.* 103: 335–341.

57 Wu, X.J., Xu, Y.J., Hu, Y. et al. (2018). Microfluidic-spinning construction of black-phosphorus-hybrid microfibres for non-woven fabrics toward a high energy density flexible supercapacitor. *Nat. Commun.* 9: 1–11.

58 Hwang, C.M., Khademhosseini, A., Park, Y. et al. (2008). Microfluidic chip-based fabrication of PLGA microfiber scaffolds for tissue engineering. *Langmuir* 24 (13): 6845–6851.

59 Lee, K.H., Shin, S.J., Kim, C.B. et al. (2010). Microfluidic synthesis of pure chitosan microfibers for bio-artificial liver chip. *Lab Chip* 10 (10): 1328–1334.

60 Lee, B.R., Lee, K.H., Kang, E. et al. (2011). Microfluidic wet spinning of chitosan-alginate microfibers and encapsulation of HepG2 cells in fibers. *Biomicrofluidics* 5 (2): 022208.

61 Onoe, H., Okitsu, T., Itou, A. et al. (2013). Metre-long cell-laden microfibres exhibit tissue morphologies and functions. *Nat. Mater.* 12 (6): 584–590.

62 Lim, D., Lee, E., Kim, H. et al. (2015). Multi stimuli-responsive hydrogel microfibers containing magnetite nanoparticles prepared using microcapillary devices. *Soft Matter* 11 (8): 1606–1613.

63 Cheng, Y., Yu, Y.R., Fu, F.F. et al. (2016). Controlled fabrication of bioactive microfibers for creating tissue constructs using microfluidic techniques. *ACS Appl. Mater. Interfaces* 8 (2): 1080–1086.

64 Bell, R.V., Parkins, C.C., Young, R.A. et al. (2016). Assembly of emulsion droplets into fibers by microfluidic wet spinning. *J. Mater. Chem. A* 4 (3): 813–818.

65 Xu, P.D., Xie, R.X., Liu, Y.P. et al. (2017). Bioinspired microfibers with embedded perfusable helical channels. *Adv. Mater.* 29 (34): 1701664.

66 Yu, Y.R., Shang, L.R., Guo, J.H. et al. (2018). Design of capillary microfluidics for spinning cell-laden microfibers. *Nat. Protoc.* 13 (11): 2557–2579.

67 Berthier, E., Dostie, A.M., Lee, U.N. et al. (2019). Open microfluidic capillary systems. *Anal. Chem.* 91 (14): 8739–8750.

68 Weng, X., Kang, Y.J., Guo, Q. et al. (2019). Recent advances in thread-based microfluidics for diagnostic applications. *Biosens. Bioelectron.* 132: 171–185.

69 Chen, C.T., Chen, X., Zhang, H. et al. (2017). Electrically-responsive core–shell hybrid microfibers for controlled drug release and cell culture. *Acta Biomater.* 55: 434–442.

70 Weerakoon-Ratnayake, K.M., O'Neil, C.E., Uba, F.I., and Soper, S.A. (2017). Thermoplastic nanofluidic devices for biomedical applications. *Lab Chip* 17 (3): 362–381.

71 Chan, H.N., Tan, M.J.A., and Wu, H.K. (2017). Point-of-care testing: applications of 3D printing. *Lab Chip* 17 (16): 2713–2739.

72 Au, A.K., Huynh, W., Horowitz, L.F., and Folch, A. (2016). 3D-printed microfluidics. *Angew. Chem. Int. Ed.* 55 (12): 3862–3881.

73 Ho, C.M.B., Ng, S.H., Li, K.H.H., and Yoon, Y.J. (2015). 3D printed microfluidics for biological applications. *Lab Chip* 15 (18): 3627–3637.

74 Bhattacharjee, N., Urrios, A., Kanga, S., and Folch, A. (2016). The upcoming 3D-printing revolution in microfluidics. *Lab Chip* 16 (10): 1720–1742.

75 Pranzo, D., Larizza, P., Filippini, D., and Percoco, G. (2018). Extrusion-based 3D printing of microfluidic devices for chemical and biomedical applications: a topical review. *Micromachines* 9 (8): 374.

76 Weisgrab, G., Ovsionikov, A., and Costa, P.F. (2019). Functional 3D printing for microfluidic chips. *Adv. Mater. Technol.* 4 (10): 1900275.

77 Amin, R., Knowlton, S., Hart, A. et al. (2016). 3D-printed microfluidic devices. *Biofabrication* 8 (2): 022001.

78 Zhang, Y.S. and Khademhosseini, A. (2017). Advances in engineering hydrogels. *Science* 356 (6337): eaaf3627.

79 Wei, K.C., Senturk, B., Matter, M.T. et al. (2019). Mussel-inspired injectable hydrogel adhesive formed under mild conditions features near-native tissue properties. *ACS Appl. Mater. Interfaces* 11 (51): 47707–47719.

80 Yang, B.G., Wei, Z., Chen, X.Y. et al. (2019). Manipulating the mechanical properties of biomimetic hydrogels with multivalent host-guest interactions. *J. Mater. Chem. B* 7 (10): 1726–1733.

81 Heo, Y.J., Shibata, H., Okitsu, T. et al. (2011). Long-term in vivo glucose monitoring using fluorescent hydrogel fibers. *Proc. Natl. Acad. Sci. U.S.A.* 108 (33): 13399–13403.

82 Daniele, M.A., Boyd, D.A., Adams, A.A., and Ligler, F.S. (2015). Microfluidic strategies for design and assembly of microfibers and nanofibers with tissue engineering and regenerative medicine applications. *Adv. Healthc. Mater.* 4 (1): 11–28.

83 Takei, T., Sakai, S., Ijima, H., and Kawakami, K. (2006). Development of mammalian cell-enclosing calcium-alginate hydrogel fibers in a co-flowing stream. *Biotechnol. J.* 1 (9): 1014–1017.

84 Takei, T., Sakai, S., Yokonuma, T. et al. (2007). Fabrication of artificial endothelialized tubes with predetermined three-dimensional configuration from flexible cell-enclosing alginate fibers. *Biotechnol. Progr.* 23 (1): 182–186.

85 Kim, B., Kim, I., Choi, W. et al. (2008). Fabrication of cell-encapsulated alginate microfiber scaffold using microfluidic channel. *J. Manuf. Sci. Eng.* 130 (2): 021016.

86 Park, D.Y., Mun, C.H., Kang, E. et al. (2014). One-stop microfiber spinning and fabrication of a fibrous cell-encapsulated scaffold on a single microfluidic platform. *Biofabrication* 6 (2): 024108.

87 Ghorbanian, S., Qasaimeh, M.A., Akbari, M. et al. (2014). Microfluidic direct writer with integrated declogging mechanism for fabricating cell-laden hydrogel constructs. *Biomed. Microdevices* 16 (3): 387–395.

88 Yu, Y., Zhang, Y.H., Martin, J.A., and Ozbolat, I.T. (2013). Evaluation of cell viability and functionality in vessel-like bioprintable cell-laden tubular channels. *J. Biomech. Eng.* 135 (9): BIO-12-1543.

89 Onoe, H., Kato-Negishi, M., Itou, A., and Takeuchi, S. (2016). Differentiation induction of mouse neural stem cells in hydrogel tubular microenvironments with controlled tube dimensions. *Adv. Healthc. Mater.* 5 (9): 1104–1111.

90 Kato-Negishi, M., Onoe, H., Ito, A., and Takeuchi, S. (2017). Rod-shaped neural units for aligned 3D neural network connection. *Adv. Healthc. Mater.* 6 (15): 1700143.

91 Lee, K.H., Shin, S.J., Park, Y., and Lee, S.H. (2009). Synthesis of cell-laden alginate hollow fibers using microfluidic chips and microvascularized tissue-engineering applications. *Small* 5 (11): 1264–1268.

92 Gao, Q., Liu, Z.J., Lin, Z.W. et al. (2017). 3D bioprinting of vessel-like structures with multilevel fluidic channels. *ACS Biomater. Sci. Eng.* 3 (3): 399–408.

93 Jeong, G.S. and Lee, S.H. (2014). Microfluidic spinning of grooved microfiber for guided neuronal cell culture using surface tension mediated grooved round channel. *Tissue Eng. Regener. Med.* 11 (4): 291–296.

94 Liberski, A.R., Delaney, J.T., Schafer, H. et al. (2011). Organ weaving: woven threads and sheets as a step towards a new strategy for artificial organ development. *Macromol. Biosci.* 11 (11): 1491–1498.

95 Attalla, R., Puersten, E., Jain, N., and Selvaganapathy, P.R. (2019). 3D bioprinting of heterogeneous bi- and tri-layered hollow channels within gel scaffolds

using scalable multi-axial microfluidic extrusion nozzle. *Biofabrication* 11 (1): 015012.

96 Yu, Y.R., Chen, G.P., Guo, J.H. et al. (2018). Vitamin metal-organic framework-laden microfibers from microfluidics for wound healing. *Mater. Horiz.* 5 (6): 1137–1142.

97 Yamada, M., Utoh, R., Ohashi, K. et al. (2012). Controlled formation of heterotypic hepatic micro-organoids in anisotropic hydrogel microfibers for long-term preservation of liver-specific functions. *Biomaterials* 33 (33): 8304–8315.

98 Yajima, Y., Lee, C.N., Yamada, M. et al. (2018). Development of a perfusable 3D liver cell cultivation system via bundling-up assembly of cell-laden microfibers. *J. Biosci. Bioeng.* 126 (1): 111–118.

99 Leng, L., McAllister, A., Zhang, B.Y. et al. (2012). Mosaic hydrogels: one-step formation of multiscale soft materials. *Adv. Mater.* 24 (27): 3650–3658.

100 Kobayashi, A., Yamakoshi, K., Yajima, Y. et al. (2013). Preparation of stripe-patterned heterogeneous hydrogel sheets using microfluidic devices for high-density coculture of hepatocytes and fibroblasts. *J. Biosci. Bioeng.* 116 (6): 761–767.

101 Yoshida, K. and Onoe, H. (2017). Functionalized core-shell hydrogel microsprings by anisotropic gelation with bevel-tip capillary. *Sci. Rep.* 7: 45987.

102 Tang, M.J., Wang, W., Li, Z.L. et al. (2018). Controllable microfluidic fabrication of magnetic hybrid microswimmers with hollow helical structures. *Ind. Eng. Chem. Res.* 57 (29): 9430–9438.

103 Fujimoto, K., Higashi, K., Onoe, H., and Miki, N. (2017). Microfluidic mass production system for hydrogel microtubes for microbial culture. *Jpn. J. Appl. Phys.* 56 (6): 06GM2.

104 Zhang, X.L., Huang, C., Zhao, Y., and Jin, X.Y. (2017). Ampicillin-incorporated alginate-chitosan fibers from microfluidic spinning and for vitro release. *J. Biomater. Sci., Polym. Ed.* 28 (13): 1408–1425.

105 Gao, G., Lee, J.H., Jang, J. et al. (2017). Tissue engineered bio-blood-vessels constructed using a tissue-specific bioink and 3D coaxial cell printing technique: a novel therapy for ischemic disease. *Adv. Funct. Mater.* 27 (33): 1700798.

106 Gao, G., Kim, H., Kim, B.S. et al. (2019). Tissue-engineering of vascular grafts containing endothelium and smooth-muscle using triple-coaxial cell printing. *Appl. Phys. Rev.* 6 (4): 041402.

107 Luo, Y.X., Lode, A., and Gelinsky, M. (2013). Direct plotting of three-dimensional hollow fiber scaffolds based on concentrated alginate pastes for tissue engineering. *Adv. Healthc. Mater.* 2 (6): 777–783.

108 Zhou, M.L., Gong, J.H., and Ma, J.H. (2019). Continuous fabrication of near-infrared light responsive bilayer hydrogel fibers based on microfluidic spinning. *e-Polymers* 19 (1): 215–224.

109 Guo, J.H., Yu, Y.R., Wang, H. et al. (2019). Conductive polymer hydrogel microfibers from multiflow microfluidics. *Small* 15 (15): 1805162.

110 Nakajima, S., Kawano, R., and Onoe, H. (2017). Stimuli-responsive hydrogel microfibers with controlled anisotropic shrinkage and cross-sectional geometries. *Soft Matter* 13 (20): 3710–3719.

111 Tamayol, A., Najafabadi, A.H., Aliakbarian, B. et al. (2015). Hydrogel templates for rapid manufacturing of bioactive fibers and 3D constructs. *Adv. Healthc. Mater.* 4 (14): 2146–2153.

112 Colosi, C., Shin, S.R., Manoharan, V. et al. (2016). Microfluidic bioprinting of heterogeneous 3D tissue constructs using low-viscosity bioink. *Adv. Mater.* 28 (4): 677–684.

113 Zhang, Y.S., Arneri, A., Bersini, S. et al. (2016). Bioprinting 3D microfibrous scaffolds for engineering endothelialized myocardium and heart-on-a-chip. *Biomaterials* 110: 45–59.

114 Liu, W.J., Zhong, Z., Hu, N. et al. (2018). Coaxial extrusion bioprinting of 3D microfibrous constructs with cell-favorable gelatin methacryloyl microenvironments. *Biofabrication* 10 (2): 024102.

115 Pi, Q.M., Maharjan, S., Yan, X. et al. (2018). Digitally tunable microfluidic bioprinting of multilayered cannular tissues. *Adv. Mater.* 30 (43): 1706913.

116 Jia, W.T., Gungor-Ozkerim, P.S., Zhang, Y.S. et al. (2016). Direct 3D bioprinting of perfusable vascular constructs using a blend bioink. *Biomaterials* 106: 58–68.

117 Costantini, M., Idaszek, J., Szoke, K. et al. (2016). 3D bioprinting of BM-MSCs-loaded ECM biomimetic hydrogels for in vitro neocartilage formation. *Biofabrication* 8 (3): 035002.

118 Yu, Y.R., Shang, L.R., Gao, W. et al. (2017). Microfluidic lithography of bioinspired helical micromotors. *Angew. Chem. Int. Ed.* 56 (40): 12127–12131.

119 Cai, J., Ye, D.D., Wu, Y.X. et al. (2019). Injectable alginate fibrous hydrogel with a three-dimensional network structure fabricated by microfluidic spinning. *Compos. Commun.* 15: 1–5.

120 Costantini, M., Testa, S., Mozetic, P. et al. (2017). Microfluidic-enhanced 3D bioprinting of aligned myoblast-laden hydrogels leads to functionally organized myofibers in vitro and in vivo. *Biomaterials* 131: 98–110.

121 Wei, S.S., Qu, G., Luo, G.Y. et al. (2018). Scalable and automated fabrication of conductive tough-hydrogel microfibers with ultrastretchability, 3D printability, and stress sensitivity. *ACS Appl. Mater. Interfaces* 10 (13): 11204–11212.

122 Wang, L.L., Zhong, C., Ke, D.N. et al. (2018). Ultrasoft and highly stretchable hydrogel optical fibers for in vivo optogenetic modulations. *Adv. Opt. Mater.* 6 (16): 1800427.

123 Liu, Y., Zhang, K.H., Ma, J.H., and Vancso, G.J. (2017). Thermoresponsive semi-IPN hydrogel microfibers from continuous fluidic processing with high elasticity and fast actuation. *ACS Appl. Mater. Interfaces* 9 (1): 901–908.

124 Sakai, S., Liu, Y., Mah, E.J., and Taya, M. (2013). Horseradish peroxidase/catalase-mediated cell-laden alginate-based hydrogel tube production in two-phase coaxial flow of aqueous solutions for filament-like tissues fabrication. *Biofabrication* 5 (1): 015012.

125 Liu, Y., Sakai, S., and Taya, M. (2012). Production of endothelial cell-enclosing alginate-based hydrogel fibers with a cell adhesive surface through simultaneous cross-linking by horseradish peroxidase-catalyzed reaction in a hydrodynamic spinning process. *J. Biosci. Bioeng.* 114 (3): 353–359.

126 Wei, D., Sun, J., Bolderson, J. et al. (2017). Continuous fabrication and assembly of spatial cell-laden fibers for a tissue-like construct via a photolithographic-based microfluidic chip. *ACS Appl. Mater. Interfaces* 9 (17): 14606–14617.

127 Sakai, S., Yamaguchi, S., Takei, T., and Kawakami, K. (2008). Oxidized alginate-cross-linked alginate/gelatin hydrogel fibers for fabricating tubular constructs with layered smooth muscle cells and endothelial cells in collagen gels. *Biomacromolecules* 9 (7): 2036–2041.

128 Cho, S., Shim, T.S., and Yang, S.M. (2012). High-throughput optofluidic platforms for mosaicked microfibers toward multiplex analysis of biomolecules. *Lab Chip* 12 (19): 3676–3679.

129 Ebrahimi, M., Ostrovidov, S., Salehi, S. et al. (2018). Enhanced skeletal muscle formation on microfluidic spun gelatin methacryloyl (GelMA) fibres using surface patterning and agrin treatment. *J. Tissue Eng. Regener. Med.* 12 (11): 2151–2163.

130 Miri, A.K., Nieto, D., Iglesias, L. et al. (2018). Microfluidics-enabled multimaterial maskless stereolithographic bioprinting. *Adv. Mater.* 30 (27): 1800242.

131 Ouyang, L.L., Highley, C.B., Sun, W., and Burdick, J.A. (2017). A generalizable strategy for the 3D bioprinting of hydrogels from nonviscous photo-crosslinkable inks. *Adv. Mater.* 29 (8): 1604983.

132 Kim, S.R., Oh, H.J., Baek, J.Y. et al. (2005). Hydrodynamic fabrication of polymeric barcoded strips as components for parallel bio-analysis and programmable microactuation. *Lab Chip* 5 (10): 1168–1172.

133 Yeh, C.H., Lin, P.W., and Lin, Y.C. (2010). Chitosan microfiber fabrication using a microfluidic chip and its application to cell cultures. *Microfluid. Nanofluid.* 8 (1): 115–121.

134 Chen, C.T., Zhang, T., Dai, B.B. et al. (2016). Rapid fabrication of composite hydrogel microfibers for weavable and sustainable antibacterial applications. *ACS Sustainable Chem. Eng.* 4 (12): 6534–6542.

135 Agnello, S., Gasperini, L., Reis, R.L. et al. (2016). Microfluidic production of hyaluronic acid derivative microfibers to control drug release. *Mater. Lett.* 182: 309–313.

136 Yamada, M. and Seki, M. (2018). Multiphase micro fluidic processes to produce alginate-based microparticles and fibers. *J. Chem. Eng. Jpn.* 51 (4): 318–330.

137 Moroni, L., Burdick, J.A., Highley, C. et al. (2018). Biofabrication strategies for 3D in vitro models and regenerative medicine. *Nat. Rev. Mater.* 3 (5): 21–37.

138 Wanjare, M., Kusuma, S., and Gerecht, S. (2013). Perivascular cells in blood vessel regeneration. *Biotechnol. J.* 8 (4): 434–447.

139 Morimoto, Y. and Takeuchi, S. (2013). Three-dimensional cell culture based on microfluidic techniques to mimic living tissues. *Biomater. Sci.* 1 (3): 257–264.

140 Caves, J.M., Kumar, V.A., Wen, J. et al. (2010). Fibrillogenesis in continuously spun synthetic collagen fiber. *J. Biomed. Mater. Res. Part B* 93B (1): 24–38.

141 Costantini, M., Colosi, C., Swieszkowski, W., and Barbetta, A. (2019). Co-axial wet-spinning in 3D bioprinting: state of the art and future perspective of microfluidic integration. *Biofabrication* 11 (1): 012001.

142 Caves, J.M., Kumar, V.A., Martinez, A.W. et al. (2010). The use of microfiber composites of elastin-like protein matrix reinforced with synthetic collagen in the design of vascular grafts. *Biomaterials* 31 (27): 7175–7182.

143 Zhang, Y., Ding, J.X., Qi, B.W. et al. (2019). Multifunctional fibers to shape future biomedical devices. *Adv. Funct. Mater.* 29 (34): 1902834.

144 Schneider, L.A., Korber, A., Grabbe, S., and Dissemond, J. (2007). Influence of pH on wound-healing: a new perspective for wound-therapy? *Arch. Dermatol. Res.* 298 (9): 413–420.

145 Huang, H.W., Sakar, M.S., Petruska, A.J. et al. (2016). Soft micromachines with programmable motility and morphology. *Nat. Commun.* 7: 1–10.

146 Sharifi, F., Sooriyarachchi, A.C., Altural, H. et al. (2016). Fiber based approaches as medicine delivery systems. *ACS Biomater. Sci. Eng.* 2 (9): 1411–1431.

147 Jiang, M.Y., Ju, X.J., Deng, K. et al. (2016). The microfluidic synthesis of composite hollow microfibers for K^+-responsive controlled release based on a host-guest system. *J. Mater. Chem. B* 4 (22): 3925–3935.

148 Sugimoto, M., Kitagawa, Y., Yamada, M. et al. (2018). Micropassage-embedding composite hydrogel fibers enable quantitative evaluation of cancer cell invasion under 3D coculture conditions. *Lab Chip* 18 (9): 1378–1387.

149 Wu, J., Chen, Q.S., Liu, W. et al. (2017). Recent advances in microfluidic 3D cellular scaffolds for drug assays. *Trends Anal. Chem.* 87: 19–31.

150 Kroplin, P., Dieling, C., Beckers, M. et al. (2017). Overview of the POF market. In: *Polymer Optical Fibres: Fibre Types, Materials, Fabrication, Characterisation and Applications.*, vol. 89 (ed. C.-A. Bunge, T. Gries and M. Beckers), 349–400. Woodhead Publishing.

151 Quandt, B.M., Braun, F., Ferrario, D. et al. (2017). Body-monitoring with photonic textiles: a reflective heartbeat sensor based on polymer optical fibres. *J. R. Soc. Interface* 14 (128): 20170060.

152 Quandt, B.M., Hufenus, R., Weisse, B. et al. (2017). Optimization of novel melt-extruded polymer optical fibers designed for pressure sensor applications. *Eur. Polym. J.* 88: 44–55.

153 Krehel, M., Wolf, M., Boesel, L.F. et al. (2014). Development of a luminous textile for reflective pulse oximetry measurements. *Biomed. Opt. Express* 5 (8): 2537–2547.

154 Guo, J.J., Yang, C.X., Dai, Q.H., and Kong, L.J. (2019). Soft and stretchable polymeric optical waveguide-based sensors for wearable and biomedical applications. *Sensors* 19 (17): 3771.

155 Kuhner, M., Tampe, R., and Sackmann, E. (1994). Lipid monolayer and bilayer supported on polymer-films-composite polymer-lipid films on solid substrates. *Biophys. J.* 67 (1): 217–226.

156 Umar, M., Min, K., and Kim, S. (2019). Advances in hydrogel photonics and their applications. *APL Photonics* 4 (12): 120901.

157 Nazempour, R., Zhang, Q.Y., Fu, R.X., and Sheng, X. (2018). Biocompatible and implantable optical fibers and waveguides for biomedicine. *Materials* 11 (8): 1283.

158 Jorfi, M., Voirin, G., Foster, E.J., and Weder, C. (2014). Physiologically responsive, mechanically adaptive polymer optical fibers for optogenetics. *Opt. Lett.* 39 (10): 2872–2875.

159 Choi, M., Humar, M., Kim, S., and Yun, S.H. (2015). Step-index optical fiber made of biocompatible hydrogels. *Adv. Mater.* 27 (27): 4081–4086.

160 Mano, J.F., Silva, G.A., Azevedo, H.S. et al. (2007). Natural origin biodegradable systems in tissue engineering and regenerative medicine: present status and some moving trends. *J. R. Soc. Interface* 4 (17): 999–1030.

161 Guo, J.J., Liu, X.Y., Jiang, N. et al. (2016). Highly stretchable, strain sensing hydrogel optical fibers. *Adv. Mater.* 28 (46): 10244–10249.

162 Jiang, N., Ahmed, R., Rifat, A.A. et al. (2018). Functionalized flexible soft polymer optical fibers for laser photomedicine. *Adv. Opt. Mater.* 6 (3): 1701118.

163 Yetisen, A.K., Jiang, N., Fallahi, A. et al. (2017). Glucose-sensitive hydrogel optical fibers functionalized with phenylboronic acid. *Adv. Mater.* 29 (15): 1606380.

164 Zhou, M.J., Guo, J.J., and Yang, C.X. (2018). Ratiometric fluorescence sensor for Fe^{3+} ions detection based on quantum dot-doped hydrogel optical fiber. *Sens. Actuators, B* 264: 52–58.

165 Zhao, L.S., Gan, J.L., Xia, T.F. et al. (2019). A luminescent metal-organic framework integrated hydrogel optical fibre as a photoluminescence sensing platform for fluorescence detection. *J. Mater. Chem. C* 7 (4): 897–904.

166 Elsherif, M., Hassan, M.U., Yetisen, A.K., and Butt, H. (2019). Hydrogel optical fibers for continuous glucose monitoring. *Biosens. Bioelectron.* 137: 25–32.

167 Guo, J.J., Luo, Y.Q., Yang, C.X., and Kong, L.J. (2018). In situ surface-enhanced Raman scattering sensing with soft and flexible polymer optical fiber probes. *Opt. Lett.* 43 (21): 5443–5446.

168 Choi, M., Choi, J., Kim, S. et al. (2013). Light-guiding hydrogels for cell-based sensing and optogenetic synthesis in vivo. *Nat. Photonics* 7 (12): 987–994.

169 Guo, J.J., Huang, H.X., Zhou, M.J. et al. (2018). Quantum dots-doped tapered hydrogel waveguide for ratiometric sensing of metal ions. *Anal. Chem.* 90 (20): 12292–12298.

170 Beckers, M., Weise, B., Kalapis, S. et al. (2017). Basics of light guidance. In: *Polymer Optical Fibres: Fibre Types, Materials, Fabrication, Characterisation and Applications*, vol. 89, 9–46.

12

Embedding Hydrogels into Microfluidic Chips: Vascular Transport Analyses and Drug Delivery Optimization

Ana M. Martins, Alexander B. Cook, Martina Di Francesco, Maria Grazia Barbato, Sayanti Brahmachari, Martina Pannuzzo, and Paolo Decuzzi

Istituto Italiano di Tecnologia, Laboratory of Nanotechnology for Precision Medicine, Via Morego 30, Genova 16163, Italy

12.1 Introduction: Microfluidic Chips for Modeling Human Diseases and Developing New Therapies

Static two-dimensional (2D) cell cultures (e.g. Petri dishes, flasks, and culture plates) are limited mainly because of their inability to simulate the complex environment of native tissue and organs, including structural and mechanical properties, composition, and dynamic interactions [1]. 2D cell cultures therefore drastically differ from the tissue microenvironment that is found *in vivo* [2]. On the other hand, current preclinical animal models have several drawbacks, including high cost, low reproducibility, low physiological similarity to humans, ethical problems, and unwanted immune responses due to their non-autologous nature. There is a great need for better predictive tools for modeling human diseases and developing new therapies including nanomedicines, such as the recently approved Alnylam siRNA lipid nanoparticle therapy [3] and the plethora of polymer nanoparticles, inorganic nanoparticles, liposomes, and polymer conjugates [4–6]. An environment that closely mimics the native tissue or organ is desirable to properly replicate biological functions *in vitro* and thus to enhance translation of nanomedicine beyond the laboratory.

The three-dimensional (3D) structural organization of cells plays an important role in the mimicking of native tissue environment. The recapitulation of tissue and organ physiology *in vitro* can be accomplished through careful design of the extracellular space, cellular components, and greater hierarchical 3D structure. However, 3D organization is often not enough. Static 3D cultures, such as transwell models, spheroids, and organoids, have some limitations such as high variability in size and shape, inconsistent cell-adhesive properties, poor circulation of medium, and absence of fluid flow. There is a large gap between 3D static cultures on one side and the animal models on the other one. The development of hydrogel-based microfluidic systems and the concept of organ-on-chip systems have emerged as a new way to address this gap.

Multifunctional Hydrogels for Biomedical Applications, First Edition.
Edited by Ricardo A. Pires, Iva Pashkuleva, and Rui L. Reis.

The first studies combining cell culture with microfluidics were developed in the early 2000s [7] and resulted in so-called organ-on-a-chip technology. Tissue- or organ-on-a-chip models have since emerged as an alternative for animal experiments in disease modeling and a new tool for developing new therapies. These chips are bioengineered 3D culture microfluidic systems that can mimic the architecture, mechanics, and physiological response of functional tissue or organ [8, 9]. In the last 10 years, many studies have been published describing different tissue-/organ-on-a-chip systems. These include vascularized tissue-engineered structures [10–12], gut [13–16], brain [17–22], lung [23–26], skin [27, 28], cancer [29–31], heart [32–39], liver [40–44], pancreas [45–47], bone [48–51], cartilage [49, 52, 53], among others.

Many different types of microfluidic chips have been used to assess biological processes and to evaluate nanomedicine performance. While these have been discussed in several reviews focusing on specific techniques or applications, in this chapter, we review the hydrogel-microfluidic chips with focus on the work developed in our laboratory. Firstly, we highlight the properties and compositions of various natural and synthetic polymers used for 3D culture in microfluidic chips. We then discuss different methods to fabricate microfluidic chips and biological applications of the same. Lastly, evaluation of different nanoparticles and nanomedicines using hydrogel-based microfluidic chips and computational methods will be introduced. Challenges and future directions for the field will end the chapter.

12.2 Hydrogels to Mimic the Extracellular Matrix (ECM)

To transform the microfabricated cell growth chambers into organ mimetic systems, it is necessary to introduce a soft cell growth platform which closely mimics the microenvironment of the targeted tissue. In a biological system, the extracellular matrix (ECM) refers to the complex environment in between cells whose composition varies from one tissue to another. The main role of the ECM is to provide structural support to the cells; however, it also plays an important role in signal transduction, modulating cell shape and polarity, regulating cell migration, and resistance to external forces [54]. In native tissue, the ECM composition is dynamic, and the three most abundant components include collagens, proteoglycans, and glycoproteins (for more details, see Chapter 1). Cell growth scaffolds with different properties can be developed by varying the ratio of these three components. The main requirements for these artificial matrices to facilitate the transformation of isolated cells into functional tissues are to allow cell adhesion, growth, maintenance and signal transduction, to support effective nutrient and metabolic transfer, such as gas exchange (i.e. O_2 and CO_2) and metabolic waste removal, and to be biocompatible.

In general, hydrogels are soft matrices usually composed of hydrophilic polymers of diverse origin. They have water contents of over 90% and have viscoelastic properties with storage moduli higher than their corresponding loss moduli [55]. The properties of hydrogels are primarily governed by the chemistry of the constituent molecules. These polymers are held together by covalent, noncovalent, or physical cross-links. In addition to the chemistry, an enormous diversity in terms of mechanical and biological properties of these materials can result in different outcomes of cell attachment, proliferation, differentiation, migration, and signaling. Depending on the nature of the targeted tissue, different kinds of hydrogels have been utilized in microfluidic chips, and these are summarized in Table 12.1. Based on the chemical features and origin, the common hydrogels used for the development of tissue chips can be classified into three categories: protein-based, mucopolysaccharides, and nonnatural polymers. In addition to providing support for the cells, these matrices are often designed to include cell growth factors that assist the formation of structured tissue. Hence, the role of the hydrogel in this realm of research is to provide optimal growth environment for the cells by providing a support matrix and nutrients to foster the evolution from isolated cell configuration into functional tissues [76]. Several ECM-like hydrogels have been shown potential toward mimicking native ECM in microfluidic devices: collagen [56, 77–79], Matrigel [31, 69], hyaluronan/hyaluronic acid (HA) [66], fibrin [64], and chitosan [80].

Collagen-based ECM mimics are described in Chapter 2. Our group has successfully applied collagen for the development of a tissue chamber chip to study the diffusion of different kinds of materials (e.g. spherical polymeric nanocontructs, liposomes, and polystyrene nanoparticles) [57]. This subject will be extensively discussed in the next section. We have also used Matrigel (presented in Chapter 1) in double-channel microfluidic chips [69, 70]. Hyaluronate hydrogels (reviewed in Chapter 10) were used to assess the vascular permeability and transport of nanoparticles in the double-channel microfluidic chip devices [66].

12.3 Fabrication of Microfluidic Chips

The fabrication of microfluidic chips requires microengineering expertise and was first reported in the 1990s [81]. Nowadays, microfabrication is becoming more accessible [82]. Most chips are processed via soft lithography methods and are made of polydimethylsiloxane (PDMS), because it is easy to use and has high optical clarity, gas permeability, and biocompatibility [83]. Microfluidic chips can also be composed of other optically clear polymers, such as polyurethanes or glass. These chips can contain one or more perfused channels, hydrogels, and cells to recapitulate *in vivo* tissue, organ physiology, and pathophysiology by creating tissue-/organ-like structure and function *in vitro* [83, 84]. Microfluidic chips can have a single channel filled with cells and usually embedded in a hydrogel. More complex devices can have two or more channels, usually connected through a permeable membrane and cells (from the same tissue or different types).

12.3.1 Single-Channel Microfluidic Chips

Microfluidic chips with a single channel are relatively simple to fabricate, yet offer controllable biomimetic parameters, such as the channel's width and length, flow conditions, and incorporation of tissue-engineered components. The processing

Table 12.1 List of different types of hydrogels used in microfluidic chips for various applications as tissue mimics.

Hydrogel	Structure	Advantages (+) /disadvantages (−)	Applications	References
Collagen	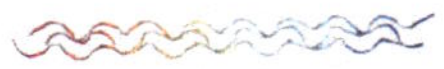	+ Mimics native ECM, adhesive and bioactive, biodegradable − Potential mechanical instability, gelation sensitive to modification	Transmigration of neutrophils in inflammation, invasion of metastatic rat mammary adenocarcinoma cells, angiogenesis	[56–60]
Alginate	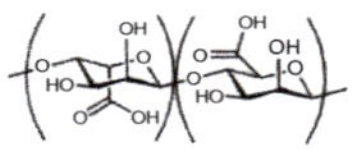	+ Fast ionic gelation, abundant, functionalizable − Nonbiodegradable, poorly adhesive Cation diffusion can lead to dissolution	Perfusable vascular networks, angiogenesis	[61, 62]
Gelatin	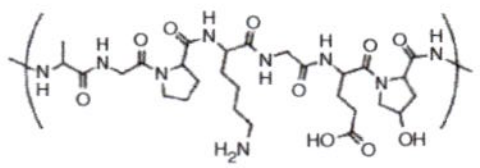	+ Adhesive and bioactive, functionalizable, abundant, biodegradable − Mechanically weak, contamination can lead to immunogenicity	Encapsulation of the hepatocarcinoma cell line	[63]
Fibrin	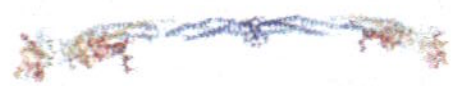	+ Low cost, inflammation, immune response, toxicity, good cell adhesion − Lengthy cross-linking, fast degradation, potential mechanical instability	Human microphysiological vascularized tissue, angiogenesis	[64, 65]
Hylaruonic acid	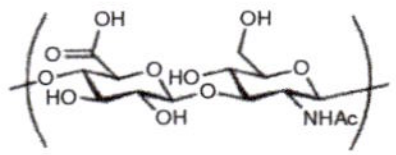	+ Bioactive, biocompatible, binds growth factors and cytokines, functionalizable − Low stability without cross-linking, fast degradation *in vivo*	Monitoring of cell alignment and migration	[66, 67]
Agarose	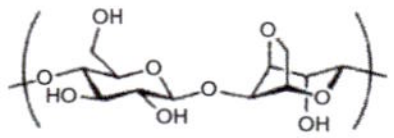	+ Simple gelation, readily functionalizable − High viscosity, requires temperature control	Biomimetic synthetic vasculature	[68]

Matrigel	Mixture of: • Collagen  • Laminin 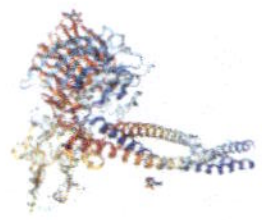 • Heparan 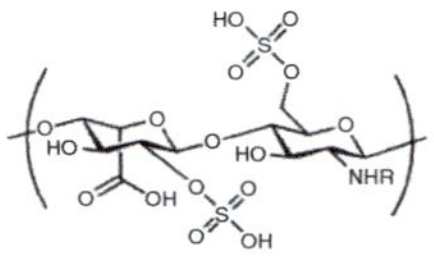	+ Close resemblance with native ECM, biocompatible, degradable, bioadhesive – Complex mixture, potentially variable gelation	Linked tumor and liver chambers on chips	[69–71]
PEGDA	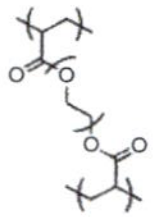	+ Variable molecular weight and cross-linking, modular gel properties – Nondegradable, potential immunogenicity	Assay for the detection of the hepatocyte growth factor	[72]
PEG peptide hybrids	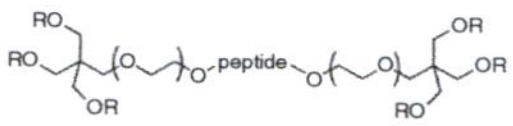	+ Tunable properties, fast gelation, cell-specific adhesion, enzyme-sensitive degradation, growth factor binding – Synthetically complex	Dynamic alteration of the three-dimensional cellular environment	[73]
poly(*N*-isopropila-crilammide) (pNIPAM)	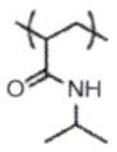	+ Temperature responsive (lower critical solution temperature (LCST)), biocompatible, low immunogenicity – Monomer cytotoxic, nondegradable	Tissue-mimicking patterned materials, microlenses	[74, 75]

The list includes the hydrogel chemical structures and common advantages and disadvantages of different hydrogels.

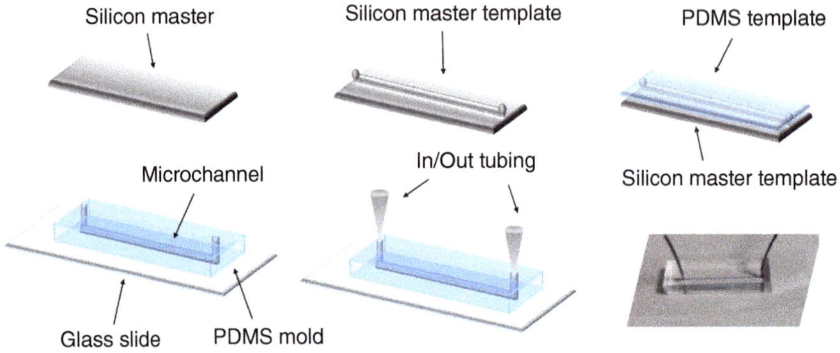

Figure 12.1 Schematic presentation of the fabrication of a single-channel microfluidic chip.

of single-channel chips, developed in our lab, is described in detail by Manneschi et al. [66] and Mollica et al. [85] and illustrated in Figure 12.1. Briefly, using lithographic techniques, a single-channel silicon master template is obtained from a negative template of SU8-50 photoresist. The silicon template is replicated using a mixture of PDMS and sealed with a glass slide. In this configuration, the obtained single-channel microfluidic chip has a length of 2.7 cm, a height of 42 μm, and a width of 210 μm.

In another configuration, a tissue chamber chip was designed to investigate the extracellular diffusivity and transport of nanoparticles and small molecules in real time [57]. This device was fabricated with $15 \times 15 \times 3.5\,\text{mm}^3$ PDMS with an empty chamber of dimensions $5 \times 5 \times 3.5\,\text{mm}^3$ created in the center (Figure 12.2). The PDMS tissue chamber was bonded to a glass slide using oxygen plasma, and an access channel with 0.8 mm diameter was generated in the side of the device. This chip has a chamber filled with collagen hydrogel, and the nanoparticles were injected through the channel.

With this chip, the dynamics of different nanoparticles was estimated within the collagen hydrogel. It was also possible to determine the diffusion coefficients and the transport of nanoparticles within the collagen hydrogel in real time with routine microscopy techniques by designing the chip to fit on top of a standard microscope slide. The tissue chamber chip can be used as a preliminary tool to analyze

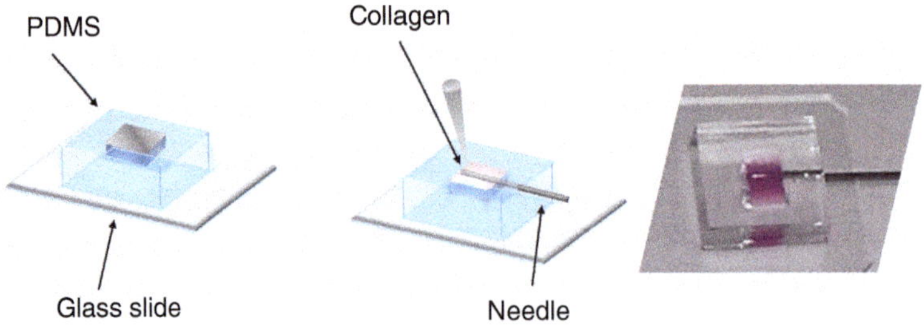

Figure 12.2 Schematic presentation of the fabrication process of a tissue chamber chip.

particles diffusion in a tissue-like environment and to test the extravascular transport of nanomedicines.

12.3.2 Double-Channel Microfluidic Chip

Higher levels of complexity can be achieved in microfluidic chip systems by incorporating networks of interconnected channels, permeable membranes, and different cell types. In 2013, Kim et al. [64] proposed a microfluidic platform to form a functional microvascular network and angiogenic sprout, where human umbilical vein endothelial cells (HUVECs) and human glioblastoma multiforme (U87 MG) cells were co-cultured on opposite sides of a central fibrin hydrogel-filled channel [64]. Nguyen et al. [56] designed a microfluidic device that enabled angiogenic sprouting morphogenesis and new vessel formation. This angiogenesis chip was filled with collagen type I where endothelial cells were cultured in one microchannel perfused with medium and, in a parallel channel, a medium supplemented with angiogenic factors (e.g. hepatocyte growth factor (HGF), basic fibroblast growth factor (bFGF), monocyte chemoattractant protein-1, vascular endothelial growth factor (VEGF), and sphingosine-1-phosphate (S1P)) was perfused [56]. Another device, containing two microfluidic channels separated by a vitrified collagen membrane, was developed by Choi et al. [86] to simulate the microarchitecture of ductal carcinoma *in situ* (DCIS) of breast cancer *in vitro*. In this two-channel chip, normal mammary epithelial cells and spheroids obtained from DCIS patients were cultured in one channel with perfused medium. In the other channel, collagen hydrogel containing human mammary fibroblasts was placed on the lower surface of the collagen membrane to create a stromal compartment. The cell growth was monitored by fluorescence labeling of different cell types, and it was shown that treatment with the anticancer drug paclitaxel prevented growth of DCIS spheroids without toxic effect on the normal mammary epithelial cells [86].

The preparation of a double-channel microfluidic chip in our laboratory is described in detail by Manneschi et al. [66] (Figure 12.3). In the first step, an optical mask of glass in conjunction with photolithography techniques is used to pattern

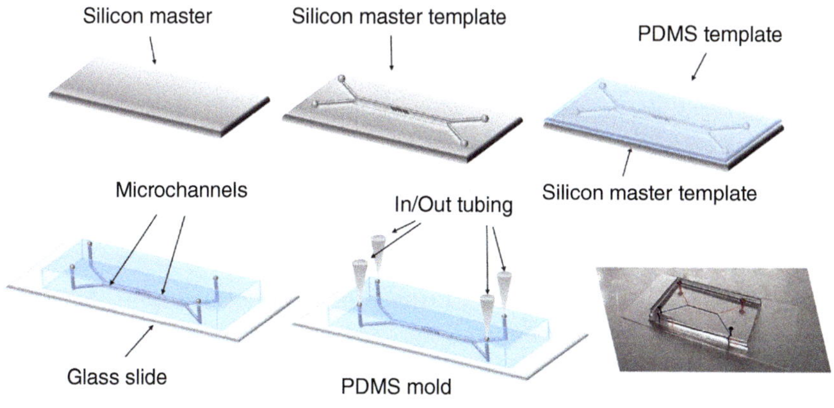

Figure 12.3 Fabrication design of a double-channel microfluidic chip. The last picture shows the vascular channel in red and the extravascular channel in blue.

the designated double channels into the silicon master chip. In the second step, the obtained silicon master template is replicated via a soft lithography approach with PDMS. The final PDMS template is composed by two microfluidic channels with a length of 27 mm, interconnected in the middle part by an array of micropillars with 500 μm in length with a gap size of 3 μm. The two channels have a height of 50 μm and a width of 200 μm. In more detail, these microfluidic chips comprise two parallel channels (upper – vascular channel and lower – extravascular channel). Each channel has one inlet and one outlet and is connected by a micropillar permeable membrane. Usually, the vascular channel is injected with drugs, active compounds, nanoparticles or seeded with cells (e.g. endothelial-like cells). While, the extravascular channel is usually injected with a hydrogel and embedded cells to mimic the 3D architecture/structure of tissue or organ.

12.4 Applications of Microfluidic Chips in Biophysical Transport Analysis

12.4.1 Single-Channel Microfluidic Chips

Our group has employed single-channel microfluidic chips to investigate the vascular adhesion of circulating tumor cells (CTCs) [85]. The use of microfluidic chips in this instance proved to be critical, as solution rheology and flow rate can greatly affect CTC deposition. Analysis of the rolling and adhesion of both colorectal (HCT-15) and breast cancer (MDA-MB-23) cells under various conditions were performed. Interestingly, with the addition of tumor necrosis factor (TNF)-α, CTC adhesion increased up to four times without the cell velocity being significantly affected. It was also found that whole blood enhanced circulating cell vascular deposition.

A single-channel microfluidic chip has also been used in our lab to simulate the 3D structure of brain tumors. As a proof of concept, Martins et al. [70] used a human glioblastoma multiforme cell line (U87 MG) and a standard potent drug, docetaxel (DTXL), known to be very efficient in the treatment of various cancers. In this case, U87 cells were embedded into Matrigel and injected into the microfluidic chips to form a tumor-like tissue-on-chip platform. Several concentrations (0.01, 0.1, 0.5, 1, and 10 μM) of DTXL were injected through the channel, and obtained results showed that only concentrations equal or higher than 0.1 μM significantly enhanced the death of U87 MG over time. However, when the highest concentrations (1 and 10 μM DTXL) were used, almost no cells were detected after 24 hours. The cell viability tremendously decreased (>80%) after one day [70].

12.4.2 Double-Channel Microfluidic Chips

To mimic better the dynamics and 3D structure of multiple coexisting biological microenvironments, as occurs *in vivo*, hydrogels and tissue-derived cells can be injected into different channels. The double-channel chip, presented in Figure 12.3, allows to simultaneously monitor the dynamics of cells within two different channels and across the permeable membrane. HA was the first hydrogel used in the double-channel chips developed by our lab [66]. This double-channel microfluidic chip resembles the interface between the vasculature walls and the extravascular matrix. To study the permeability between both channels, the extravascular channel was filled with HA hydrogel, while polystyrene beads or dextran molecules were injected in the vascular channel. Transport experiments on chips using different size beads within the HA hydrogel was monitored in real time via optical microscopy. The permeability between both channels was reduced with molecular weight of dextran and the size of beads [66].

Mollica et al. [69] used the double-channel chip to replicate *in vitro* the processes of cell intravasation, vascular transport, cell adhesion, extravasation, and invasion – all of which are key steps of the tumor metastatic cascade. One of the channels, acting as a vascular compartment, was coated with HUVECs, forming a confluent layer over the micropillars (Figure 12.4). The other channel was filled with Matrigel and breast cancer cells (MDA-MB-231) to replicate the tumor tissue.

Tumors are highly vascularized to support the greater metabolic rates of tumor tissue compared to normal tissue. Simulation of vasculature in microfluidics

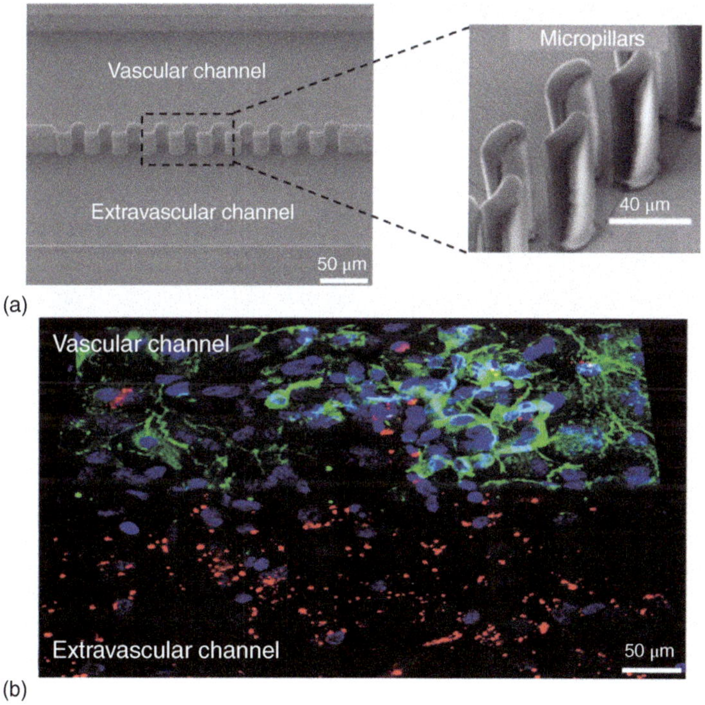

Figure 12.4 (a) Scanning electron microscopy images of the permeable membrane between the two channels of a double-channel microfluidic chip; (b) confocal image of the double-channel chip showing the vascular compartment seeded with a HUVEC cells (cell nuclei stained with 4′,6-diamidino-2-phenylindole (DAPI) – blue, VE-Cadherin – adherents junction, green) and MDA-MB-231 breast cancer cells embedded in Matrigel in the extravascular compartment (cell membrane stained with 1,1′-dioctadecyl-3,3,3′,3′-tetramethylindocarbocyanine perchlorate (DIL) – red). Source: Mollica et al., (2019), [69], Figure1, Pg 02 / with permission of American Chemical Society.

chips allows the investigation of the metastatic potential of cells and tissues. In addition, the use of cancer-on-a-chip devices which can model metastasis are also able to assess new nanomedicines in a fast and optimized manner and evaluate their subsequent toxicities. Martins et al. [70] used double-channel microfluidic chips to investigate several anticancer therapies. Human glioblastoma multiforme (U87 MG) cells were embedded into Matrigel and injected into the avascular channel and cultured for 72 hours. Free DTXL with different concentrations, spherical polymeric nanoconstructs with loaded DTXL (docetaxel (DTXL)-loaded spherical polymeric nanoconstructs (SPNs) (DTXL-SPNs)), and a novel compound named *N*-(fluorenylmethoxycarbonyl)-glucosamine-6-phosphate (Fmoc-Glc6P) were added to the vascular channel. Results showed that only the highest concentration of DTXL (10 μM) was effective to induce U87 MG cell death but after 48 hours. DTXL-SPNs presented the same trend, showing a significant decrease in cell viability (≈40%) after 48 hours, without changing after 72 hours. The most promising result was obtained with Fmoc-Glc6P. This compound was previously used to control cancer cell fate, namely with osteosarcoma cells (SaOs2), where the compound formed a cytotoxic nanonet/hydrogel "cage" surrounding the cells to eventually induced cell death [87]. When U87 MG cells were embedded in Matrigel and Fmoc-Glc6P was injected into the extravascular channel the following day, approximately 50% of cells died. After 48 hours, cell viability gradually decreases, and after 72 hours only 20% of cells remained viable [70].

12.5 Nanoparticle Transport Analyses

Microfluidic chips combined with hydrogel materials, as described in this chapter, provide a valuable platform for the analysis of vascular and extravascular environments and idealized processes [88, 89]. However, they also provide a promising method for the analysis of various physicochemical properties and size/shape design parameters of nanoparticles and nanomedicines. Conventionally, nanomedicines have been evaluated in static 2D systems, either cell culture plates for cell studies or other static systems for permeation studies. Microfluidic chips offer the advantage of including flow conditions, which improve *in vitro* tests to more closely mimic the *in vivo* situation.

Microfluidic chips have been used to study the effect of size on nanomedicine ability to cross a semi-permeable membrane – mimicking extravasation [66]. Spherical polystyrene nanoparticles of 200 nm, 5 μm, and 10 μm were infused through the upper channel of the chip, and permeation to the bottom channel through micropillar membrane was studied. Larger particles of 5 and 10 μm remained in the upper channel and after some time blocked the membrane, while 200-nm nanoparticles were found distributed throughout the two channels. The bottom channel was also filled with a hyaluronic acid hydrogel to mimic the ECM, and spherical nanoparticles of 200 nm, 0.75 μm, and 1.5 μm were studied. This configuration mimics better biological environment, and the penetration depth of the nanoparticles was reduced. The 200-nm particles penetrated 50 μm into the hydrogel channel, while the larger particles penetrated very little and appeared to adhere to the hydrogel surface.

While polystyrene nanoparticles are useful to study size-related parameters, they are usually not realistic options for use as nanomedicines. Our group has progressed to the analysis of more complex nanoparticles in tissue-mimicking collagen chips [57]. Spherical polymeric nanoparticles were formed by an emulsion method and had a hydrodynamic size of 186 ± 13 nm and a zeta potential of -45.9 ± 0.79 mV, with two different degrees of polyethylene glycol (PEG) surface functionalization. In addition, lipid bilayer liposomes with an aqueous core were formed and coated with hyaluronic acid and had a hydrodynamic size of 138.5 ± 4.8 nm with a zeta potential of -37 ± 4 mV. These nanoparticles were then compared to 200-nm polystyrene, in the previously described tissue chamber chip. It was found that nanoparticle diffusion through the collagen hydrogel increased with increasing surface functionalization with PEG chains. Increases in particle diffusivity with PEGylation have also been seen in the literature [90]. While in the case of hyaluronic acid-coated nanoparticles, increasing surface functionalization caused a reduction in permeation through the hydrogel chip device. This trend was attributed to either attractive electrostatic forces or specific hyaluronic acid–collagen interactions.

The role of nonspherical particles in microfluidic chip systems has also been investigated [91, 92]. These particles are of significance to microfluidic systems for particle analysis, as they typically behave differently under flow conditions, e.g. tend to marginate toward channel walls. Colasuonno et al. [92] fabricated poly(lactic-co-glycolic acid) (PLGA)-based discoidal polymeric nanoconstructs (DPNs) with diameters of 1000 nm and height of 400 nm and conjugated tissue plasminogen activator (tPA) to the particle surface (Figure 12.5a,b). Using a double-channel chip as an *in vitro* model, fibrin blood clots were formed at the interface between the two channels (Figure 12.5c), and tissue plasminogen activator (tPA)- loaded discoidal polymeric nanoconstructs (DPN) (tPA-DPN) used as a new therapeutic agent to more effectively dissolve clots under flow conditions (Figure 12.5d). After 60 minutes, the clot area reduced by $57\% \pm 8\%$, with tPA-DPNs, while for free tPA it takes 90 minutes to reach this value (Figure 12.5e). These results were confirmed in an *in vivo* model for thrombotic events.

12.6 Computer Simulations of Nanoparticle and Cell Transport

The role of vascular and extravascular transport of particles and cells is often an overlooked aspect of both understanding disease and evaluation of nanomedicines and cell therapies. By combining predictive computer simulations with experimental microfluidic systems, researchers aim to facilitate faster development of effective therapies and possibly enhance translation.

Chemical–physical properties such as size and deformability are known to significantly affect the vascular and extravascular transport of cells or systemically injected particles. Given the large space of tunable parameters, it is unfeasible to experimentally screen all the possible combinations for testing the therapeutic efficacy of the latter. In this context, computational tools are available to refine hypotheses and support nanoconstructs' design, helping to reduce the overall experimental workload.

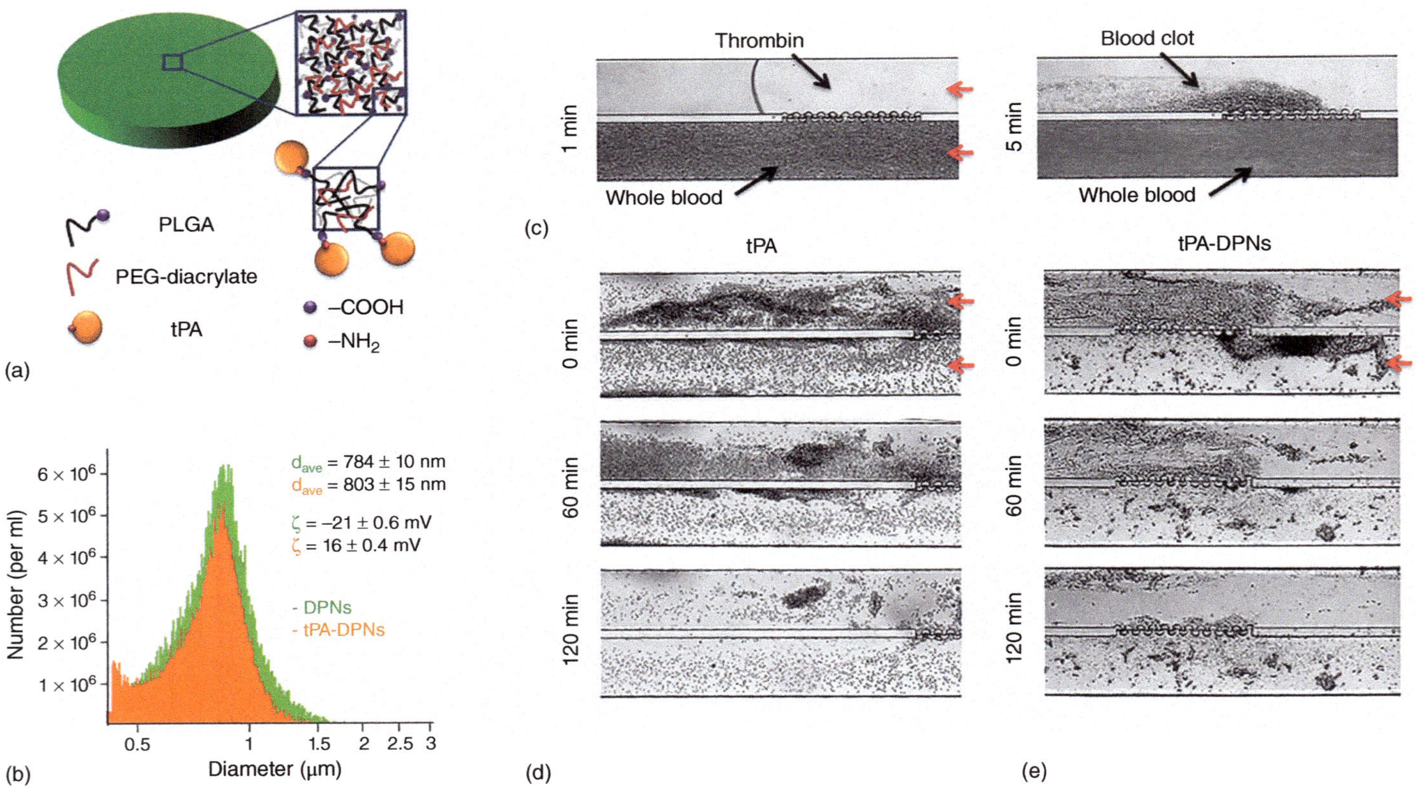

Figure 12.5 (a) Schematic representation of tPA-DPNs, and their direct conjugation with tPA, (b) multisizer analysis of DPNs (green) and tPA-DPNs (orange), (c) representative images of a blood clot forming spontaneously within the chambers of a microfluidic chip upon mixing of whole blood (bottom channel) and a thrombin solution (upper channel), (d) representative images of a blood clot taken at 0, 60, and 120 minutes post-injection of free tPA, (e) representative images of a blood clot taken at 0, 60, and 120 minutes post-injection of tPA-DPNs. Source: Colasuonno, M., et al. (2018), [92], Figure 05, Pg 07 / with permission of American Chemical Society.

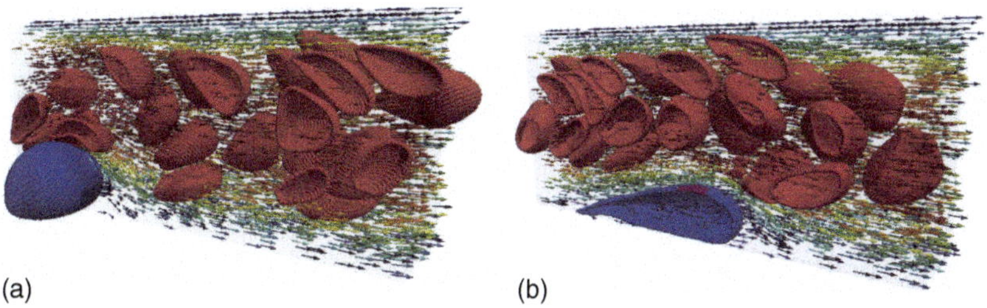

Figure 12.6 The left panel (a) shows a CTC (in blue) firmly adhering to the wall of a capillary; on the right panel (b) represents a less sticking CTC rolling along the bottom of the capillary. Source: From Lenardaet al. [93]/with permission from Springer Nature.

Similar approaches can be used to predict how vascular dynamics enables CTCs to establish metastatic niches, thus allowing the development of preventive strategies (e.g. Figure 12.6).

Several computational approaches have been developed to mimic blood flow and simulate the transport of cells or particles within several vascular domains, namely: (i) Direct numerical simulations (DNS) [94], (ii) immersed boundary methods (IBMs) [95], (iii) isogeometric analysis (IA) [96], and (iv) immersed finite element methods (IFEMs) [97]. However, these methods, all based on the discretization and numerical integration of the Navier–Stokes and continuity equations, are computationally expensive, restricting their use for simulating multiple particles or accounting for complex shapes or deformability. Recently, particle-based techniques such as the lattice Boltzmann method (LBM) emerged as an alternative approach due to their easier implementation and the advantage of being parallelizable. Among other applications, this method has been successfully employed to model deformable red blood cells (RBCs) and leukocytes and predict their aggregation propensities in narrow capillaries [98] or the role of RBCs on the dynamics of leukocytes [99]. Considering that extravasation is preceded by the adhesion of particles or cells to the vascular endothelium, a combined lattice Boltzmann-immersed boundary (LB-IB) model was used in our lab to investigate particles sticking to the capillary wall via specific ligand receptor bonds [100], as a function of particle shape, surface ligand density, ligand receptor binding strength, and fluid viscosity, both in 2D [101] and 3D [93]. Computational predictions helped to identify different adhesive regimes and explain experimental observations on compartmentalized chips [85].

12.7 Conclusions and Future Directions

Recent advances indicate that 3D cultures with integrated flow resemble *in vivo* function much more closely than static 2D culture conditions. Microfluidic technology is one of the most effective tools that we have to reproduce the physiological environment of tissue/organs *in vitro* and address the limitations of current cell and animal models. Microfluidic devices with embedded 3D hydrogels (mimicking the structure of tissues and organs) are powerful tools for the further development of nanomedicines. For instance, one particularly promising future direction combining microfluidic systems and nanomedicines will be their application in the development and testing of personalized nanomedicines. This will be possible by the easy production of microfluidic chips and the ability to incorporate patient-derived cells, while also having the ability to test formulations in parallel chip setups. These systems will be able to optimize dosages and combination therapies on personalized organ-on-chip devices, but more importantly with also allow the high-throughput screening of large libraries of different nanoparticle therapies with different sizes, shapes, and chemical compositions to identify efficient personalized nanomedicines. Combining high-throughput microfluidic chip devices, patient-derived cells, and nanomedicines with machine learning will improve our understanding of biophysical processes and support the development of more effective medications.

References

1 Lee, J., Cuddihy, M.J., and Kotov, N.A. (2008). Three-dimensional cell culture matrices: state of the art. *Tissue Eng. Part B Rev.* 14 (1): 61–86.

2 Breslin, S. and O'Driscoll, L. (2013). Three-dimensional cell culture: the missing link in drug discovery. *Drug Discovery Today* 18 (5, 6): 240–249.

3 Garber, K. (2018). Alnylam launches era of RNAi drugs. *Nat Biotechnol.* 36 (9): 777–778.

4 Boraschi, D., Italiani, P., Palomba, R. et al. (2017). Nanoparticles and innate immunity: new perspectives on host defence. *Semin. Immunol.* 34: 33–51.

5 Nam, J., Son, S., Park, K.S. et al. (2019). Cancer nanomedicine for combination cancer immunotherapy. *Nat. Rev. Mater.* 4 (6): 398–414.

6 Cook, A.B. and Perrier, S. (2019). Branched and dendritic polymer architectures: functional nanomaterials for therapeutic delivery. *Adv. Funct. Mater.* 30: 1901001.

7 Park, T.H. and Shuler, M.L. (2003). Integration of cell culture and microfabrication technology. *Biotechnol. Progr.* 19 (2): 243–253.

8 Zhang, B.Y. et al. (2018). Advances in organ-on-a-chip engineering. *Nat. Rev. Mater.* 3 (8): 257–278.

9 Ronaldson-Bouchard, K. and Vunjak-Novakovic, G. (2018). Organs-on-a-chip: a fast track for engineered human tissues in drug development. *Cell Stem Cell* 22 (3): 310–324.

10 Trkov, S. et al. (2010). Micropatterned three-dimensional hydrogel system to study human endothelial – mesenchymal stem cell interactions. *J. Tissue Eng. Regener. Med.* 4 (3): 205–215.

11 Cimetta, E., Yeager, K., and Vunjak-Novakovic, G. (2012). Spatial and temporal regulation of signaling pathways in hESCs using microfluidic technologies. *J. Tissue Eng. Regener. Med.* 6: 249–249.

12 Cimetta, E. et al. (2010). Microfluidic device generating stable concentration gradients for long term cell culture: application to Wnt3a regulation of beta-catenin signaling. *Lab Chip* 10 (23): 3277–3283.

13 Kim, H.J. et al. (2012). Human gut-on-a-chip inhabited by microbial flora that experiences intestinal peristalsis-like motions and flow. *Lab Chip* 12 (12): 2165–2174.
14 Villenave, R. et al. (2017). Human gut-on-a-chip supports polarized infection of coxsackie B1 virus in vitro. *PLoS One* 12 (2): e0169412.
15 Trietsch, S.J. et al. (2017). Membrane-free culture and real-time barrier integrity assessment of perfused intestinal epithelium tubes. *Nat. Commun.* 8: 262.
16 Sidar, B. et al. (2019). Long-term flow through human intestinal organoids with the gut organoid flow chip (GOFlowChip). *Lab Chip* 19 (20): 3552–3562.
17 Adriani, G. et al. (2017). A 3D neurovascular microfluidic model consisting of neurons, astrocytes and cerebral endothelial cells as a blood-brain barrier. *Lab Chip* 17 (3): 448–459.
18 Marino, A. et al. (2018). A 3D real-scale, biomimetic, and biohybrid model of the blood-brain barrier fabricated through two-photon lithography. *Small* 14 (6): https://doi.org/10.1002/smll.201702959.
19 Osaki, T., Sivathanu, V., and Kamm, R.D. (2018). Engineered 3D vascular and neuronal networks in a microfluidic platform. *Sci. Rep.* 8: 5168.
20 Maoz, B.M. et al. (2018). A linked organ-on-chip model of the human neurovascular unit reveals the metabolic coupling of endothelial and neuronal cells. *Nat. Biotechnol.* 36 (9): 865–874.
21 Park, T.E. et al. (2019). Hypoxia-enhanced blood-brain barrier chip recapitulates human barrier function and shuttling of drugs and antibodies. *Nat. Commun.* 10: 2621.
22 Osaki, T., Uzel, S.G.M., and Kamm, R.D. (2018). Microphysiological 3D model of amyotrophic lateral sclerosis (ALS) from human iPS-derived muscle cells and optogenetic motor neurons. *Sci. Adv.* 4 (10): eaat5847.
23 Humayun, M., Chow, C.W., and Young, E.W.K. (2018). Microfluidic lung airway-on-a-chip with arrayable suspended gels for studying epithelial and smooth muscle cell interactions. *Lab Chip* 18 (9): 1298–1309.
24 Benam, K.H. et al. (2016). Small airway-on-a-chip enables analysis of human lung inflammation and drug responses in vitro. *Nat. Methods* 13 (2): 151–157.
25 Benam, K. et al. (2016). Human small airway-on-a-chip: a novel microphysiological system to model lung inflammation, accelerate drug development and enable inhalational toxico-analysis. *Eur. Respir. J.* 48: OA4542.
26 Huh, D. et al. (2010). Reconstituting organ-level lung functions on a chip. *Science* 328 (5986): 1662–1668.
27 van den Broek, L.J. et al. (2017). Progress and future prospectives in skin-on-chip development with emphasis on the use of different cell types and technical challenges. *Stem Cell Rev. Rep.* 13 (3): 418–429.
28 Sriram, G. et al. (2018). Full-thickness human skin-on-chip with enhanced epidermal morphogenesis and barrier function. *Mater. Today* 21 (4): 326–340.
29 Marturano-Kruik, A. et al. (2018). Human bone perivascular niche-on-a-chip for studying metastatic colonization. *Proc. Natl. Acad. Sci. U.S.A.* 115 (6): 1256–1261.

30 Lai, B.F.L. et al. (2017). InVADE: Integrated vasculature for assessing dynamic events. *Adv. Funct. Mater.* 27 (46): 1703524.

31 Carvalho, M.R. et al. (2019). Colorectal tumor-on-a-chip system: a 3D tool for precision onco-nanomedicine. *Sci. Adv.* 5 (5): eaaw1317.

32 Chramiec, A. and Vunjak-Novakovic, G. (2019). Tissue engineered models of healthy and malignant human bone marrow. *Adv. Drug Delivery Rev.* 140: 78–92.

33 Parsa, H., Wang, B.Z., and Vunjak-Novakovic, G. (2017). A microfluidic platform for the high-throughput study of pathological cardiac hypertrophy. *Lab Chip* 17 (19): 3264–3271.

34 Zhao, Y.M. et al. (2019). A multimaterial microphysiological platform enabled by rapid casting of elastic microwires. *Adv. Healthc. Mater.* 8 (5): e1801187.

35 Au, H.T.H. et al. (2009). Cell culture chips for simultaneous application of topographical and electrical cues enhance phenotype of cardiomyocytes. *Lab Chip* 9 (4): 564–575.

36 Zhang, B.Y. et al. (2016). Biodegradable scaffold with built-in vasculature for organ-on-a-chip engineering and direct surgical anastomosis. *Nat. Mater.* 15 (6): 669–678.

37 Conant, G. et al. (2017). High-content assessment of cardiac function using heart-on-a-chip devices as drug screening model. *Stem Cell Rev. Rep.* 13 (3): 335–346.

38 Nunes, S.S. et al. (2013). Biowire: a platform for maturation of human pluripotent stem cell-derived cardiomyocytes. *Nat. Methods* 10 (8): 781–787.

39 Marsano, A. et al. (2016). Beating heart on a chip: a novel microfluidic platform to generate functional 3D cardiac microtissues. *Lab Chip* 16 (3): 599–610.

40 Lee, K.H. et al. (2010). Microfluidic synthesis of pure chitosan microfibers for bio-artificial liver chip. *Lab Chip* 10 (10): 1328–1334.

41 Prot, J.M. et al. (2012). Predictive toxicology using systemic biology and liver microfluidic "on chip" approaches: application to acetaminophen injury. *Toxicol. Appl. Pharmacol.* 259 (3): 270–280.

42 Zhou, Q. et al. (2015). Liver injury-on-a-chip: microfluidic co-cultures with integrated biosensors for monitoring liver cell signaling during injury. *Lab Chip* 15 (23): 4467–4478.

43 Gori, M. et al. (2016). Investigating nonalcoholic fatty liver disease in a liver-on-a-chip microfluidic device. *PLoS One* 11 (7): e0159729.

44 Du, Y. et al. (2017). Mimicking liver sinusoidal structures and functions using a 3D-configured microfluidic chip. *Lab Chip* 17 (5): 782–794.

45 Kovachev, N., Canals, A., and Escarpa, A. (2010). Fast and selective microfluidic chips for electrochemical antioxidant sensing in complex samples. *Anal. Chem.* 82 (7): 2925–2931.

46 Nguyen, T.T. et al. (2017). Endocrine system on chip for a diabetes treatment model. *Biofabrication* 9 (1): 015021.

47 Jiang, K. et al. (2019). 3-D physiomimetic extracellular matrix hydrogels provide a supportive microenvironment for rodent and human islet culture. *Biomaterials* 198: 37–48.

48 Shi, X.T. et al. (2012). Directing osteogenesis of stem cells with drug-laden, polymer-microsphere-based micropatterns generated by teflon microfluidic chips. *Adv. Funct. Mater.* 22 (18): 3799–3807.

49 Shi, X.T. et al. (2013). Gradient-regulated hydrogel for interface tissue engineering: steering simultaneous osteo/chondrogenesis of stem cells on a chip. *Adv. Healthc. Mater.* 2 (6): 846–853.

50 Ma, H.P. et al. (2018). A microfluidic chip-based co-culture of fibroblast-like synoviocytes with osteoblasts and osteoclasts to test bone erosion and drug evaluation. *R. Soc. Open Sci.* 5 (9): 180528.

51 Leclerc, E. et al. (2006). Study of osteoblastic cells in a microfluidic environment. *Biomaterials* 27 (4): 586–595.

52 Li, M. et al. (2018). Microfluidic-based screening of resveratrol and drug-loading PLA/Gelatine nano-scaffold for the repair of cartilage defect. *Artif. Cells Nanomed. Biotechnol.* 46: S336–S346.

53 Occhetta, P. et al. (2019). Hyperphysiological compression of articular cartilage induces an osteoarthritic phenotype in a cartilage-on-a-chip model. *Nat. Biomed. Eng.* 3 (7): 545–557.

54 Geckil, H. et al. (2010). Engineering hydrogels as extracellular matrix mimics. *Nanomedicine (Lond)* 5 (3): 469–484.

55 Weng, L., Chen, X., and Chen, W. (2007). Rheological properties of in situ crosslinkable hydrogels from dextran and chitosan derivatives. *Biomacromolecules* 8: 1109–1115.

56 Nguyen, D.H. et al. (2013). Biomimetic model to reconstitute angiogenic sprouting morphogenesis in vitro. *Proc. Natl. Acad. Sci. U.S.A.* 110 (17): 6712–6717.

57 Lusi, V. et al. (2019). A tissue chamber chip for assessing nanoparticle mobility in the extravascular space. *Biomed. Microdevices* 21 (2): 41.

58 Han, S. et al. (2012). A versatile assay for monitoring in vivo-like transendothelial migration of neutrophils. *Lab Chip* 12 (20): 3861–3865.

59 Abhyankar, V.V. et al. (2008). A platform for assessing chemotactic migration within a spatiotemporally defined 3D microenvironment. *Lab Chip* 8 (9): 1507–1515.

60 Zheng, Y. et al. (2012). In vitro microvessels for the study of angiogenesis and thrombosis. *Proc. Natl. Acad. Sci. U.S.A.* 109 (24): 9342–9347.

61 Wang, X.Y. et al. (2014). Engineering interconnected 3D vascular networks in hydrogels using molded sodium alginate lattice as the sacrificial templatet. *Lab Chip* 14 (15): 2709–2716.

62 Fischbach, C. et al. (2009). Cancer cell angiogenic capability is regulated by 3D culture and integrin engagement. *Proc. Natl. Acad. Sci. U.S.A.* 106 (2): 399–404.

63 Billiet, T. et al. (2014). The 3D printing of gelatin methacrylamide cell-laden tissue-engineered constructs with high cell viability. *Biomaterials* 35 (1): 49–62.

64 Kim, S. et al. (2013). Engineering of functional, perfusable 3D microvascular networks on a chip. *Lab Chip* 13 (8): 1489–1500.

65 Hsu, Y.H. et al. (2013). A microfluidic platform for generating large-scale nearly identical human microphysiological vascularized tissue arrays. *Lab Chip* 13 (15): 2990–2998.

66 Manneschi, C. et al. (2016). A microfluidic platform with permeable walls for the analysis of vascular and extravascular mass transport. *Microfluid. Nanofluid.* 20 (8): 1–12.

67 Lee, K.H. et al. (2014). Integration of microfluidic chip with biomimetic hydrogel for 3D controlling and monitoring of cell alignment and migration. *J. Biomed. Mater. Res. A* 102 (4): 1164–1172.

68 Ling, Y. et al. (2007). A cell-laden microfluidic hydrogel. *Lab Chip* 7 (6): 756–762.

69 Mollica, H. et al. (2019). Two-channel compartmentalized microfluidic chip for real-time monitoring of the metastatic cascade. *ACS Biomater. Sci. Eng.* 5 (9): 4834–4843.

70 Martins, A.M., Barbato, M.G., Felici, A., et al., (2022). Efficacy of Molecular and Nano-Therapies on Brain Tumor Models in Microfluidic Devices

71 Sung, J.H. and Shuler, M.L. (2009). A micro cell culture analog (mu CCA) with 3-D hydrogel culture of multiple cell lines to assess metabolism-dependent cytotoxicity of anti-cancer drugs. *Lab Chip* 9 (10): 1385–1394.

72 Son, K.J. et al. (2017). Detecting cell-secreted growth factors in microfluidic devices using bead-based biosensors. *Microsyst. Nanoeng.* 3: 17025.

73 DeForest, C.A. and Anseth, K.S. (2011). Cytocompatible click-based hydrogels with dynamically tunable properties through orthogonal photoconjugation and photocleavage reactions. *Nat. Chem.* 3 (12): 925–931.

74 Tekin, H. et al. (2011). Responsive micromolds for sequential patterning of hydrogel microstructures. *J. Am. Chem. Soc.* 133 (33): 12944–12947.

75 Dong, L. et al. (2006). Adaptive liquid microlenses activated by stimuli-responsive hydrogels. *Nature* 442 (7102): 551–554.

76 Fedorovich, N.E. et al. (2007). Hydrogels as extracellular matrices for skeletal tissue engineering: state-of-the-art and novel application in organ printing. *Tissue Eng.* 13 (8): 1905–1925.

77 Puleo, C.M. et al. (2009). Integration and application of vitrified collagen in multilayered microfluidic devices for corneal microtissue culture. *Lab Chip* 9 (22): 3221–3227.

78 Sung, K.E. et al. (2009). Control of 3-dimensional collagen matrix polymerization for reproducible human mammary fibroblast cell culture in microfluidic devices. *Biomaterials* 30 (27): 4833–4841.

79 Jeong, S.Y. et al. (2016). Co-culture of tumor spheroids and fibroblasts in a collagen matrix-incorporated microfluidic chip mimics reciprocal activation in solid tumor microenvironment. *PLoS One* 11 (7): e0159013.

80 Adibnia, V. et al. (2019). Chitosan hydrogel micro-bio-devices with complex capillary patterns via reactive-diffusive self-assembly. *Acta Biomater.* 99: 211–219.

81 Harrison, D., Fluri, K., Seiler, K. et al. (1993). Micromachining a miniaturized capillary electrophoresis-based chemical analysis system on a chip. *Science* 261: 895–897.

82 Chen, C. et al. (2016). 3D-printed microfluidic devices: fabrication, advantages and limitations – a mini review. *Anal. Methods* 8 (31): 6005–6012.

83 Bhatia, S.N. and Ingber, D.E. (2014). Microfluidic organs-on-chips. *Nat. Biotechnol.* 32 (8): 760–772.

84 Sontheimer-Phelps, A., Hassell, B.A., and Ingber, D.E. (2019). Modelling cancer in microfluidic human organs-on-chips. *Nat. Rev. Cancer* 19 (2): 65–81.

85 Mollica, H. et al. (2018). Deciphering the relative contribution of vascular inflammation and blood rheology in metastatic spreading. *Biomicrofluidics* 12 (4): 042205.

86 Choi, S. et al. (2016). Microfluidic-based non-enzymatic glycation enhances cross-linking of human scleral tissue compared to conventional soaking. *Scanning* 38 (5): 421–426.

87 Pires, R.A. et al. (2015). Controlling cancer cell fate using localized biocatalytic self-assembly of an aromatic carbohydrate amphiphile. *J. Am. Chem. Soc.* 137 (2): 576–579.

88 He, Z., Ranganathan, N., and Li, P. (2018). Evaluating nanomedicine with microfluidics. *Nanotechnology* 29 (49): 492001.

89 Albanese, A. et al. (2013). Tumour-on-a-chip provides an optical window into nanoparticle tissue transport. *Nat. Commun.* 4: 2718.

90 Zhang, C. et al. (2017). Convection enhanced delivery of cisplatin-loaded brain penetrating nanoparticles cures malignant glioma in rats. *J. Controlled Release* 263: 112–119.

91 Kolhar, P. et al. (2013). Using shape effects to target antibody-coated nanoparticles to lung and brain endothelium. *Proc. Natl. Acad. Sci. U.S.A.* 110 (26): 10753–10758.

92 Colasuonno, M. et al. (2018). Erythrocyte-inspired discoidal polymeric nanoconstructs carrying tissue plasminogen activator for the enhanced lysis of blood clots. *ACS Nano* 12 (12): 12224–12237.

93 Lenarda, P., Coclite, A., and Decuzzi, P. (2019). Unraveling the vascular fate of deformable circulating tumor cells via a hierarchical computational model. *Cell. Mol. Bioeng.* 12 (6): 543–558.

94 Joseph, D.D. and Ocando, D. (2002). Slip velocity and lift. *J. Fluid Mech.* 454: 263–286.

95 de Tullio, M.D. et al. (2007). An immersed boundary method for compressible flows using local grid refinement. *J. Comput. Phys.* 225 (2): 2098–2117.

96 Hossain, S.S., Hughes, T.J., and Decuzzi, P. (2014). Vascular deposition patterns for nanoparticles in an inflamed patient-specific arterial tree. *Biomech. Model. Mechanobiol.* 13 (3): 585–597.

97 Lee, T.R. et al. (2013). On the near-wall accumulation of injectable particles in the microcirculation: smaller is not better. *Sci. Rep.* 3: 2079.

98 McWhirter, J.L., Noguchi, H., and Gompper, G. (2009). Flow-induced clustering and alignment of vesicles and red blood cells in microcapillaries. *Proc. Natl. Acad. Sci. U.S.A.* 106 (15): 6039–6043.

99 Sun, C., Migliorini, C., and Munn, L.L. (2003). Red blood cells initiate leukocyte rolling in postcapillary expansions: a lattice Boltzmann analysis. *Biophys. J.* 85 (1): 208–222.

100 Coclite, A. et al. (2016). A combined lattice Boltzmann and immersed boundary approach for predicting the vascular transport of differently shaped particles. *Comput. Fluids* 136: 260–271.

101 Coclite, A. et al. (2017). Predicting different adhesive regimens of circulating particles at blood capillary walls. *Microfluid. Nanofluid.* 21 (11): 1–15.

13

Multifunctional Granular Hydrogels for Tissue-Specific Repair

Rui J. Almeida, Ana Fernandes, Vítor M. Gaspar, and João F. Mano

Department of Chemistry, CICECO – Aveiro Institute of Materials, University of Aveiro, Campus Universitário de Santiago, 3810-193 Aveiro, Portugal

13.1 Introduction

Traditional tissue engineering and regenerative medicine (TERM) strategies aim to repair or replace damaged tissues by stimulating or mimicking the inherent bioactivity of key fundamental building blocks encountered in human organs, including (i) multiple cell types, (ii) signaling biomolecules (e.g. growth factors, cytokines), (iii) extracellular vesicular bodies (e.g. exosomes, microvesicles, etc.), and (iv) tissue-specific supporting extracellular matrix (ECM) [1–4]. Adding to these elements, organogenesis and tissue repair processes are also naturally dependent on the establishment of intra/intercellular communication networks, on cell–ECM dynamic interactions, as well as on the build-up of human-scale cytoarchitectures and biomechanics, which altogether ultimately dictate tissue functionality [5]. To emulate or stimulate such intricate events, researchers have increasingly pursued the bioengineering of different types of biomaterial-based platforms (e.g. nano/microparticles, fibers, hydrogels, etc.), as a strategy to promote stem cells cell delivery, endogenous cells migration, and/or the release of bioactive molecules for bioinstructing cellular differentiation and guide functional repair processes.

Among the diverse tri-dimensional (3D) scaffolds for biomedical applications, hydrogels are commonly employed owing to their high water content and ability to replicate native ECM physicochemical and bioactive features (i.e. cell adhesive motifs presentation, growth factors depot, etc.) and thus to function as unique supports for cellular attachment and proliferation. Other advantages of hydrogels, including their chemical versatility, tunable mechanical properties, *in situ* injectability, self-healing, capability to accommodate therapeutic molecules, that could be delivered at the implantation site, fit-to-shape properties, as well as ease of processing into human-scale static/stimuli-responsive constructs (e.g. via 3D/4D (four-dimensional) bioprinting), make them excellently fitted for TERM applications [4, 6, 7]. Despite their widespread use, hydrogels have also some disadvantages, particularly when envisioning the assembly of large micro/macrosized

Multifunctional Hydrogels for Biomedical Applications, First Edition.
Edited by Ricardo A. Pires, Iva Pashkuleva, and Rui L. Reis.

cell-rich structures (c.a. >500 μm, up to several millimeters) – as they generally fail to provide optimal nutrients/metabolites diffusion and gas exchange, originating a marked decrease in cell viability, and ultimately failing in sustaining long-term biofunctionality [8, 9]. Bulk hydrogel networks also exhibit nanometer scale mesh sizes (10–100 nm range) [10], being generally less permissive to endogenous cells infiltration following implantation in damaged host tissues, a key aspect that is also dependent on scaffolds cross-linking, mechanical properties and biodegradability [11]. To overcome these limitations, different approaches for creating microporosity in hydrogel networks have been materialized through different techniques such as solvent/particle leaching [12], freeze–drying/gradient freezing [13], by exploring gas foaming/air bubbles injection [10], or via additive manufacturing techniques like 3D Printing/Bioprinting [14]. However, the majority of these methodologies are laborious, require specialized equipment, are unsuitable for cells encapsulation due to organic solvents usage, and/or involve subsequent top–down strategies where a low number of adhered cells is obtained after seeding in 3D scaffolds, thus limiting their final biomedical applications. Apart from this, the generated porosity is often highly random across hydrogels volume and significant batch-to-batch variability is obtained.

Seeking for alternatives to the diffusional barriers present in bulk viscoelastic hydrogels, researchers have been recently focusing on bottom–up engineering of granular hydrogel-based constructs build-up from multi-hydrogel microparticles (HMPs), i.e. microgels building blocks in an optimal jammed state [9, 15]. In these systems, the particulated units generally present a size range that overcomes the cellular uptake threshold while remaining suitable for supporting cellular attachment (HMPs size range typically >10–1000 μm) [16]. Interestingly, in granular platforms designed for biomedical applications, microgels may act both as structural and biofunctional elements that modulate the surrounding microenvironment at a tissue and unicellular level. Under specific conditions, gravitational and interparticle interactions force HMPs to reside in a spatially packed organization that ultimately generates a full particle-based structure with interstitial void spaces [17]. These interconnected microsized pores formed between adjacent microgels can ensure the necessary space for nutrients metabolites and gas exchange and enable the assembly of living 3D scaffolds which surpass cell-rich bulk hydrogels diffusional limitations [16].

Despite behaving as a self-assembled bulk material under specific conditions, granular hydrogels are also intrinsically dynamic since externally applied forces can disrupt the jammed state and immediately trigger particles rearrangement [9, 16, 18]. Granular hydrogels unit elements endows them with self-assembly, self-healing, and shear-thinning features, which render these systems highly amenable for oral administration or for intratissue administration through via minimally invasive injection [19–21]. Owing to these properties, granular hydrogels have also been recently explored as supporting baths or as biomaterial inks for suspension 3D bioprinting [17]. Since granular gels also immediately adopt a bulk-like configuration following injection *in situ*, they constitute excellent tissue fillers and present valuable defect filling properties for TERM applications.

From a bottom–up multiscale engineering perspective, different classes of unitary microgel blocks can be exploited to imprint further functionality into granular platforms since HMPs can be fabricated from a wide range of biocompatible synthetic, nature-derived (e.g. marine, human-origin), or hybrid biomaterials exhibiting different physicochemical properties [22, 23]. This expands granular hydrogels applicability beyond cell supporting/recruiting platforms, enabling them to also function as advanced delivery systems for promoting spatiotemporally controlled release of key bioactive molecules (e.g. growth factors, cytokines, etc.) *in situ* [24–27].

Recent advances in particle manufacturing technologies (e.g. microfluidics, lithography, electrohydrodynamic spraying, etc.) have also opened new avenues for fabricating microgels with tailored bioactivity/biodegradability, homogeneous and controlled sizes, programmable morphologies (e.g. spheres, rods, and polygons), as well as tuneable mechanical properties [21]. This adds further degrees of freedom and modularity to granular systems allowing researchers to tailor particle heterogeneity and complexity from the bottom–up. Notably, microgel building blocks have also been chemically programmed or stimulated on-demand to become interlinked following injection *in situ*, forming stable microporous annealed particles (MAPs) scaffolds. Such interlinked 3D granular infrastructures [28, 29] have been assembled by exploiting numerous chemical cross-linking routes (e.g. click-chemistry [30], guest–host interactions [31], enzymatic cross-linking, etc.) and have already demonstrated promising potential for being used in numerous TERM applications owing to their interconnected microporosity and tuneable physicochemical properties [16, 21].

In this chapter, we will discuss granular hydrogels key properties, namely chemical and biophysical features, as well as their assembly into interlinked scaffolds. Finally, the application of interlinked microporous particle scaffolds in tissue-specific repair and biofabrication of tailored 3D constructs will be discussed. The overall goal is to demonstrate the most recent advances and numerous applications of granular hydrogels, as well as to provide key features/design aspects and identify opportunities to build-up innovative scaffolds.

13.2 Granular Hydrogels – Functional Features and Design

The physicochemical properties and versatility of HMPs have prompted their widespread use in numerous biomedical applications spanning from drug/nucleic acids delivery, sensing, bioimaging, to cell encapsulation and *in vitro* 3D cell culture, among several others [22, 32]. In many of these approaches, HMPs are exploited as single entities; one can thus envision to leverage these unit-associated features and transpose them into biomaterial platforms that take advantage of HMPs as collective particle swarms. This combinatorial bottom–up concept is in the genesis of granular hydrogel platforms in which single HMPs properties are augmented when they function as a joint supraparticle structure.

Granular hydrogels are hierarchic, multiscale systems comprised by multiple microgels packed in an ideal "jammed state" where the existence of interparticle interactions (e.g. via van der Walls forces or hydrogen bonds, etc.), and void spaces are favored. This setting generally occurs at a specific particle-volume fraction (ϕ)/particle packing ratio, where the continuous phase is reduced, but still present [19, 25, 33]. In these systems, the desired jamming condition for monodispersed formulations of spherical microgels can be normally achieved at $\phi \approx 0.58$ (i.e. so termed random loose packing configuration) and is generally established under specific stress and temperature conditions [9]. Such key parameters mostly govern the minimally stable jamming state in granular hydrogels. Further concentration of spherical HMP-based systems into particle-to-volume fractions close to $\phi \approx 0.64$ (i.e. so termed random closed packing configuration), results in the establishment of bulk granular scaffolds which exhibit similar features to those of their standard bulk hydrogel counterparts. This regime ($0.58 < \phi < 0.64$) theoretically offers suitable spatial configurations for TERM applications since the highly desired void spaces can still be present in the final scaffold. Additionally, increasing particle agglomeration to limit values ($\phi \rightarrow 1$) leads to ultra-close packing arrangements where interstitial spaces collapse and microgels morphology becomes irreversibly deformed [28]. However, these are somewhat merely theoretical thresholds, and it is important to notice that several other factors, such as particle shape, size, viscoelasticity/deformation, friction/repulsion, surface topography, swelling, protein corona, and biodegradation in biological medium, must be taken into consideration during design stages. In this sense, advanced computational modeling approaches are rapidly emerging as highly valuable *in silico* tools for aiding researchers in simulating, understanding, and manipulating these parameters in a particle-to-particle and particle-to-cell interaction basis [34–39]. Recently, computational analysis was exploited for optimizing jammed gelatin microgels behavior when processed by advanced 3D manufacturing techniques enabling researchers to successfully predict extruded filament cross-sectional morphology, adding further relevance to these approaches for TERM applications [40].

The transition of microgel formulations into the optimal jammed state for obtaining granular hydrogels with desirable features can be performed using different methodologies including: (i) continuous phase removal/particle concentration by vacuum, (ii) gravity-mediated microgel sedimentation, (iii) centrifugation-assisted packing, and (iv) particle vortexing, among others [16, 31]. Precisely tuning the experimental conditions and the underlying concepts pertaining to particle-to-volume parameters allow the formulation of granular gels that can take full advantage of microgels intrinsic properties, of the void spaces formed during their controlled jamming, and ultimately, of the multiscale/hierarchical features of these systems.

From a thermodynamic perspective, granular hydrogels are far-from-equilibrium in the jamming state, since upon external stimulation this arrangement may be readily disrupted [41–43]. Such un-jamming event, occurs when local constraints can no longer be satisfied when externally applied forces exceed a given particle slipping threshold. From another perspective, when the generally weak particle–particle

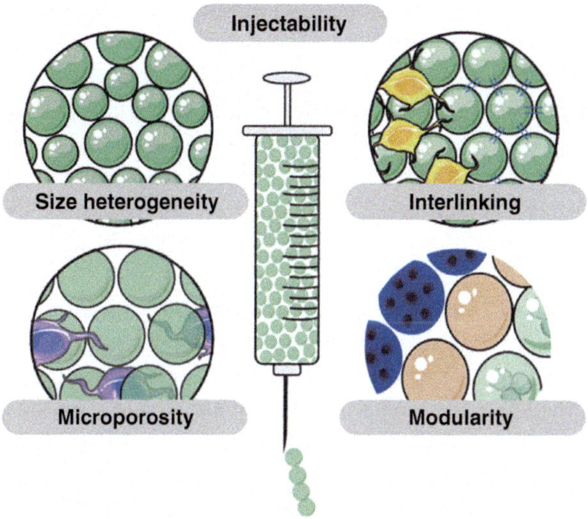

Figure 13.1 Multifunctionality and processability of granular hydrogel platforms assembled from the combination of unitary hydrogel microparticle building blocks. Heterogeneity/modularity can be easily imprinted through the introduction microgel blocks with different features (i.e. bioactivity, biodegradability, nano-porosity, loaded bioactive molecules, surface topography, etc.).

bonding interactions are disrupted, the granular hydrogel will in turn acquire a disordered, more liquid-like behavior [33], which is then restored when the applied forces cease to exist. For granular systems to reach mechanical equilibrium, Coulombic conditional restriction (i.e. charge), as well as force and torque balance (i.e. static equilibrium), must be assured. In a jammed state, force balancing is satisfied by microgel blocks network self-arrangement, suggesting that this state is dependent on the properties of the biomaterial selected for microgels fabrication, as well as on HMPs density, stiffness, surface charge, and interparticle friction, etc. [21]. The collective dynamics of multimicrogel blocks ultimately imprints multiple functionalities to granular scaffolds (Figure 13.1) including tissue filling, shear-thinning, and self-healing properties that unlock their implantation through various administration routes (e.g. topical/transdermal, oral, ocular, nasal, etc.), being highly advantageous for TERM applications.

13.2.1 Injectability

Granular hydrogels can be easily administered in the desired location via well-established and minimally invasive medical procedures comprising particles focalized injection through hypodermic needles, catheter systems or high-pressure liquid jet injection devices. Contrariwise, pre-assembled bulk hydrogel 3D scaffolds are generally difficult to be administered by injection, either requiring the inclusion of specific shear-thinning compatible network cross-linking chemistries or demanding to be injected as viscous precursor formulations which are then cross-linked *in situ*. The facility for injectability of granular hydrogels is a highly desirable feature that broadens their potential to be used as off-the-shelf pre-packed systems, since they can be readily administered in diseased/damaged tissues without requiring complex open body surgeries performed by specialized medical personnel.

Holistically, granular scaffolds injectability features arise from a synergic combination of their relatively small-sized microgel building blocks and the dynamic interparticle interactions that are at play in the optimal jammed state. When injection forces are applied, jammed microgels collectively behave more as fluid-like formulations that return into a viscoelastic solid-like state *in situ* post injection [21]. Particle jamming inside the syringe upon plunger compression during injection also minimizes the turbulent flow that can arise during the procedure, with particles generally being expelled as compacted viscoelastic microgel masses, reducing ejected volume dispersion at the injection site, and enabling a more precise/continuous microgel delivery. Syringe loading is generally very straightforward and effortlessly achieved by simple pipetting granular hydrogels into the syringe barrel. Leveraging on this methodology, researchers have recently fabricated spatially patterned hydrogels through sequential loading three layers of modified hyaluronan (HA)-based particle hydrogels combined with peptide substrates for factor XIIIa (FXIIIa) and arginine-glycine-aspartic acid (RGD) peptides, into a syringe [44]. Bioactive hydrogels *in vivo* injection into different tissues (i.e. skin, brain stroke model) at specific flow rates upkeeps the user programmed layered structure. This elegant, yet simple strategy, is extremely attractive for exploring interfacial tissue engineering methodologies that can be applied in several types of multilayered tissues in the human body. This sequential layering feature can also be explored to fabricate chemical or biological gradient-like biomaterial scaffolds which are highly desirable for spatially instructing tissue microenvironments which naturally exhibit this heterogeneity [45]. Moreover, this process may be automated via combination with fluid-handling robotic pipetting systems and artificial intelligence (AI) algorithms, providing a step toward improving reproducibility and scalability [46].

When injected, and similarly to standard hydrogels/hydrogel precursor solutions, jammed HMPs readily rereorganize into a favorable configuration and fit-to-tissue defect shape post-delivery. Hence, functioning as fluid-flow permissive platforms and also as protective physical and thermal barriers, potentially contributing to further restore homeostasis in environmentally exposed tissues (e.g. skin, eyes, hears, nasal cavity, etc.). This extrudability profile may also be leveraged for processing granular hydrogels through additive manufacturing techniques, such as freeform or standard extrusion 3D bioprinting that can be performed in loco in a more clinical setting, expanding bioactive 3D granular scaffolds personalization toolbox.

13.2.2 Inter-particle Annealing Toward MAPs Assembly

Throughout life and during repair processes, living tissues are constantly in contact with a myriad of biofluidic and biochemical signals and subjected to biomechanical stress; it is therefore of utmost importance that granular hydrogels jammed configuration can be steadily maintained post administration into damaged tissues [47]. In fact, despite granular microgels behave as solid-like multiparticle plugs at the needle tip, if the tissue microenvironment is under relatively high fluidic pressure as in the case of fluid filled cysts, effusion events (i.e. fluid build-up in the knee joints, exudates in full-thickness wounds, etc.), or in fluid filled stroke areas, the administered particulated systems may be readily dispersed across the tissue volume, with jammed granular structures then failing to self-assemble [21]. Delivery into very confined spaces or to actively moving organs, such as the heart or lungs, can also result in rapid microgels dispersion off-site. Adding to preexisting mechanical stress, the dysregulated microenvironment of injured tissues is often crowded with complex biomolecules (e.g. enzymes, antibodies, denaturated proteins, etc.), cellular debris, nano/microsized vesicles and may present nonphysiological pH/redox conditions that can all affect particle–particle interactions and jamming state stability [41–43]. Assuring granular platforms stability is critical to exploit their potential for promoting cellular invasion, cell–cell interactions and cellular differentiation toward tissue-precursor phenotypes [48]. Nevertheless, it is important to emphasize that particulated systems displacement under stress conditions is intrinsically dependent on microgels properties and multiparticle interactions, hence it should be investigated in an application-based perspective. Thus, the design should consider a careful selection of microgel precursor biomaterials and/or their chemical modification with functional groups (e.g. thiol, norbornene, acrylate, tetrazine, azide, etc.) to enable a precise control over jammed particles interlinking, fully surpassing the low stability limitations of these systems [16, 17, 21]. In the endpoint, the resulting MAPs scaffolds should be stable and exhibit the interstitial spaces among packed microgels.

Several chemical routes involving noncovalent, covalent, and dynamic/reversible chemistries have been explored to generate interlinked microgel particle scaffolds [16, 17, 21, 49]. A particular importance has been given to on-demand multiparticle annealing via light-triggered chemical reactions owing to their robustness, speed, and reactivity in physiological environments [50]. This approach has been applied successfully to obtain photo-cross-linked gelatin-methacrylate (GelMA)-based granular scaffolds [50]. Yet, such ligh-based cross-linking still requires specialized UV/blue light sources, the presence of additional photo-initiators, and operator-dependent manipulation, which can hinder its wide application in a clinical setting. Moreover, the generation of highly reactive radical species and the inhibition of photoinduced methacrylate polymerization by the presence of oxygen constitute additional limitations [51]. Supramolecular reversible guest–host interactions established between complementary host (e.g. cyclodextrin, cucurbituril [CB[6]]) and guest (e.g. adamantane, tyrosine, benzene, etc.) moieties display valuable features to overcome some of the previous bottlenecks. Dynamic granular hydrogels comprising HA-adamantane microgels and HA cyclodextrin taking advantage of this unique chemistry have been previously assembled. The natural reversibility of guest–host interactions provides shear thinning and self-healing properties, enabling prepacked microgels to flow during injection and then to reassemble *in situ*, fully recovering native hydrogel like properties [18].

Apart from its relevance to scaffolds stability, interparticle chemical linkages also impact granular platforms mechanical properties and biodegradability [9]. Ideally, engineered granular scaffolds should exhibit a spatiotemporal biodegradation profile that matches organ-specific cellular infiltration, mass transport requirements, and ultimately *de novo* tissue formation kinetics during repair. To better model this characteristic, it is important to perceive granular platforms biodegradability as a consequence of their intrinsic multicomponent, hierarchic nature. In fact, the overall biodegradability of MAP scaffolds is a multifactorial parameter resulting from individual microgel biomaterials biodegradation, from particle–particle interlinking bonds type and jamming density. A rationale selection of stimuli-responsive microgel precursor biomaterials operating as logic-gate elements that respond to external/endogenous stimuli has enabled the production of granular scaffolds with tailored degradability and controlled release of multiple bioactive molecules, as recently demonstrated in collagenase enzyme-responsive two-component microgel scaffolds [18]. Controlling MAPs biodegradation at the multimicrogel interlinking chemistry level (e.g. type of stimuli-responsiveness and particle–particle interlinks density) has been less explored to date and significant advances are envisioned on this topic in the future, especially considering the broad range of chemical tools that can be leveraged to imprint stimuli-responsive linkages in hydrogel biomaterials [52].

Providing suitable mechanical support and biophysical cues to cells and to tissue-specific microenvironments during repair is critical to activate key mechanosensing biomolecular mechanisms that instruct cellular secretome/phenotype and assure biofunctionality [53, 54]. Alike other hierarchic MAP scaffold features, mechanical properties can be controlled by modulating individual microgel building blocks, or by manipulating interparticle bridging chemistry and packing density (i.e. void space fraction). Selecting different interlinking chemistries (e.g. click-chemistry, supramolecular, etc.) can influence overall scaffold mechanics without directly modifying individual microgels mechanical features, meaning that MAPs can provide cells/damaged tissues with distinct structural support and biophysical cues at multiple length scales [21]. In fact, recent reports indicate that MAPs stiffness increases by increasing the cross-linking density enhances human dermal fibroblasts (HDFs) cells spreading and transfection, but not their proliferation [55]. Also, researchers have demonstrated that MAPs with higher storage moduli (~970 Pa), simultaneously stimulate cell adhesion and proliferation in comparison to lower storage moduli substrates (~222 Pa) [55]. However, further studies regarding the effect of MAPs cross-linking density in microporosity and its effect on cell proliferation may be required in the future to fully understand these correlations in an individual basis for each type of platform [55, 56]. Controlling mechanical properties at the individual microgels level has also been investigated by exploiting the versatility of Michael-type vinyl sulfone-thiol chemistry to cross-link poly(ethylene) glycol–vinyl sulfone (PEG–VS) precursor formulations (Figure 13.2A) [56]. The manipulation of the reaction conditions, such as polymer and cross-linker concentration (dithiothreitol) and pH, yielded PEG microgels with different stiffness (i.e. 0.5, 5.5, and 13.5 kPa, Figure 13.2C). Such enzymatically cross-linkable MAPs of varying mechanical properties were then used as testing platforms to evaluate HDFs adhesion and proliferation. A clear increase in HDFs

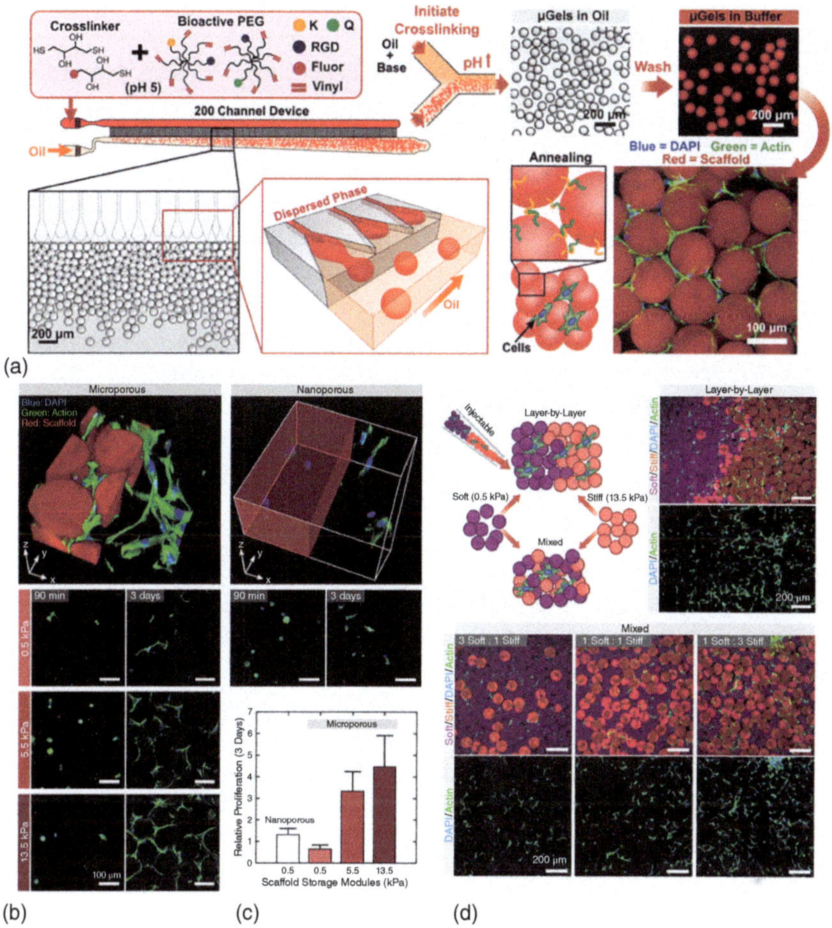

Figure 13.2 High-throughput fabrication of PEG–VS/peptide microgel precursors for modular MAPs assembly. (A) Schematic overview of microfluidic-assisted microgels fabrication and MAPs annealing/interlinking. (B and C) Formulation of MAPs with variable mechanical properties and their influence in human dermal fibroblasts (HDFs) cellular adhesion and proliferation. (D) Schematic and confocal microscopy imaging of mechanically heterogeneous modular scaffolds modular assembly via layer-by-layer deposition or mixing. HDFs adhesion, spatial distribution, and spreading analysis via actin staining (green channel) observed after 12 hours in culture. Source: De Rutte, et al. (2019), [56], Figure 04, Pg 06 / with permission of JOHN WILEY & SONS, INC.

cells adhesion and 3D network formation were observed for MAP platforms with the higher stiffness (5.5 and 13.5 kPa Figure 13.2B) when comparing to both their softer (0.5 kPa) and nanoporous counterparts, indicating the importance of controlling mechanical properties at the building block level [56]. Further insights into mechanical properties tunning in MAPs scaffolds were provided by assembling mechanically heterogeneous scaffolds with PEG–VS microgels of varying stiffness across the platform. Such mechanical modulation had a profound effect on HDFs cellular adhesion, with a higher cellular density being observed in stiffer hydrogel regions (Figure 13.2D).

Engineering MAPs scaffolds with spatially encoded mechanical properties is highly desirable not only considering that various interconnected human tissues display different biomechanics but also that directed cellular migration can be controlled by (and is highly dependent on) the substrate mechanics [50, 57]. Elegant approaches to create stiffness gradients in granular hydrogels may also be further materialized by employing the sequential packing strategy in syringe barrels that was described before [44]. One can also hypothesize that innovations pertaining to the development of mechanoresponsive materials and the fabrication of mechanically tunned microgels/granular scaffolds that evolve their physico-chemical properties according to tissue-specific microenvironments along time (e.g. pH, temperature, biofluids presence, etc.) may provide further developments in microgel-based biomaterials field.

13.2.3 Void Spaces and Microporosity

The unique void space-rich microarchitecture of interlinked MAP scaffolds arises from particles packing and provides considerable advantages in comparison to standard bulk hydrogels. The voids/microporous elements in granular scaffolds are not only key for enabling mass transport of critical nutrients/metabolites/gases but also to support and guide cellular infiltration, to promote cell–cell contacts, the establishment of 3D multicellular networks, and to instruct cellular behavior [56]. In contrast, cellular migration in bulk hydrogels is generally achieved though cellular-mediated degradation (e.g. via matrix metalloproteinases (MMPs) secretion) [58]. *In vivo* evidences that blood vessels (BVs) infiltration is more effectively obtained in implanted MAPs in comparison to their bulk counterparts, further adds to their translational potential, especially considering that vascular infiltration is a highly sought-after feature in biomaterials for TERM applications [28, 59]. It is important to emphasize that strategies for imparting porosity in hydrogel biomaterials have been widely investigated and materialized in the form of macroporous single/multiphasic cryogels [60], as hydrogel foams [10], or as photocaged/photopaternable functional hydrogels [61], among others. The latter is particularly advantageous, as a directional control over cellular migration in 3D hydrogels volume may be obtained. Despite presenting some advantages over standard hydrogels, the manufacture of some of these platforms still requires highly specialized equipment, often involves laborious steps, as well as encompasses a poor control over pore size homogeneity and spatial distribution.

In granular scaffolds, microporosity is mostly influenced by microgel building blocks size, morphology, mechanical properties, and packing density. Generally, upon implantation and endogenous cell infiltration the natural cellular movement across MAPs void spaces does not trigger microgel deformation/movement. However, depending on microgels stiffness, natural tissue motility or externally applied forces may lead to irreversible particle collapse. Tunning stiffness at a multiscale level (i.e. microgel units and bulk MAP) and according to tissue-specific requirements is critical to assure interconnected micropores maintenance and hence structural stability at early stages of cellular infiltration. Microgels size and morphology also influence pore size, being observed that larger sized spherical microgels (average diameter ~120 μm, PDI = 0.29) often yields larger average pore size when compared to that obtained with smaller microgel building blocks (average diameter ~15 μm, PDI = 0.11). Interestingly in both platforms the existing pores exhibited heterogeneous shapes, i.e. for larger microgels an average pore aspect ratio of 2.1 was obtained [62]. Further evidences that larger void spaces improve cellular infiltration, spreading, proliferation, cell–cell clustering and well-defined actin fibers production in comparison to smaller pores, provide valuable design guidelines for controlling and advancing the assembly of tissue-specific living microenvironments [25, 48, 62].

In a different perspective, one must consider that porosity also impacts MAPs scaffolds degradability and a precise control over this parameter is key to match tissue-specific kinetics during repair, enabling tissue ingrowth and remodeling [48, 49]. Adding to this, other additional tissue-specific microenvironment factors that may impact individual microgels degradation or MAPs interlinking bridges disruption, including the presence of enzymes, pH/redox/temperature deregulation and biological effusions/exudates, are also key factors to consider when designing MAPs for tissue-specific engineering.

13.2.4 Modularity and Multifunctionality in Granular Systems

The hierarchic and modular nature of granular scaffolds enables the fabrication of highly sophisticated and more complex heterogeneous granular systems, with multiple functionalities imprinted in a single platform. Modularity can be explored both at the single intraparticle level or at MAPs interlinked particle scale. Owing to unitary microgels physicochemical versatility, one can envision that granular hydrogels can be designed to include multiple units with varying chemistries or surface topographies, or to be constituted by microgels loading different protein cocktails, drugs, or nanoparticles (NPs) [63, 64]. Such systems can also comprise different types of biomaterials (e.g. nature, human-based, synthetic), or single/multiple stimuli-responsive features [65] since all of these have been reported for standalone microgels used for TERM applications [66]. Several of these approaches have already been implemented in modular granular hydrogels fabrication to impart multibiofunctionality. Recently, MAPs scaffolds heterogeneity at the building blocks level was successfully accomplished by combining different transforming growth factor β1 (TGF-β1) loaded gelatin microgels and bone morphogenetic protein-2 (BMP-2) loaded mineral-coated hydroxyapatite microparticles [67]. This combinatorial strategy was exploited for bioinstructing human mesenchymal stem cells (hMSCs) assembled into ring like structures toward chondrogenic lineages via spatiotemporally controlled presentation of morphogens during *in vitro* maturation [67]. The possibilities are virtually endless and imprinting heterogeneity into naturally modular systems such as MAPs scaffolds could be as simple as switching the chirality of MMP-responsive peptide microgels. This elegant approach enhanced innate and adaptive immune system type 2 pro-regenerative responses in *in vivo* wound healing models, accelerating wound closure and sustaining high quality tissue repair [68].

The recent advances in biomaterials processing, microgels assembly methodologies, and chemical tools for their interlinking provide unique opportunities to create evermore modular and multiactive scaffolds that are better suited for stimulating and guiding repair in a tissue-oriented mode.

13.2.5 Bioactive Molecules Delivery

Exploiting microgel building blocks as controlled delivery systems apart from their role as structural supporting units adds another layer of biofunctionality to MAPs scaffolds, especially considering that these platforms are mostly exploited as acellular biomaterials. Adding further features to favor endogenous cells recruitment to the injury site or to locally modulate injured tissues microenvironment components can ultimately improve the overall regenerative outcome.

Microgels have been widely employed as carriers for drugs, proteins, nucleic acids, and their combinations thereof, enabling their spatiotemporally controlled release and focalized presentation at the target site [66, 69–71]. Bioactive molecules release profile modulation has been accomplished by varying particles size, shape, polymer mesh degradability/cross-linking, or by installing responsivity to different stimuli, among other strategies. To date few granular scaffolds have been exploited as bioactive molecule delivery systems and several opportunities in this focus remain to be explored [72–76].

Granular hydrogel unit elements have also been leveraged as multibioactive and multicomponent nano-in-micro drug reservoirs for cardiac tissues repair following myocardial infarction (MI). In an elegantly designed approach, hydrophobic drug-loaded nanoparticles were incorporated in 4-arm PEG–VS/SH-MMP Q and K-peptide spherical microgels during assembly in a microfluidic device (Figure 13.3A). This rationale aimed to surpass polymeric microgels well-recognized low encapsulation efficacy of small hydrophobic compounds. The in-house designed microfluidic-assisted nanoparticle-in-microparticle incorporation enabled high loading efficacy and the expedite manufacture of highly homogeneous multicomponent spherical microgel units that were then employed by the authors to

Figure 13.3 Multifunctional drugMAPs formulation and application as scaffolds for cardiac repair. (A) Schematic overview of microfluidic generation of drug-loaded nano-in-micro microgel precursors and drugMAPs endogenously controlled assembly following injection *in situ*. (B) Fluorescence microscopy micrographs of pristine (μGel) and nanoparticle-loaded microgels (NPs-μGel). (C) Characterization of Forskolin – F and RepSox – R, cumulative release profile from different platforms. Nanoparticles (FR/NPs) and drugMAP. (D) Histological analysis of Masson's trichrome-stained rat infarcted heart sections after five weeks. PBS, Phosphate buffered saline; FR/NPs, drug-loaded nanoparticles; MAP, microporous-annealed particles; FR/drugMAP, drug-loaded MAP platform. Source: J. Fang, et al, (2020), Fig 02, Pg 04 / with permission of JOHN WILEY & SONS, INC.

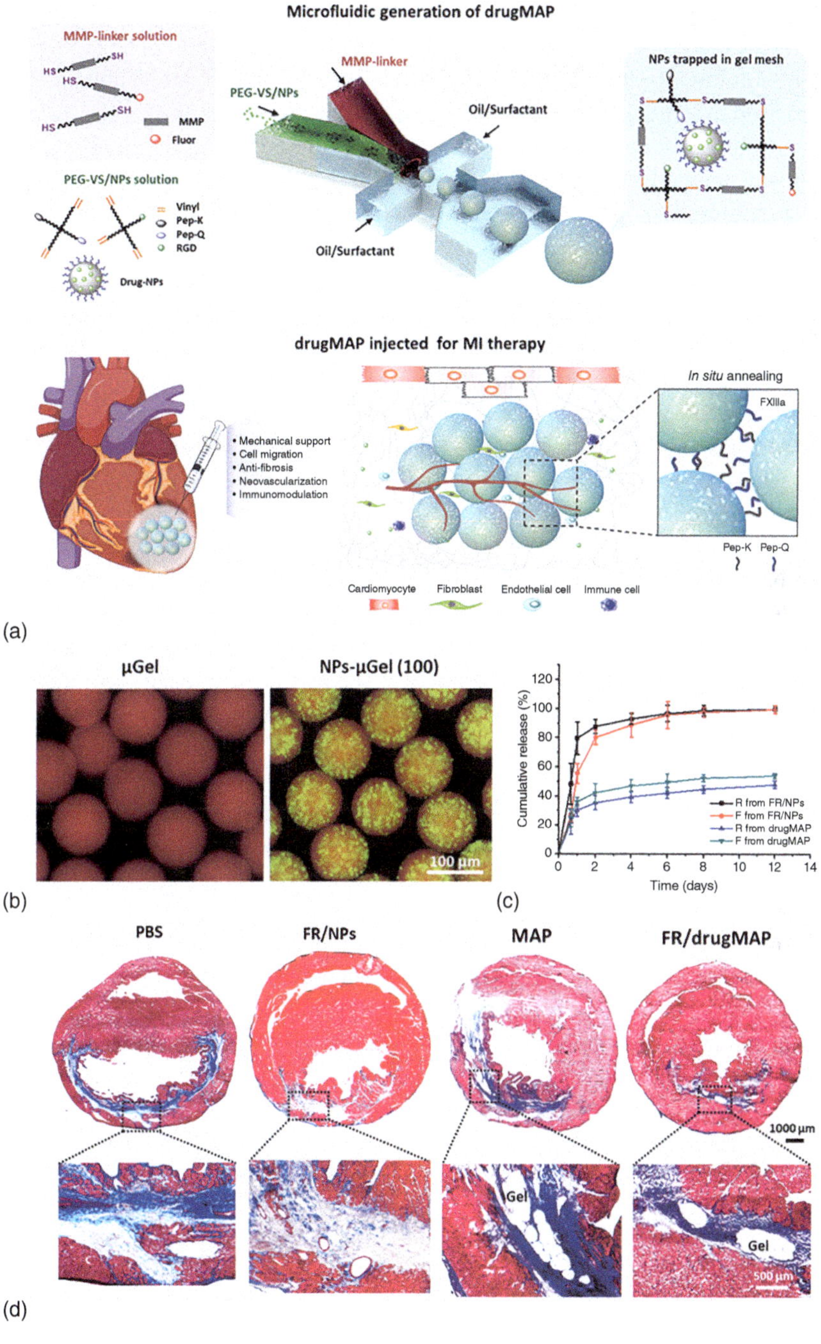
Microfluidic generation of drugMAP
MMP-linker solution
MMP
Fluor
PEG-VS/NPs solution
Vinyl
Pep-K
Pep-Q
RGD
Drug-NPs
MMP-linker
PEG-VS/NPs
Oil/Surfactant
Oil/Surfactant
NPs trapped in gel mesh
drugMAP injected for MI therapy
• Mechanical support
• Cell migration
• Anti-fibrosis
• Neovascularization
• Immunomodulation
In situ annealing
FXIIIa
Pep-K
Pep-Q
Cardiomyocyte
Fibroblast
Endothelial cell
Immune cell
(a)
μGel
NPs-μGel (100)
100 μm
(b)
Cumulative release (%)
Time (days)
R from FR/NPs
F from FR/NPs
R from drugMAP
F from drugMAP
(c)
PBS
FR/NPs
MAP
FR/drugMAP
1000 μm
Gel
Gel
500 μm
(d)

assemble an interlinked drugMAP (Figure 13.3B). Importantly, cardiac dysfunction and MI-remodeling drugs – Forskolin (F, cAMP antagonist) and RepSox (selective TGF-β inhibitor) – release kinetics from drugMAPs was significantly attenuated in comparison to standalone nanoparticle systems, suggesting that microgels jamming and annealing poses an additional barrier to drugs diffusion (Figure 13.3C).

Following nano-in-microgels intramyocardial injection *in vivo,* drugMAP scaffolds were cross-linking via endogenous FXIIIa without requiring further catalysts of operator manipulation. After five weeks of implantation, this multifunctional platform was shown to successfully increase angiogenesis, reduce fibrotic scar tissue, attenuate cardiac wall thinning, and improve injection faction, overall ameliorating tissue-specific remodeling and dysfunction (Figure 13.3D). Such relevant findings further emphasize the advantages of granular systems modular and hierarchic nature and its potential to be used for regenerating major tissue injuries.

Gathering on the immense possibilities offered by multifunctional granular hydrogel platforms in the following sections advances on the use of MAPs scaffolds for promoting tissue-specific repair in several scenarios will be showcased and discussed in light of future advances and opportunities. Unconventional systems based on cell-mediated microgels/microparticles assembly rather than chemically mediated annealing of MAPs scaffolds will also be emphasized. Additionally, relevant microparticulated formulations that may be leveraged as building blocks for granular scaffolds assembly owing to their unique properties as standalone systems will also be discussed so as to provide a broader overview of the combinatorial possibilities in this field.

13.3 Granular Hydrogels for Tissue-Specific Repair

13.3.1 Vascularization Strategies

Tissue-specific (re)vascularization is crucial for functional regeneration, since the vascular system is utterly responsible for providing nutrients/metabolites and gases exchange to the majority of tissues in the human body [77]. Stimulating *de novo* formation of highly vascularized perfusable networks in injured tissues and promoting blood vessels ingrowth in engineered biomaterials have remained two of the greatest challenges in TERM [78]. To date, several tissue graft-based, biomaterial-based and/or cell-based approaches have been explored for promoting functional vascularization [77, 79–81].

Recently, different types of MAP systems have been employed for tissue-specific repair of various tissues (e.g. neuronal, cardiac, skin). In several of these examples apart from stimulating native tissue repair as it will be further discussed, MAPs platforms also stimulate vascular cells infiltration and tissue re-vascularization *in vitro* and *in vivo* [20, 49]. This is a highly valuable outcome considering that most of these systems are mostly acellular and that are not specifically designed for vascular tissues repair. Such evidences indicate that they enclose a vast potential to be used as cell-instructive platforms and for stimulating/activating multiple endogenous tissue repair pathways [16, 60]. These observations are associated to various MAP intrinsic factors including, but not limited to (i) biomaterial bioactivity (i.e. surface chemistry, presence of cell adhesion/cell recruiting motifs, immune system modulatory properties), (ii) architecture associated aspects (i.e. microporous networks size/interconnectivity, biodegradability), and/or (iii) loading of proregenerative bioactive/bioinstructive molecules (i.e. small molecule drugs and/or growth factors), among others [18, 20, 49, 62]. In all these strategies, *in vivo* implanted MAPs generally provide the required space and permissive microenvironment to promote multiple vascular progenitor cells recruitment, adhesion, and proliferation as recently evidenced by the presence of endothelial cells (platelet endothelial cell adhesion molecule [PECAM-1+]) and pericytes (i.e. NG2+ and PDGFRβ+ cell populations), after a short five days period following MAP implantation [49]. In another approach focusing on cardiac repair, drugMAPs scaffolds further enhanced human umbilical vein endothelial cells (HUVECs) vascular networks formation, where junctions, cell meshes, and tube-like structures were clearly visible (Figure 13.4A,B) [20]. Adding to these acellular platforms, MAPs scaffolds ability to delivery hMSCs and also promote tissue ingrowth and vascularization when implanted subcutaneously has also been explored and demonstrated (Figure 13.4C–E) [28]. This is a really seminal report that has validated MAPs as cellular delivery platforms while remaining stable as well as bioactive, and further adds to the already well-established MAPs use as acellular platforms.

Such preclinical data provide important evidences on MAPs scaffolds realistic potential in comparison to other technologies solely based on nonporous bulk hydrogels.

Gathering on insights from various studies comprising microgels and microcapsules for tissue engineering, several other aspects for promoting vascularization could be further explored in MAPs, particularly considering that their modular and heterogeneous nature is easily tuneable. In line with this, HMPs that function as MAPs building blocks have provided several evidences of their standalone versatility for (re)vascularization applications. In the context of vascularization/angiogenesis promotion microgels have been extensively employed as delivery systems for spatiotemporally controlled release of vascular instructing elements (e.g. via the encapsulation of key GFs/GF-encoding nucleic acids) [82, 83], and as platforms for promoting vascular GFs protease triggered release *in vitro* and *in vivo* [84]. Furthermore, rationally designed microgels have also been exploited as cell-anchoring supporting platforms or as devices for encapsulating vascular precursor cells. In an interesting report, unitary microporous gelatin microcryogels served as cellular priming microniches for managing critical hindlimb ischemia [85]. Such cell-adhesive microniches enabled *in vitro* prestimulation of cultured hMSCs, leading to improved deposition of ECM proteins (e.g. Collagen I, IV, and laminin) and to the establishment of cell–cell interactions, aiming to further potentiate cellular therapies biological performance and proangiogenic potential postimplantation *in vivo*. The resulting living microtissue assemblies protected hMSCs from mechanical stress while increased cellular retention *in situ* and sustained long-term cell survival in comparison to freely administered hMSCs. Most importantly, cell-rich microporous microniches

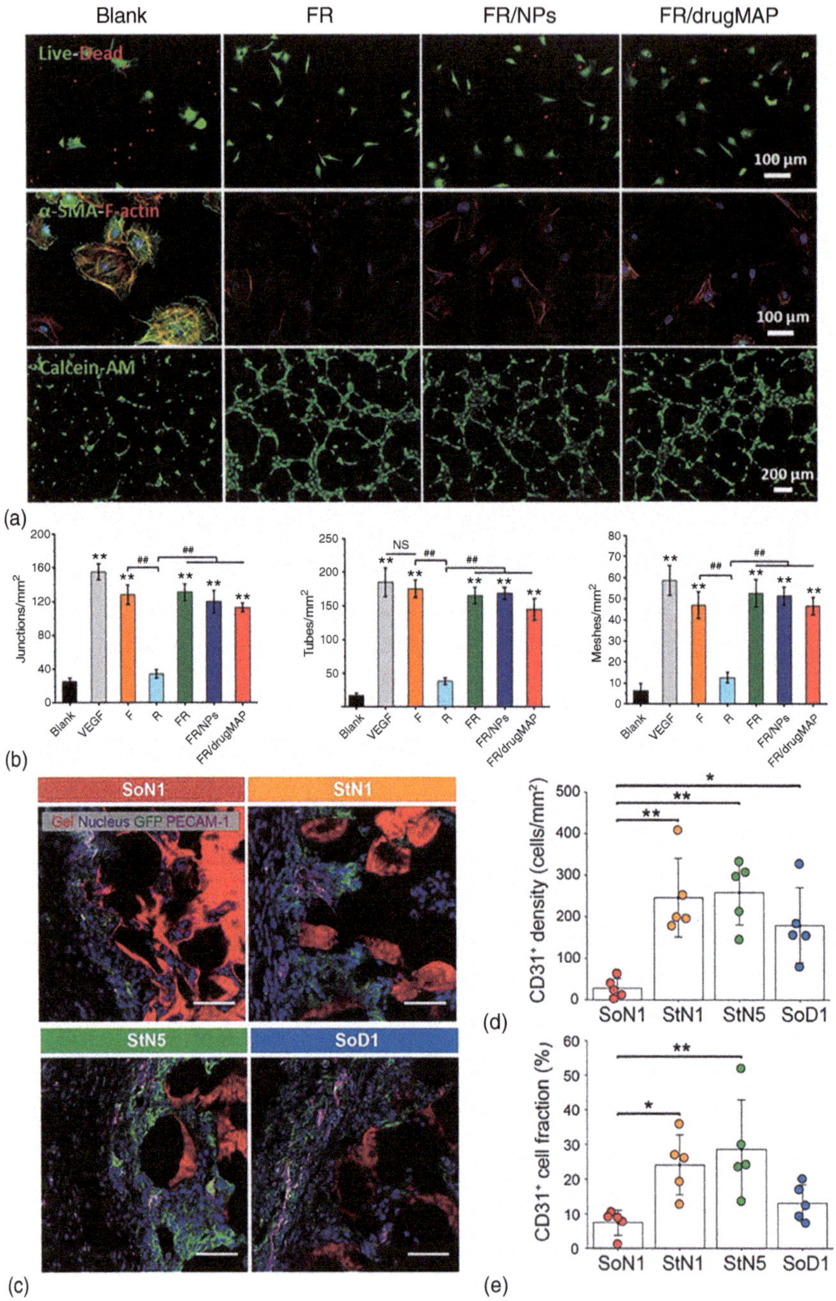

Blank
FR
FR/NPs
FR/drugMAP
Live-Dead
100 µm
α-SMA-F-actin
100 µm
Calcein-AM
200 µm
(a)
Junctions/mm²
Tubes/mm²
Meshes/mm²
NS
Blank
VEGF
F
R
FR
FR/NPs
FR/drugMAP
(b)
SoN1
StN1
StN5
SoD1
Gel Nucleus GFP PECAM-1
(c)
CD31⁺ density (cells/mm²)
(d)
CD31⁺ cell fraction (%)
(e)

Figure 13.4 *In vitro* and *in vivo* evidences of MAPs potential for promoting vascularization. (A) *In vitro* evaluation of multifunctional drugMAPs platforms comprising microgel building blocks impregnated with nanoparticles (NPs) loading beneficial drugs (Forskolin – F; RepSox – R) for cardiac tissue repair following myocardial infarction (MI). Live/dead staining of neonatal cardiomyocytes, at day 3, top-row; Myo-differentiation of neonatal cardiac fibroblasts, day 5, middle row; human umbilical vein endothelial cells (HUVECs) vascular network formation analysis through Calcein-AM, bottom-row. (B) Quantification of junction numbers, tube numbers, and mesh numbers. Data shown as mean ± s.d. $^{*}p < 0.05$. $^{**}p < 0.01$ refers to comparisons against blank. $^{\#\#}p < 0.01$ refers to comparisons against R experimental condition. NS refers to non-significant difference. (C) Fluorescence microscopy micrographs of platelet endothelial cell adhesion molecule (PECAM-1) and GFP-MSCs indicating the presence of endothelial cells growing in from surrounding tissue. Scale bar: 50 μm. (D and E) $CD31^{+}$ cells per area and ratio of $CD31^{+}$ cells to all cells present in the scaffolds, at two weeks after implantation, respectively. Data shown as mean ± s.d. $^{*}p < 0.05$ and $^{**}p < 0.01$. Source: Koh, J., et al. (2019), [28], Figure 04c, pg 07 / with permission of JOHN WILEY & SONS, INC.

significantly enhanced angiogenesis as demonstrated by *de novo* formed microvessels networks and also improved blood perfusion/angiogenesis factors expression in mice ischemic hindlimbs, greatly surpassing the poor bioperformance observed with simple free cell injections [85].

It becomes clear from these evidences that protecting tissue progenitor and angiogenesis modulating cells during implantation is a critical aspect for attaining a successful therapeutic outcome. Such results support the rapidly emerging concepts of cellular encapsulation in microgels or liquefied microcapsule systems as means to promote cellular protection and assure long-term residence at target site, as we and others demonstrated [86].

Alternative combinatorial strategies leveraging hybrid cell-rich microgel platforms loaded with bioactive molecules may also enclose the desired therapeutic outcome as recently demonstrated [87]. Adding to the vascularization technological toolbox, nucleic acid-modulated strategies based on vascular endothelial growth factor (VEGF) genetic-based priming of HUVECs laden in gelatin microgels have demonstrated to further contribute for stimulating cellular polarization/neovascularization, leading to increased capillaries formation in comparison to single/nonprimed injected cells [88]. Concerning the delivery of vascularization-specific MAPs scaffolds that take advantage of microenvironment modulating features, the development of annealing processes triggered by reactive oxygen species generally present in injured tissues may be explored in the future.

To date MAPs designed to accommodate such findings and possibilities are yet to be fully explored.

13.3.2 Skin Tissues Repair

Skin is the largest human tissue and a master regulator of internal organs protection against several environmental factors (i.e. pollution, microorganisms, and radiation), including temperature fluctuations. Owing to its externally oriented facet, skin is subjected to a number of diseases such as melanoma, psoriasis, and to a number of acute injuries including cuts and burns [89]. Despite human skin is able to naturally self-regenerate, damage beyond repair is frequently observed in numerous scenarios including full thickness burns and diabetes-induced keloids, all of which are extremely challenging to repair from a TERM perspective [90]. Several approaches involving a myriad of biomaterials, small molecules, and cells have been explored to accelerate wound repair and generate fully functional tissue [91–93].

MAPs platforms for skin tissue repair have also been widely explored, especially owing to the ease of administration of these platforms in skin injuries. On the other hand, considering that wound closure is intrinsically a cell-mediated process that involves cellular migration, cell–cell interactions, and vascular vessels infiltration, MAPs unique features render them highly attractive platforms for such applications. One of the earliest reports on MAPs for skin tissue repair leveraged a microfluidic platform for fabricating 4-arm PEG–VS/SH-MMP-SH peptide/peptide-Q/peptide-K spherically shaped microgels via water-in-oil emulsion [49]. Microfluidic production in a droplet generating chip yielded highly homogeneous microgels with controlled sizes and potential for scalability. MAPs scaffolds were readily obtained upon cross-linking with FXIIIa and the granular networks exhibited the tuneable microporosity (range ~10–35 μm) according to the size of the selected microgel precursor units, as well as governed degradability. Remarkably, *in vitro* data revealed that cellular adhesion and spreading of different cell types including hMSCs (i.e. bone and adipose-derived cells), as well as HDFs, could be observed as early as 90 minutes after annealing [49]. Most importantly, owing to the injectability features of unitary PEG microgel building blocks, researchers were able to cover the wound bed and promote particle interlinking *in situ* through FXIIIa administration. MAP scaffolds intrinsic physicochemical properties accelerated wound closure and enabled wound bed re-epithelialization, while eliciting a significantly lower immune response in comparison to standard bulk hydrogel.

In a follow-up approach, the same researchers engineered spatially patterned granular hydrogels based on HA microgel building blocks. Taking advantage on the unique processability and modularity inherent to granular systems, spatial patterning was easily implemented through sequential pipetting into a syringe [44]. Sequentially packed granular gels were then injected in a full thickness wound defect, and the distinct layered architecture was observed after three days post-injection. Considering the unique layered architecture of human skin, one can hypothesize that this approach could provide valuable improvements in the future.

Apart from enabling endogenous tissue repair, vascular cells infiltration and easy processing into highly hierarchical user-programmed architectures, granular scaffolds timely mechanical support/biodegradation, and immune system activation are major parameters that must be addressed in wound repair, and in fact, in most TERM applications, where *de novo* tissue ingrowth is required. To address these important parameters, MAPs scaffolds with tuneable degradation and selective immune system activation features were recently developed [68]. In an elegant strategy, MAP precursor microgels cross-linking via D- or L-amino acid interlinking peptide species with distinct enzyme-mediated degradation rates was optimized. Amino acids chirality is well recognized to stimulate the immune system in a number of ways, with mounting evidences indicating that D-enantiomers are mostly considered poorly immunogenic species [94]. The effect of swapping peptide cross-linkers chirality kinetics in immune system activation and in overall wound regeneration performance was then evaluated *in vivo*. Interestingly, a clear-cut correlation between cross-linking species chirality and MAPs degradation kinetics was readily observed after collagenase I treatment, with D-chiral microgel-based MAPs presenting a higher resistance to degradation, a finding that was also observed *in vivo* after 21 days. Of note, D-MAPs scaffolds induced proregenerative adaptive immune responses and exhibited neogenic hair follicles formation in full thickness wounds, a major finding since it is well recognized that full thickness wounds are highly prone to scar tissue formation and follicles loss [68]. This seminal study provides a major leap forward in understanding the relationship between biomaterials chemistry, biodegradation, immune system activation and the key factors required to promote virtually fully functional wound repair. Nevertheless, since the repair process is a highly complex process involving a myriad of cellular, acellular, and biomolecular effectors, the influence of exogenous bioactive molecules delivery could provide additional improvements in would closure time. In fact, a recent report adding to the body of knowledge on MAPs potential for wound healing evidences the importance and the advantage of biomolecular effectors spatiotemporal controlled release (i.e. platelet-derived growth factor [PDGF]) in the wound bed [95]. Further studies addressing such approaches are thus highly desirable to bring forth the full potential of MAPs for wound repair.

13.3.3 Bone Tissue Repair

Critical bone loss arising from traumatic events or bone diseases like osteoporosis and cancer remains a significant medical challenge that affects millions of people worldwide. Currently, the gold-standard medical treatment for such non-healing scenarios is still based on the use of autologous implants that are poised by their limited availability and low dimensionality, as well as by significant donor site morbidity [96]. TERM-based approaches and biomaterials designed specifically for bone tissue engineering (BTE) have been intensively investigated as an alternative to bone grafts [97]. Despite significant advances regarding the understanding of bone tissues hybrid organic/inorganic composition and physiology, as well as of the underlying biomolecular mechanisms activated in endogenous repair processes, the discovery of an "ideal" biomaterial, cellular therapy, or combinations thereof that can be readily translated to bone repair at clinic setting still remains challenging [98]. Granular hydrogels present several advantages for BTE due to their modular microporous structure, programmable geometry, cellular recruitment ability, and tunable mechanical properties.

Recent advances in engineering MAPs for bone tissue-specific repair have been materialized through microfluidic-assisted manufacture of photocrosslinked PEG-norbornene microgel based building blocks using a bi-functional di-thiol cross-linker [99]. Unlike other reports focused on leveraging assembling size controlled homogeneous microgels dispersions, in this inspired approach, the microfluidic assembly process was additionally exploited as a processing tool to assemble spatially patterned granular scaffolds on the fly during particle recovery stages from the microchip. This ingenious approach enabled the sequential manufacture of spatially patterned granular gels through layer-by-layer packing into a 1 ml syringe. Such methodology further enabled the assembly of continuous gradient profiles or step gradients according to processing conditions (i.e. number/layer thickness). Granular hydrogels were then interlinked by including a photocross-linkable PEG-dithiol linker and a photoinitiator (i.e. lithium phenyl-2,4,6-trimethylbenzoylphosphinate (LAP)), resulting in MAPs assembly. MAPs exhibiting spatial gradients were then successfully injected into a mouse femoral defect. The straightforward gradients assembly in combination with MAPs softer-to-stiffer mechanical tunability, and the reported hMSCs cell adhesion/proliferation across microgels gradients, renders these platforms highly attractive for BTE [99]. The full osteogenic differentiation of seeded hMSCs, and MAPs ability to release bone morphogens/small pro-regenerative compounds, remains to be evaluated, but promising results toward improving bone tissue repair are envisioned. Fundamental studies evaluating the influence of cell adhesion ligands inclusion in PEG microgels, as well as the influence of microgels surface topography in hMSCs bioactivity will be pivotal to validate these biomaterials as suitable candidates for BTE. Recently, hMSCs response to different microgel surfaces (i.e. wrinkled or rigged), comprising differential cell adhesion ligands (i.e. c(RRETAWA), RGDS) installed in PEG microgels with different MMP-mediated degradation rates, was reported [100]. Gathered evidences indicated a major influence of PEG microgels degradation in hMSCs ECM deposition, proliferation, and responsivity to different adhesion cues. Interestingly, hMSCs exhibited a higher BMP-2 expression when cultured in c(RRETAWA) peptide functionalized MAPs, but a higher VEGF expression was obtained when hMSCs were cultured in RGDS-peptide MAPs. Hence, a possible combinatorial approach of both platforms could eventually prove useful for BTE [100].

Selecting a suitable microgel annealing chemistry is also a critical step as these interlinks are the “life-line” of MAPs scaffolds and ultimately determine their bioperformance. Recently, the formulation of microgel units equipped with biorthogonal annealing chemistries and its influence in the resulting MAPs properties/modularity in the context of BTE were investigated. By leveraging tetrazine-norbornene click-chemistry MAP scaffolds, so termed TzMAPs were assembled with high speed, selectivity, and totally under catalyst-free conditions [101, 102]. This unique approach not only surpasses the limitations of enzyme or light-based MAP cross-linking regarding the requirement for intermediators (i.e. photoinitiator, FXIIIa enzymes), but mostly does so by augmenting the chemical selectivity of microgel–microgel binding in complex environments such as those of injured tissues. Such is only possible owing to the unique bioorthogonal nature of the selected chemistry [103]. The advantages of this approach are further evidenced by the ability for promoting site-selective conjugation of recombinant proteins to MAPs platforms, as demonstrated by selective immobilization of a histidine-tagged recombinant human bone morphogenetic protein-2 (His-BMP2), expanding the possibility to used MAPs for selective conjugation of protein therapeutics [102].

This opens great opportunities for bioinstructing living microenvironments in a spatially controlled mode where selected proteins may be displayed only to desired cells according to tissues cytoarchitecture.

The formulation of MAPs from microgels containing unconventional nanofibrous surface topographies has also been demonstrated, gathering on the rationale that both nanoscale cues and microporosity are important for promoting functional bone tissue repair [104]. Nanofibrous hydrogel building blocks were formulated by spray freezing technology (i.e. liquid N_2) in contrast to the widely used microfluidics-based techniques. This approach enabled the production of gelatin microparticles cross-linked by EDC/NHS, exhibiting in-particle nanofibrous structures with diameters ranging from 100 to 300 nm, matching those of native collagen nanofibers. Such is a highly desirable feature considering that ECM physical and architecture-mediated cues are recognized to influence cellular bioactivity [105]. Nanofibrous microparticles were then combined by photocrosslinking to generate so termed microparticle assembled nanofibrous (MANF) hydrogels (Figure 13.5). The assembled MAPs exhibited a microporous structure with average interparticle pore diameter ~15 μm, fit-to-shape properties and elastic modulus of ~55 kPa. *In vitro* the assembled platforms were able to fully sustain hMSCs cells viability, adhesion/spreading/proliferation. Most importantly, MANF cultured hMSCs displayed an increased alkaline phosphatase (ALP) activity and expression of key osteocalcin and Runx2 classical biomarkers (Figure 13.5B–F). Furthermore, *in vivo* administration of MANF hydrogels in a rat calvarial defect model stimulated 83% higher new bone volume formation in comparison to standard gelatin-microparticle annealed hydrogel (MA). Interestingly, histological analysis further revealed that *de novo* bone tissue formation was observed throughout all the defect area (Figure 13.5G–I).

MAPs applications in bone tissue repair remains widely open to be investigated and further advances in upcoming years are expected. It is envisioned that most of these will be supported by numerous multifunctional microgel platforms with unique physicochemical, mechanical, morphological, and stimuli-responsive properties that are currently being developed [25].

A remaining challenge in bone regeneration is (re)vascularization; however, in most approaches, this factor is not yet sufficiently addressed. In this context, VEGF-alginate microparticles incorporation in porous collagen–hydroxyapatite scaffolds led to an extend release of this morphogen (~35 days) and enhanced *in vivo* blood vessels formation, ultimately improving the repair of a rat calvarial defect. Strategies that leverage the same underlying concepts in combination with other MAPs properties could be valuable for future endeavors. Inducing mechanical loading during the healing process may also be beneficial, particularly considering the natural motility that bone tissues are subjected to during lifetime. In this sense, TGF-β1, loaded gelatin microspheres combined with hMSCs cells sheets, proved beneficial for stimulating neovascularization, as well as induced endochondral bone formation *in vivo*. Interestingly, mechanical loading has demonstrated to induce similar regeneration to that obtained with the gold-standard BMP-2 based treatment [106]. Additional advances in bone tissue-specific repair by exploring

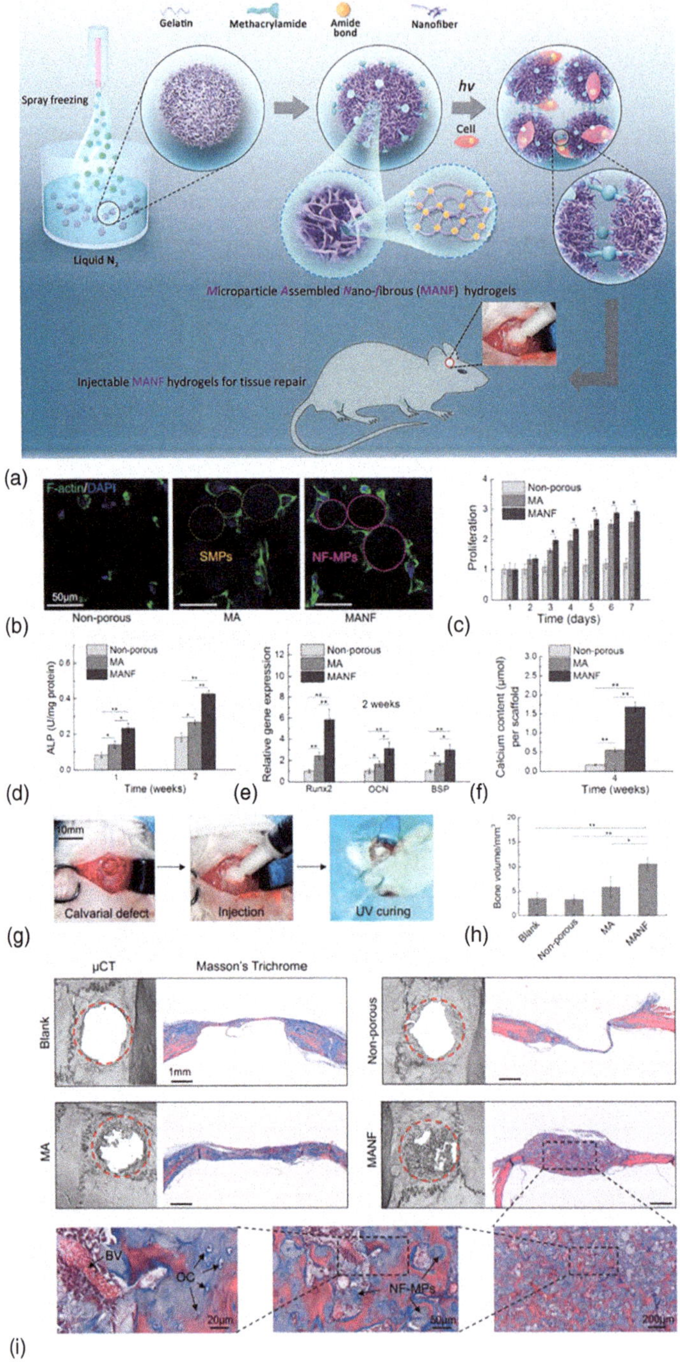
Gelatin
Methacrylamide
Amide bond
Nanofiber
Spray freezing
Liquid N2
hv
Cell
Microparticle Assembled Nano-fibrous (MANF) hydrogels
Injectable MANF hydrogels for tissue repair
(a)
F-actin/DAPI
SMPs
NF-MPs
50μm
Non-porous
MA
MANF
(b)
Non-porous
MA
MANF
Proliferation
Time (days)
(c)
ALP (U/mg protein)
Time (weeks)
(d)
Relative gene expression
2 weeks
Runx2
OCN
BSP
(e)
Calcium content (μmol) per scaffold
Time (weeks)
(f)
10mm
Calvarial defect
Injection
UV curing
(g)
Bone volume/mm3
Blank
Non-porous
MA
MANF
(h)
μCT
Masson's Trichrome
Blank
Non-porous
MA
MANF
1mm
BV
OC
NF-MPs
20μm
50μm
200μm
(i)

Figure 13.5 Microparticle-assembled nanofibrous (MANF) hydrogels for bone tissue-specific repair. (A) Schematic illustration of MANF hydrogels fabrication and application. (B and C) *In vitro* evaluation of hMSCs cell adhesion (five days) and time-course proliferation analysis. MA – gelatin-microparticle annealed hydrogel. Nonporous hydrogel control. (D–F) Analysis of ALP expression, osteogenic biomarkers expression, and calcium content in hydrogels at different time points, respectively. Data presented as mean ± s.d., $n \geq 3$. $^{*}p < 0.05$; $^{**}p < 0.01$. (G) MANFs *in vivo* injection procedure. (H) Micro-CT (μCT) quantitative analysis of *de novo* formed bone volume for all experimental groups. Blank – nontreated group – saline. (I) *Ex vivo* histomorphological Masson's trichrome-based analysis of rat calvarial defects after eight weeks. Arrows indicate the locations of nanofibrous microparticles (NF-MPs), osteocyte-like cells (OC), and blood vessels (BV) in regenerated bone tissues. Source: Hou, S., et al. (2019), [104], Figure 07, Pg 09 / with permission of American Chemical Society.

the potential of other key cellular players such as hematopoietic stem cells or by including piezoelectric cues naturally present in bone tissue are being investigated.

13.3.4 Emerging Trends and Applications

MAPs with unconventional physicochemical features for TERM application have emerged recently owing to the requirement to imprint exotic features in biomaterials such as sensing, imaging, and also other important biophysiological cues, such as electrical conductivity capabilities, that are naturally present in the human body and that may be advantageous in the context of tissue-specific engineering. In this context, conductive granular hydrogels were recently developed by conjugating gallol-modified hyaluronic acid with silver nanoparticles [106]. Functionalized granular hydrogels successfully exhibited fivefold higher conductive properties, when compared with their bulk hydrogel counterpart. Such has been hypothesized to be a by-product of the higher amount of silver nanoparticles in granular hydrogels due to their higher surface area. Successful muscle contractility was also demonstrated in this platform. This characteristic will be extremely useful for repairing different muscle lesions but can also be envisioned to be applied in cardiac tissues. On a different route, granular hydrogels have also begun to be leveraged as gene transfer platforms [55, 107]. This adds to the already reported drug and protein delivery capabilities and may open an untapped potential to use MAPs as multicellular microenvironment modulators in injured tissue niches if, for example, cell-specific gene expression is accomplished. Several other granular hydrogel-related advances are envisioned in coming years in several areas ranging from 3D/4D additive manufacturing to soft-robotic actuators.

13.4 Conclusions and Future Perspectives

In this chapter, we have showcased granular hydrogels unique multifunctionalities and key features that render them unique biomaterials for TERM applications. Such hierarchic platforms are highly chemically versatile, modular, and easily combined with numerous bioactive entities such as cells, protein cocktails, specific growth factors, nucleic acids, and/or nanoparticles. Their ability to conjugate key elements of TERM (i.e. biomaterials, cells, growth factors) and inherent scaffold microporosity undoubtedly renders granular hydrogels highly promising platforms for improving tissues repair. On this focus one can envision that size-controlled microgel/microcapsule building blocks containing encapsulated cells may be leveraged to assemble living microporous granular scaffolds where resident cells may function as tissue precursors and as recruiting agents. This approach remains relatively underexplored to date and significant advances are expected. Improvements in *in silico* modeling of MAPs annealing from microgel unit blocks are also expected to provide critical information on how structure, function, and mechanical resistance may be connected. Such approaches will be pivotal for increasing MAPs design rationale at early stages and in a tissue-specific mode. Recent advances in biomaterials high-throughput screening platforms will surely contribute to expedite the identification of most promising MAPs scaffolds. Moreover, the rapid advance of drug designing technologies and stem cells bioengineering tools (e.g. CRISPR/CAS-9, etc.) will contribute to increase MAPs bioperformance and broaden their TERM applications.

Acknowledgments

This work was developed within the scope of the project CICECO – Aveiro Institute of Materials, UIDB/50011/2020 and UIDP/50011/2020, financed by national funds through the Portuguese Foundation for Science and Technology/MCTES. This work was also supported by the Programa Operacional Competitividade e Internacionalização (POCI), in the component FEDER, and by national funds (OE) through FCT/MCTES, in the scope of the project MARGEL (PTDC/BTM-MAT/31498/2017). The authors acknowledge the financial support by the Portuguese Foundation for Science and Technology (FCT) through a Junior Researcher contract (CEEC/1048/2019, Vítor M. Gaspar).

References

1 Lee, K.Y. and Mooney, D.J. (2001). *Chem. Rev.* 101: 1869.
2 Shin, H., Jo, S., and Mikos, A.G. (2003). *Biomaterials* 24: 4353.
3 Koh, C.J. (2004). *J. Am. Soc. Nephrol.* 15: 1113.
4 Vacanti, J.P. and Langer, R. (1999). *Lancet* 354: S32.
5 Gaspar, V.M., Lavrador, P., Borges, J. et al. (2020). *Adv. Mater.* 32: 1903975.
6 Mano, J.F. (2015). *Mater. Lett.* 141: 198.
7 Wang, L.-S., Chung, J.E., Pui-Yik Chan, P., and Kurisawa, M. (2010). *Biomaterials* 31: 1148.
8 Hsu, R., Chen, P., Fang, J. et al. (2019). *Adv. Sci.* 6: 1900520.
9 Riley, L., Schirmer, L., and Segura, T. (2019). *Curr. Opin. Biotechnol.* 60: 1.
10 Salvador, T., Oliveira, M.B., and Mano, J.F. (2020). *Adv. Healthc. Mater.* 9: 2000543.

11 Ehrbar, M., Sala, A., Lienemann, P. et al. (2011). *Biophys. J.* 100: 284.
12 Judawisastra, H., Nugraha, F.R., and Wibowo, U.A. (2020). *Macromol. Symp.* 391: 1900187.
13 Bodenberger, N., Kubiczek, D., Abrosimova, I. et al. (2016). *Biotechnol. Rep.* 12: 6.
14 Ying, G., Jiang, N., Maharjan, S. et al. (2018). *Adv. Mater.* 30: 1805460.
15 Wyss, C.S., Karami, P., Bourban, P.-E., and Pioletti, D.P. (2020). *Soft Matter* 16: 3769.
16 Qazi, T.H. and Burdick, J.A. (2021). *Biomater. Biosyst.* 1: 100008.
17 Cheng, W., Zhang, J., Liu, J., and Yu, Z. (2020). *View* 1: 20200060.
18 Mealy, J.E., Chung, J.J., Jeong, H. et al. (2018). *Adv. Mater.* 30: 1705912.
19 Alzanbaki, H., Moretti, M., and Hauser, C.A.E. (2021). *Micromachines* 12: 45.
20 Fang, J., Koh, J., Fang, Q. et al. (2020). *Adv. Funct. Mater.* 30: 2004307.
21 Daly, A.C., Riley, L., Segura, T., and Burdick, J.A. (2020). *Nat. Rev. Mater.* 5: 20.
22 Neto, M.D., Oliveira, M.B., and Mano, J.F. (2019). *Trends Biotechnol.* 37: 1011.
23 Oliveira, M.B. and Mano, J.F. (2011). *Biotechnol. Progr.* 27: 897.
24 Shahin, H.I., Vinjamuri, B.P., Mahmoud, A.A. et al. (2019). *J. Controlled Release* 302: 126.
25 Caldwell, A.S., Aguado, B.A., and Anseth, K.S. (2020). *Adv. Funct. Mater.* 30: 1907670.
26 Du, J., Du, P., and Smyth, H.D.C. (2013). *Ther. Delivery* 4: 1293.
27 Xin, S., Chimene, D., Garza, J.E. et al. (2019). *Biomater. Sci.* 7: 1179–1187.
28 Koh, J., Griffin, D.R., Archang, M.M. et al. (2019). *Small* 15: 1903147.
29 Nih, L.R., Sideris, E., Carmichael, S.T., and Segura, T. (2017). *Adv. Mater.* 29: 1.
30 Darling, N.J., Xi, W., Sideris, E. et al. (2020). *Adv. Healthc. Mater.* 9: 1.
31 Widener, A.E., Bhatta, M., Angelini, T.E., and Phelps, E.A. (2021). *Biomater. Sci.* 9: 2480.
32 Jenjob, R., Phakkeeree, T., and Crespy, D. (2020). *Biomater. Sci.* 8: 2756.
33 Newsom, J.P., Payne, K.A., and Krebs, M.D. (2019). *Acta Biomater.* 88: 32.
34 Liu, A.J. and Nagel, S.R. (2010). *Annu. Rev. Condens. Matter Phys.* 1: 347.
35 van Hecke, M. (2009). *J. Phys.: Condens. Matter* 22: 33101.
36 Yuan, Y., Liu, L., Zhuang, Y. et al. (2018). *Phys. Rev. E* 98: 42903.
37 Haustein, M., Gladkyy, A., and Schwarze, R. (2017). *SoftwareX* 6: 118.
38 Sun, Q., Jin, F., Liu, J., and Zhang, G. (2010). *Int. J. Mod. Phys. B* 24: 5743.
39 Dias, C.S., Custódio, C.A., Antunes, G.C. et al. (2020). *ACS Appl. Mater. Interfaces* 12: 48321.
40 Song, K., Zhang, D., Yin, J., and Huang, Y. (2021). *Addit. Manuf.* 41: 101963.
41 Bi, D. and Chakraborty, B. (2009). *Philos. Trans. R. Soc. A Math. Phys. Eng. Sci.* 367: 5073.
42 Ramola, K. and Chakraborty, B. (2016). *J. Stat. Mech.: Theory Exp.* 2016: 114002.
43 Behringer, R.P. and Chakraborty, B. (2018). *Rep. Prog. Phys.* 82: 12601.
44 Darling, N.J., Sideris, E., Hamada, N. et al. (2018). *Adv. Sci.* 5: 1801046.
45 Li, C., Ouyang, L., Armstrong, J.P.K., and Stevens, M.M. (2021). *Trends Biotechnol.* 39: 150.

46 Eggert, S., Mieszczanek, P., Meinert, C., and Hutmacher, D.W. (2020). *HardwareX* 8: e00152.
47 Gilbert, P.M. and Weaver, V.M. (2017). *Semin. Cell Dev. Biol.*, Elsevier 141–152.
48 Caldwell, A.S., Rao, V.V., Golden, A.C., and Anseth, K.S. (2020). *Biomaterials* 232: 119725.
49 Griffin, D.R., Weaver, W.M., Scumpia, P.O. et al. (2015). *Nat. Mater.* 14: 737.
50 Sheikhi, A., de Rutte, J., Haghniaz, R. et al. (2019). *Biomaterials* 192: 560.
51 Ligon, S.C., Husar, B., Wutzel, H. et al. (2014). *Chem. Rev.* 114: 557.
52 Lavrador, P., Esteves, M.R., Gaspar, V.M., and Mano, J.F. (2021). *Adv. Funct. Mater.* 31: 2005941.
53 Cipitria, A. and Salmeron-Sanchez, M. (2017). *Adv. Healthc. Mater.* 6: 1700052.
54 Trujillo, S., Dobre, O., Dalby, M.J., and Salmeron-Sanchez, M. (2019). Mechanotransduction and growth factor signaling in hydrogel-based microenvironments. In: *Encyclopedia of Tissue Engineering and Regenerative Medicine* (ed. R.L. Reis), 87–101. Elsevier.
55 Truong, N.F., Kurt, E., Tahmizyan, N. et al. (2019). *Acta Biomater.* 94: 160.
56 de Rutte, J.M., Koh, J., and Di Carlo, D. (2019). *Adv. Funct. Mater.* 29: 1900071.
57 Roca-Cusachs, P., Sunyer, R., and Trepat, X. (2013). *Curr. Opin. Cell Biol.* 25: 543.
58 Yu, S., Duan, Y., Zuo, X. et al. (2018). *Biomaterials* 180: 193.
59 Rouwkema, J., Rivron, N.C., and van Blitterswijk, C.A. (2008). *Trends Biotechnol.* 26: 434.
60 Kühn, S., Sievers, J., Stoppa, A. et al. (2020). *Adv. Funct. Mater.* 30: 1908857.
61 Mosiewicz, K.A., Kolb, L., Van Der Vlies, A.J. et al. (2013). *Nat. Mater.* 12: 1072.
62 Caldwell, A.S., Campbell, G.T., Shekiro, K.M.T., and Anseth, K.S. (2017). *Adv. Healthc. Mater.* 6: 1700254.
63 Zhang, Y., Fang, C., Zhang, S. et al. (2021). *ACS Appl. Mater. Interfaces* 13: 7051.
64 Jooybar, E., Abdekhodaie, M.J., Karperien, M. et al. (2020). *Int. J. Biol. Macromol.* 144: 837.
65 Secret, E., Kelly, S.J., Crannell, K.E., and Andrew, J.S. (2014). *ACS Appl. Mater. Interfaces* 6: 10313.
66 Agrawal, G. and Agrawal, R. (2018). *Small* 14: 1801724.
67 Herberg, S., Varghai, D., Cheng, Y. et al. (2018). *Nanotheranostics* 2: 128.
68 Griffin, D.R., Archang, M.M., Kuan, C.-H. et al. (2021). *Nat. Mater.* 20: 560.
69 Nguyen, A.H., McKinney, J., Miller, T. et al. (2015). *Acta Biomater.* 13: 101.
70 Bysell, H., Månsson, R., Hansson, P., and Malmsten, M. (2011). *Adv. Drug Delivery Rev.* 63: 1172.
71 Li, J. and Mooney, D.J. (2016). *Nat. Rev. Mater.* 1: 1.
72 Cheng, J., Amin, D., Latona, J. et al. (2019). *ACS Nano* 13: 5493.
73 Williams, D.F. (2019). *Front. Bioeng. Biotechnol.* 7: 127.
74 Elkhoury, K., Russell, C.S., Sanchez-Gonzalez, L. et al. (2019). *Adv. Healthc. Mater.* 8: 1.
75 Chen, W., Liang, X., Nong, Z. et al. (2019). *Med. Chem.* 15: 459.

76 Palmese, L.L., Thapa, R.K., Sullivan, M.O., and Kiick, K.L. (2019). *Curr. Opin. Chem. Eng.* 24: 143.
77 Fu, J. and Wang, D.-A. (2018). *Trends Biotechnol.* 36: 834.
78 Zhang, B. and Radisic, M. (2020). *J. Thorac. Cardiovasc. Surg.* 159: 2003.
79 Phelps, E.A. and García, A.J. (2010). *Curr. Opin. Biotechnol.* 21: 704.
80 Yang, G., Mahadik, B., Choi, J.Y., and Fisher, J.P. (2020). *Prog. Biomed. Eng.* 2: 12002.
81 Xie, R., Zheng, W., Guan, L. et al. (2020). *Small* 16: 1902838.
82 Impellitteri, N.A., Toepke, M.W., Levengood, S.K.L., and Murphy, W.L. (2012). *Biomaterials* 33: 3475.
83 Madrigal, J.L., Sharma, S.N., Campbell, K.T. et al. (2018). *Acta Biomater.* 69: 265.
84 Foster, G.A., Headen, D.M., González-García, C. et al. (2017). *Biomaterials* 113: 170.
85 Li, Y., Liu, W., Liu, F. et al. (2014). *Proc. Natl. Acad. Sci. U.S.A.* 111: 13511.
86 Torres, A.L., Bidarra, S.J., Vasconcelos, D.P. et al. (2020). *Biomaterials* 228: 119554.
87 Zhang, R., Xie, L., Wu, H. et al. (2020). *Acta Biomater.* 113: 305.
88 Choi, Y.H., Kim, S.-H., Kim, I.-S. et al. (2019). *Acta Biomater.* 95: 285.
89 Eming, S.A., Martin, P., and Tomic-Canic, M. (2014). *Sci. Transl. Med.* 6: 265sr6.
90 Gurtner, G.C., Werner, S., Barrandon, Y., and Longaker, M.T. (2008). *Nature* 453: 314.
91 Kosaric, N., Kiwanuka, H., and Gurtner, G.C. (2019). *Expert Opin. Biol. Ther.* 19: 575.
92 Stejskalová, A. and Almquist, B.D. (2017). *Biomater. Sci.* 5: 1421.
93 Castano, O., Pérez-Amodio, S., Navarro-Requena, C. et al. (2018). *Adv. Drug Delivery Rev.* 129: 95.
94 Seia, M. and Zisman, E. (1997). *FASEB J.* 11: 449.
95 Hou, S., Lake, R., Park, S. et al. (2018). *ACS Appl. Bio Mater.* 1: 1430.
96 Qu, H., Fu, H., Han, Z., and Sun, Y. (2019). *RSC Adv.* 9: 26252.
97 Koons, G.L., Diba, M., and Mikos, A.G. (2020). *Nat. Rev. Mater.* 5: 584.
98 Armiento, A.R., Hatt, L.P., Sanchez Rosenberg, G. et al. (2020). *Adv. Funct. Mater.* 30: 1909874.
99 Xin, S., Dai, J., Gregory, C.A. et al. (2020). *Adv. Funct. Mater.* 30: 1907102.
100 Xin, S., Gregory, C.A., and Alge, D.L. (2020). *Acta Biomater.* 101: 227.
101 Isaac, A., Jivan, F., Xin, S. et al. (2019). *ACS Biomater. Sci. Eng.* 5: 6395.
102 Jivan, F. and Alge, D.L. (2020). *Adv. Ther.* 3: 1900148.
103 Oliveira, B.L., Guo, Z., and Bernardes, G.J.L. (2017). *Chem. Soc. Rev.* 46: 4895.
104 Hou, S., Niu, X., Li, L. et al. (2019). *Biomaterials* 223: 119458.
105 Padhi, A. and Nain, A.S. (2020). *Ann. Biomed. Eng.* 48: 1071.
106 McDermott, A.M., Herberg, S., Mason, D.E. et al. (2019). *Sci. Transl. Med.* 11: eaav7756.
107 Truong, N.F., Lesher-Pérez, S.C., Kurt, E., and Segura, T. (2018). *Bioconjugate Chem.* 30: 476.

14

Injectable Hydrogels as a Stem Cell Delivery Platform for Wound Healing

Qian Xu, Sigen A., and Wenxin Wang

University College Dublin, The Charles Institute of Dermatology, School of Medicine, Belfield, D04 V1W8 Dublin 4, Ireland

14.1 Wound Healing

14.1.1 Clinical Needs for Wound Healing

The healing of skin wound is one of the most complex physiological processes that involve cellular and molecular mechanisms [1]. Normal wound healing after skin injury relies on an well-orchestrated integration of complex biological and molecular events of cell recruitment, cell proliferation and migration, and extracellular matrix (ECM) deposition [1]. When the normal repair process is interrupted or deregulated in one or more phases, nonhealing or chronic wounds occur. Chronic wounds are defined as defects that are sustained for over 30 days or failed to heal through orderly and timely normal healing phases to regain structural and functional integrity [2].

Usually, the impaired wound healing is due to multiple reasons, which is challenging for the development of novel and efficient wound management. Currently, clinicians follow different strategies for the treatment of lesions and aiding wound healing, as well as to prevent recurrence (Figure 14.1). However, none of these therapies has proven to be enough efficient and thus, new, multifaceted therapeutic approaches are urgently needed to heal hard for treatment wounds. Given the complexity of the wound repair processes, better understanding and manipulation of pathophysiological and pathogenic factors and advanced therapeutic tools would give new hope for the management of hard to treat wounds.

14.1.2 Wound Healing Pathology

The skin acts as a protective barrier between the interior of the organism and the external environment. It prevents invasion by pathogens and defends interior soft tissue from environmental traumas [1, 3–11]. The typical healing process works to maintain this most important function when the skin barrier is breached by injury. There is a sequence of tightly regulated and overlapping phases that represent important steps in the wound healing process. These phases are hemostasis, inflammation, proliferation, and remodeling (Figure 14.2). The ultimate aims of each of these

Multifunctional Hydrogels for Biomedical Applications, First Edition.
Edited by Ricardo A. Pires, Iva Pashkuleva, and Rui L. Reis.

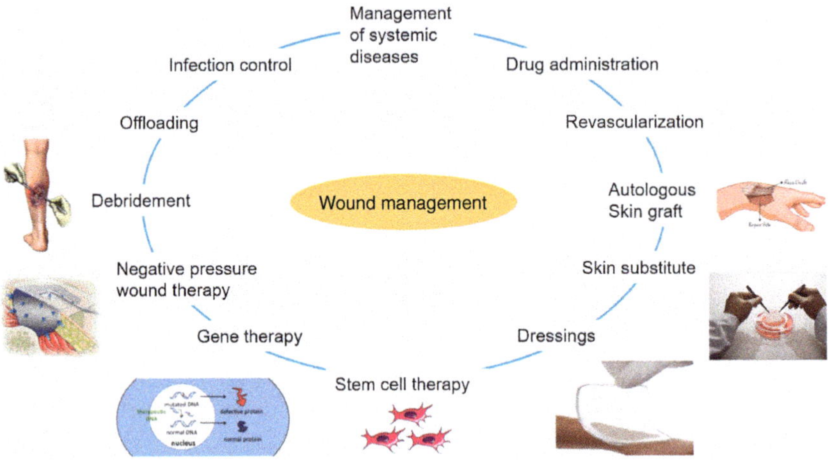

Figure 14.1 Wound management strategies. Source: Organogenesis Inc.

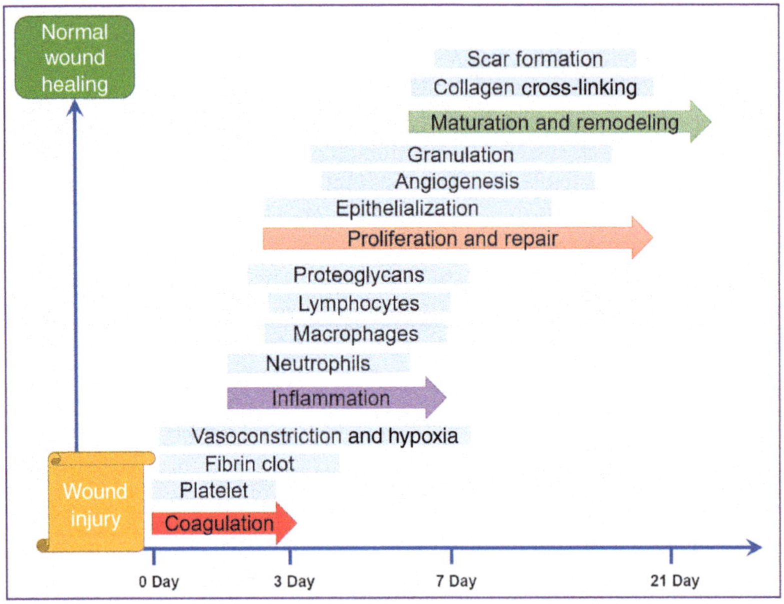

Figure 14.2 An overview of the normal wound healing and approximate times of different phases.

phases are to reduce blood loss, protect the organism from infection, rebuild and repair lost cellular structures (e.g. blood vessels), and replace lost ECM, respectively [1, 9, 12–15]. When an element of this complex and tightly regulated process is disrupted, the wound can be transformed into a chronic wound (Figure 14.3). As an example, burns can cause formation of a chronic wound depending on the severity and state of the burn.

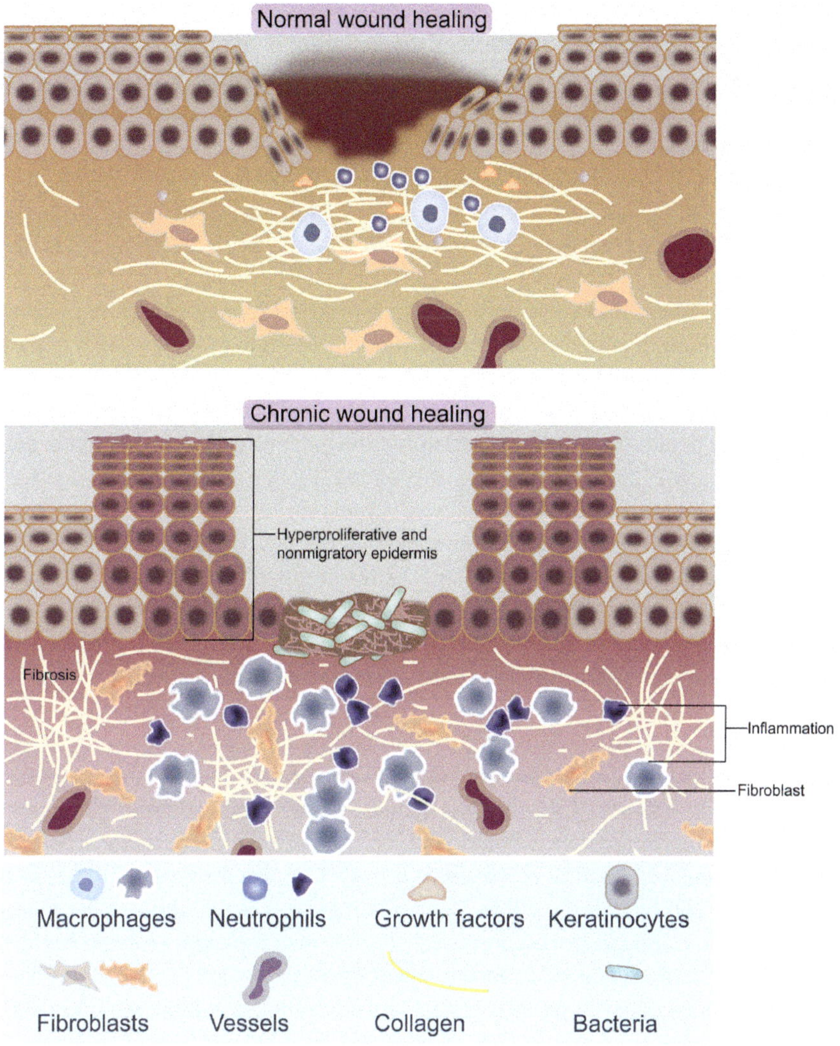

Figure 14.3 Molecular and cellular differences between normal and diabetic skin wound healing. Normal healing shows proper proliferation and migration after the inflammation stage. Diabetic wound shows increased and abnormal inflammation response (misshaped cells and unproper cell functions), presence of infection (bacteria residence and biofilm formation), reduction of angiogenesis and proliferation, hyperproliferative and nonmigratory epidermis (delayed wound closure), and fibrosis (scar).

14.1.2.1 Hemostasis

The purpose of hemostasis is to reduce the quantity of blood lost from the injury by restricting blood flow to the wound site as quickly as possible, and so it is heavily dependent on the coagulation cascade [9, 16–19]. Soon after the infliction of the injury, blood vessels begin to contract around the defect and platelets begin their coagulation activity to form blood clots. These clots may act as provisional matrices that allow inflammatory cells to invade and perform their function at the wound site. These clots also release chemotactic cues that induce the recruitment of inflammatory cells [20].

14.1.2.2 Inflammation

Inflammation processes typically result in protecting the microenvironment from pathogenic infection and clearing foreign debris and damaged tissue from the wound site. This is achieved by the recruitment of neutrophils and monocytes into the wound environment. Neutrophils act as the rapid first responders in inflammation [1, 21–24]. They act to kill invading microbes and produce cytokines and growth factors that initiate healing. Upon the recruitment of monocytes, they extravasate from the blood vessel and invade the wound environment [23, 24], where they transit to a macrophage phenotype [7, 16, 21]. Macrophages release cytokines and growth factors to aid the progress of inflammation and promote the production and deposition of new ECM components [1, 9, 16, 25–27]. They also phagocytose potential pathogens and foreign bodies. When inflammation has reached an appropriate stage, the M1 (pro-inflammatory) phenotype macrophages differentiate toward an M2 (anti-inflammatory) phenotype to aid the resolution of the inflammation stage and the induction of the proliferation stage [9, 16, 21, 24, 26, 27].

While both neutrophils and macrophages are crucial for the healing process, if their presence at the wound site is excessive and persistent, they can prolong the inflammatory state and contribute to the pathology of delayed (chronic) wound healing and hypertrophic scarring [1, 9, 24, 28, 29]. In these cases, several key proinflammatory cytokines are deregulated, such as interleukin-1β (IL-1β) and tumor necrosis factor-α (TNF-α). The increased expression of proinflammatory cytokines lead to an excessive expression of matrix metalloproteinases (MMPs) that contribute to delayed healing or excessive fibrosis [30]. Persistent inflammation is also characterized by supraphysiological oxidative stress resulting from the excessive production of reactive oxygen species (ROS) by macrophages and neutrophils. Excessive ROS can induce keratinocyte injury, dysfunction, apoptosis [31], and an impaired defense capability against antioxidants in response to hyperglycemia [32].

14.1.2.3 Proliferation

Typically, this stage occurs between two days and two weeks after the onset of injury. Throughout this phase, the cellular components of lost tissue are rebuilt, and ECM proteins are deposited within the site [1, 33–37]. Angiogenesis occurs, further contributing to the healing process with the provision of oxygen and nutrients toward cells proliferation and activation. Both fibroblasts and keratinocytes migrate to and proliferate within the wound environment and contribute to ECM production and deposition. The aim of proliferation is the re-epithelialization and therefore closure of the wound, thereby reinstating the skin with its protective barrier function. Fibroblasts and keratinocytes extend from granulation tissue around the wound edges in the form of "epithelial tongues" [38]. Granulation tissue is soft, pink, and richly vascularized tissue with newly produced ECM proteins, fibroblasts, and keratinocytes [9].

The processes of angiogenesis and vasculogenesis are promoted by the hypoxic microenvironment in the wound site, notably via the production and signaling of hypoxia-inducible factor-1 (HIF-1) [26, 39–42]. This essential requirement of the wound healing process is induced by the response of stromal cells in an ischemic environment to release angiogenic factors like vascular endothelial growth factor (VEGF), transforming growth factor-β (TGF- β), fibroblast growth factor (FGF), and platelet-derived growth factor (PDGF) [9, 14, 43]. The stromal cells include keratinocytes, fibroblasts, endothelial cells, and macrophages (likely those of the M2-phenotype).

Inadequate and aberrant vascular formation has been considered as a very important contributor to impaired healing. The abnormalities include inadequate capillary number, reduced vessel size, and pathological vascular structure. Except for the above-mentioned changes (local hyperglycemia, abnormal expression of HIF-1α, and VEGF), other pro-angiogenic mediators and vascular maturation factors show different expression levels compared with those of normal wound healing [44]. Unbalanced proteases will degrade and interface with their bioactivity in the harsh diabetic wound environment [45]. Aberrant endothelial cells in diabetic animals show a lesser amount of number and impaired function, leading to deficient angiogenesis [46]. Besides, patients who developed diabetic foot ulcers (DFUs) suffer from more severe neuropathy, inducing impaired neurovascular response and loss of protective sensation [47]. High risk of increased unnoticed trauma and vascular diseases are critical intermediates of the formation and chronicity of DFUs [48].

Within the dermis, fibroblasts are the predominant mesenchymal cell type that performs important functions throughout all the overlapping healing phases. The initial release of inflammation-induced chemo-attractants (i.e. IL-1β, PDGF, and TNF-α) from the wound site promotes the incoming recruitment of fibroblasts within 24–48 hours of the inception of injury [9, 20, 37]. These fibroblasts invade the fibrin clot and contribute to the production of growth factors and ECM components, like collagen, hyaluronic acid, fibronectin, and proteoglycans. They also secrete MMPs to degrade the fibrin clot that is gradually replaced with the new ECM, which facilitate cell migration and growth [20, 49, 50]. This new ECM gradually re-establishes the mechanical strength of the defected region. When fibroblasts are stimulated by applying mechanical stress and supplementation of TGF- β ligands, they undergo differentiation and transition into myofibroblasts. This differentiation bestows them with potent contractile capabilities due to the increased expression of α-smooth muscle actin (α-SMA) [51–54]. As the wound healing process approaches its terminal stage, fibroblasts number gradually decreases [9]. However, when the function of fibroblasts is disturbed, ECM production and contraction in wound healing will be influenced. For example, fibroblasts isolated from diabetic wounds show a decreased proliferative response to the above-mentioned growth factors [1, 55]. Diabetic wounds demonstrate malformation of ECM produced by abnormal fibroblasts under hyperglycemic conditions [56].

The skin barrier can be eventually restored. This is typically viewed as the result of the overlapping keratinocyte functions: migration, proliferation, and differentiation [57, 58]. Re-epithelialization begins within hours after injury when the cells undergo marked phenotypic alteration under favorable conditions [59, 60]. The epidermal defect first initiates the early migration of keratinocytes from the edges of the wound and a migrating epithelial tongue forms [30, 59]. The process of migration is coordinated by a number of growth factors and interactions between keratinocytes and stroma. For example, epidermal growth factor (EGF) family enhance re-epithelialization by accelerating keratinocyte migration [61]. At the nonhealing edge of diabetic wounds, keratinocytes show thickened, hyperproliferative, and nonmigratory characteristics [62, 63]. Dysregulated cytokine/growth factor networks lead to severe retardation of re-epithelialization.

14.1.2.4 Remodeling

The last phase of wound healing is the remodeling of the wound site. Typically, this phase begins two or three weeks post injury [7]. While this is the final stage of wound healing, it is also the phase with the longest duration, as it may last from several months to years, depending on the nature and size of the injury [2, 9, 19, 37]. The majority of active cells (i.e. fibroblasts, endothelial cells, and inflammatory cells) either gradually migrate from the repaired region or undergo controlled cell death (apoptosis). It is during this phase that ECM deposition is most prevalent. There is also a replacement of collagen III, initially deposited throughout the proliferation phase, with collagen I. The collagen I : collagen III ratio is considered a good indicator of wound healing quality, with a higher amount of collagen I being viewed as a beneficial sign [8, 52, 64–67]. Typically, an approximate 80% of the skin's mechanical strength is recovered after several months of remodeling [68].

Deregulated levels of proteases, such as MMPs, collagenases, and gelatinases, contribute to nonhealing wounds as they degrade matrix components and key growth factors required for remodeling of ECM [45, 69]. Moreover, altered ECM composition in nonhealing wounds and an enhanced ECM degradation rate, caused by elevated MMP levels, can impair keratinocyte attachment, leading to aberrant cell signaling and impaired migration. Keratinocytes also show senescence in diabetic wounds and secrete detrimental factors. The interactions between keratinocytes and fibroblasts can be destroyed in diabetic wounds, which results in disturbed wound healing [70].

14.2 Stem Cells for Skin Wound Healing

14.2.1 Stem Cell Overview

Stem cells have been the subject of much research and are currently under extensive investigation in multiple clinical trials [71–75]. They are multipotent cells that are capable of self-renewal and differentiation into cells that compose different types of tissue, like bone, adipose, cartilage, muscle, etc. These stem cells properties are appealing for the development of improved cell-based therapies for wound healing applications. In the last decades, numerous studies have been performed to evidence the beneficial therapeutic effects of stem cells on tissue repair and wound healing models. The therapeutic potential of stem cells is based on three widely accepted mechanisms: (i) differentiation, (ii) secretion, and (iii) homing [14, 76]. Stem cells can differentiate into a variety of cell types and directly participate in structural wound repair [77]. The undifferentiated stem cells contribute to the wound healing process by the secretion of paracrine signaling factors that induce pro-regenerative and immunomodulatory effects [78]. Homing is recruitment of innate systemic stem cells to injury site [79]. Among the used stem cells, embryonic and induced pluripotent stem cells (iPSCs) are well-known promising types of stem cell, but they have some limitations. Ethical issues and difficulties to control the differentiation toward a targeted application are main concerns about the embryonic stem cells for regenerative therapies [73, 80, 81]. For iPSCs, there are challenges associated with their genetic manipulation [14, 73, 80]. On the other hand, adult stem cells exist in abundant supply within a variety of tissues and the ethical issues for their translational application are resolvable. Bone marrow-derived MSCs (BMSCs) have been the focus of a numerous mesenchymal stem cell (MSC)-related studies [75, 82]. Recent research studies and clinical trials suggest that topical or systemic administration of BMSCs accelerate the wound closure, promote neovascularization, and increase collagen deposition for various wound types [83, 84]. For examples, one study on BMSCs subcutaneous injection into diabetic wound margin in rat by Kuo et al. suggested that enhanced wound healing is associated with suppressing inflammatory response and increasing wound epithelialization and neovascularization by means of increased expression of growth factor such as EGF and VEGF [85]. However, BMSCs are harvested from donors via a painfully invasive procedure which generates a small yield [14, 80, 86, 87]. The donor site then also carries the risk of morbidity [14, 88–90]. It is within the interest of clinicians and health science researchers to identify, harvest, and translate adult BMSCs that are safe, effective, and easy to harvest in high yields with minimum discomfort for the donor. As mentioned above, adult stem cells may be derived from several tissues, not just from bone marrow. One example of an adult MSC that has gained recent attention is the adipose-derived stem cell (ADSC).

14.2.2 Adipose-Derived Stem Cells for Wound Healing

In comparison to BMSCs, ADSCs are available in higher yields in more accessible fat tissue via a less invasive procedure (liposuction) [14, 75]. Isolations from adipose tissue typically yield about 40 times the amount of MSCs yielded from bone marrow [14]. Culture of the isolated ADSC populations can yield between 100- and 1000-fold more progenitor cells than those isolated from bone marrow [91]. ADSCs have fibroblastic morphology [92]. BMSCs and ADSCs have similar functionality. ADSCs, like BMSCs, promote angiogenesis, secrete growth factors, differentiate into multiple lineages, and modulate the immune response. However, the potent promotion of angiogenesis by ADSCs is highly recognized in soft tissue regeneration studies [34, 93, 94]. ADSCs also have a greater proliferative capacity than BMSCs [14]. These advantages make ADSCs more suitable, practical, and cost-effective choice of stem cell for application in dermal wound regeneration than BMSCs.

Recent preclinical studies demonstrated the beneficial effect of ADSCs application in promoting wound healing by secreting factors, accelerating repair and differentiating into the various types of skin cell, and recruiting and stimulating endogenous stem cells to participate in the healing process [95, 96]. Numerous studies have shown that ADSCs produce active soluble factors, e.g. growth factors, cytokines, immunomodulatory factors, ECM molecules, ECM proteases, etc., that significantly alter the wound healing process as evidenced by data with ADSCs, adipose-derived stem cells in conditioned medium (ADSC-CM), or ADSC exosomes (ADSC-Exo). For example, Zhao et al. proved that migration and proliferation of skin fibroblasts cultured in conditioned medium of ADSCs were significantly enhanced [97]. They found that EGF, PDGF-AA, VEGF, and basic fibroblast growth factor (bFGF) secreted by ADSCs in the CM contributed to this effect.

Differentiation of ADSCs into fibroblasts, keratinocytes, and endothelial cells has an efficient therapeutic potential. As an example, ADSCs injected to skin flaps during ischemia/perfusion injury by Pu et al. significantly increased flap survival and capillary density. The mechanism of this outcome includes differentiation of ADSCs into endothelial cells and secretion of IL-6 from ADSCs [98].

Cell sheets can provide a three-dimensional microenvironment for stem cells and accelerate wound repair. Kato et al. reported that ADSC sheet combining artificial skin transplantation accelerates diabetic wound healing by paracrine activity including section of angiogenic growth factors and differentiation into perivascular cells [99]. Trottier et al. replaced fibroblasts with ADSCs in a bilayered skin substitute and reconstructed a more intact trilayered structure consisting of the epidermis, dermis, and hypodermis [100]. Hamada et al. also reported similar study by transplantation with ADSCs sheets along with artificial skin accelerates wound healing and angiogenesis.

14.2.3 Current Limitations and Future Directions of SCs for Wound Healing

Despite the preclinical and clinical studies that validate the utility of stem cell therapy for wound healing through direct local injection or intradermal injection of cell suspensions, many critical questions still remain open. Cell engraftment efficiency is a critical problem that should be addressed prior to the widespread clinical application, since function within the wound sites is highly correlated with the number of cells retained. Studies have uniformly reported high death rate of the transplanted cells and poor engraftment efficacy after being introduced into the injured area [101]. Therefore, current therapeutic approaches are either inefficient or impractical dependent on the development of advanced administration approaches for improving engraftment and viability of transplanted SCs.

14.3 Injectable Hydrogel Dressing as a Delivery Platform

Wound management by dressing is a proper and effective method to protect long-term healing wounds. The primary dressing design was for the local wound environment. A dressing can prevent contamination or trauma, provide a moist environment that is desired by wound closure, and release bioactive substances and avoid their rapid degradation to encourage healing (see also Chapter 9). Numerous biomaterials have been manufactured for fabricating dressings in attempts to regenerate different tissues and organs. For the specific application of skin wound healing, hydrogels have emerged as the most promising option. The moist environment provided by hydrogels is ideally suited for wounds with minimal to moderate levels of exudate to avoid excess hydration and dry wounds that need to be rehydrated [102–105]. This moist environment also provides a cooling effect for the patient, diminishing their pain and providing comfort [102, 106–108]. A mechanical barrier is promptly established upon their application. In addition to these characteristics, hydrogels are typically soft and flexible, affording it to be well suited for the treatment of soft tissues, like skin [4, 106]. Due to these unique features, hydrogels have been widely investigated as promising materials for tissue engineering applications.

There are several drawbacks of conventional hydrogels in tissue engineering driving the needs of investigating new technologies for hydrogel fabrication. These include lack of homogeneous cell distribution, compromised cell viability, uncontrolled shape, and requirement of complicated surgical implantation [109]. One development that has become an exciting prospect of hydrogels is the notion of making them "injectable" [110].

Recent studies have focused on developing gels or gel precursors that upon application at the defect site can conform its irregular shape and then undergo gelation to establish a scaffold structure over that defect site [111, 112]. Injectable hydrogels possess almost all the advantages of hydrogels in biological and biomedical applications and own unique properties which makes them more promising [113]. Some of the advantages are listed below.

(1) Cell culture system. Hydrogels can provide immuno-isolation and mimic salient elements and mechanics similar to the environment of native tissues while still allowing nutrients, oxygen, and cell secretion products to diffuse into the hydrogel [114, 115]. These advantages endow hydrogels with the capabilities of improving cell retention and viability after encapsulation and delivery at the tissue site of interest. In addition to cell encapsulation, hydrogels also influence stem cell fate and function through biophysical and biochemical interactions [113, 116]. A substrate with physical stiffness echoing that of the native ECM

tissue is desirable for stem cells and is vital to influence stem cell stemness or differentiation status [117, 118]. For example, mechanical properties of the hydrogels regulate MSC differentiation direction when encapsulated in alginate hydrogels at different moduli. A previous study reported that when MSCs loaded in an alginate hydrogel, adipogenic differentiation is achieved at moduli between 2.5 and 5 kPa and osteogenic differentiation between 11 and 30 kPa [119].

(2) Drug release. Hydrogel-based drug-releasing technologies show broad advantages not only by controlled release of the biomolecules but also by avoiding the potential harm of local administration to targeting sites due to the short duration of action of the biomolecules [120, 121].

(3) Wound healing materials. The moist environment provided by hydrogels is ideally suited for wounds with minimal to moderate levels of exudate to avoid excess hydration and dry wounds that need to be rehydrated [102–105]. Another key benefit of hydrogels is the painless and minimal discomforting application and removal to the injury sites. Due to the marked cooling effects, patients may experience pain relief with hydrogel dressings. The moisture effect of hydrogels also promotes autolytic debridement in necrotic or sloughy wounds [122]. In addition, hydrogels allow oxygen and nutrient diffusion to the wounds.

(4) Moldable and minimal invasion. The major advantages of injectable hydrogels over the conventional prefabricated hydrogels include reduced cell damage during injection, easy manipulation during the applications, and the minimal invasive procedures [110, 123]. Moreover, injectable hydrogels are very effective and of great value when transplanting and localizing the cells to a desired anatomic site.

Injectable hydrogel formation can be achieved through either physical (non-covalent assembly) or chemical gelation (covalent cross-linking) which involves a sol–gel phase transition (Figure 14.4) [125]. There are essential properties that must be considered when designing hydrogels for tissue engineering applications, including biocompatibility, biodegradability, mechanical strength, and porosity. It is also important to understand and modulate these characteristics as they influence the utility of hydrogels for biological and biomedical applications.

14.3.1 Types of Injectable Hydrogels

A variety of biomaterials have been used for producing injectable hydrogels, including naturally derived materials (hyaluronic acid, collagen, fibrin, chitosan, alginate, etc.), synthetic materials (poly(ethylene glycol) [PEG], poly-L-lactic acid [PLLA], polyglycolic acid [PGA], and poly(vinyl alcohol) [PVA]), and hybrid hydrogels that combine both synthetic and natural materials (see also Chapter 1). Injectable hydrogel formation can be achieved through either physical (noncovalent assembly) or chemical gelation (covalent cross-linking) which involves a sol–gel phase transition (Figure 14.4) [125]. Physically cross-linked hydrogels exhibit advantages of easy process, no requirement of cross-linkers, and easy to reverse. However, physical hydrogels are heterogeneous and have poor mechanical

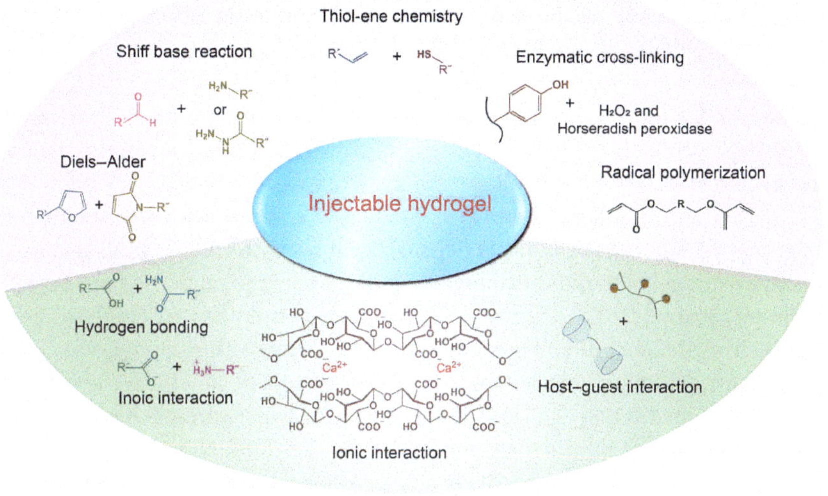

Figure 14.4 Representative methods for preparation of injectable hydrogels including chemical cross-linking approaches (the upper) and physical cross-linking approaches (the lower). Source: Based on Li et al. [110], Yang et al. [124].

properties which may limit their tissue engineering applications. Chemically cross-linked hydrogels can be obtained by covalent bond formation through chemical reactions, radical polymerization, photo-cross-linking, etc. Such hydrogels have higher mechanical strength and homogeneous structure. However, there might be residual chemical cross-linkers, organic solvents, or photo-initiators that may cause poor biocompatibility. Thus, it is important to investigate a biocompatible and chemical cross-linking approach for hydrogel creation. There are a number of key properties that are essential when designing the hydrogels for tissue engineering applications, including biocompatibility, biodegradability, mechanical strength, and porosity. It is also important to understand and modulate these characteristics as they influence the utility of hydrogels for biological and biomedical applications. Several commonly used hydrogels are discussed by summarizing the advantages and disadvantages for tissue engineering.

Naturally derived hydrogels are appealing for biological applications as they are biodegradable and biologically active due to cell signaling and interactive properties. Synthetic hydrogels possess good mechanical properties, tailored architecture, and controllable degradation, but these gels also lack biological activity and many of them are made using harsh chemistry. Thus, hydrogels based on the combination of biological macromolecules and synthetic polymers (so-called hybrid hydrogels [126, 127]) have drawn significant attention for biological and biomedical applications, because individual limitations of single material scaffolds (e.g. poor mechanical properties or lack of bioactivity or biomimetic features) are often overcome by their composite nature, which present a wide range of mechanical and chemical features [118].

14.3.1.1 Naturally Derived Injectable Hydrogels

Naturally derived hydrogels are appealing for biological applications as they are biodegradable and biologically active due to cell signaling and interactive properties. Representative materials are listed below.

Collagen and Gelatin Collagen is the most commonly existed protein of the native tissues. Type I collagen is the major strength and structural supporting component of many tissues which makes collagen an attractive material for tissue engineering (see Chapter 2). Gelatin is a hydrolysis product of collagen with the same amino acid sequence and absence of triple helical structure. Both collagen and gelatin are attractive hydrogel materials attributed to their biomimetic properties and easy formation physically [115]. Collagen can be chemically modified to facilitate chemical cross-link ability, while this usually leads to decreased bioactivity of collagen. Chemical cross-linking collagen–gelatin hydrogels can be obtained when treated with glutaraldehyde [128] or carbodiimide [129]. Collagen hydrogels have been used for wound healing [130], cartilage repair [131], osteochondral defect repair [132], and 3D cell culture [133]. Despite its benefits on cell culture and tissue repair, collagen hydrogels suffer from important drawbacks, including poor mechanical properties, limited long-term stability, and poor reproducibility which hinder its successful clinical translation [125].

Hyaluronic Acid Hyaluronic acid or hyaluronan (HA) is a non-sulfated linear immunoneutral polysaccharide consisting of a repeating disaccharide unit – (β-1,4)D-glucuronic acid and (β-1,3)*N*-acetyl-D-glucosamine (see also Chapter 10) [134]. HA is found ubiquitously throughout the body and is an essential component of the ECM [135]. HA performs an important function in a variety of biological processes, such as intracellular signaling and behavior, cell differentiation and cell growth, angiogenesis, tumor development and metastasis, and inflammation [136]. Due to its highly hydrophilic and polyanionic features, HA can absorb abundant quantities of water, forming a hydrated network. Due to the design flexibility, HA has been extensively modified to alter the properties of the resulting derivatives to meet the needs of tissue engineering and regenerative medicine [137]. HA scaffolds have been widely used for skin wound care [138], bone and cartilage defects repair [139, 140], and biomolecules and cell delivery [141, 142]. For example, the self-renewal and an undifferentiated status of human embryonic stem cells (ESCs) was maintained when encapsulated in a hydrogel entirely generated by HA [143]. Several hurdles exist when applying HA into biomedical use, such as poor mechanical strength [144] and short half-lives ranging from hours to days [145].

Fibrin Fibrin is another naturally derived ECM material that has shown great promising in tissue engineering as a cell or drug laden hydrogel scaffold [115]. Traditionally, fibrin is formed from fibrinogen and thrombin, key components involved in blood coagulation [20]. Beyond its role in hemostasis after injury, fibrin also functions as a reservoir for growth factors and cytokines and a matrix scaffold for the recruitment of tissue cells (monocytes, fibroblasts, endothelial cells, etc.) to an injured site for wound healing [146]. The primary usage of fibrin is mainly to stop bleeding and adhere tissue during surgeries [147]. In a porcine excised full-thickness burn wound model, the use of fibrin sealant demonstrated reduced skin graft dislocation and increased adherence [148]. In recent years, fibrin hydrogel has proved significant advancement in the field tissue repair and regeneration. A major advantage is that fibrin hydrogel is a feasible niche for cell adhesion and supporting cell proliferation, migration, and differentiation, such as being a vascular network formation platform [149–151]. However, its fast degradation and low mechanical properties may result in the poor long-term performance. Multicomponent hydrogel networks were designed by incorporation of synthetic polymers or ECM molecules with fibrin through chemical cross-linking methods to control the degradation rate and tune the stiffness of such hydrogels [152].

14.3.1.2 Synthetic Injectable Hydrogels

Synthetic hydrogels can be generated through various chemical reactions with high control and efficacy, such as radical polymerization and click reactions. Synthetic hydrogels possess good mechanical properties, tailored architecture, and controllable degradation, but these gels also lack biological activity and many of them are made using harsh chemistry. Examples of frequently used materials are listed below.

Poly(2-Hydroxyethyl Methacrylate) Poly(2-hydroxyethyl methacrylate) (PHEMA) is a well-studied hydrogel system first described by Wichterle and Lim and obtained by chemical polymerization with cross-linking agents such as ethylene glycol dimethacrylate [153]. Later on, copolymerization of PHEMA, 2-hydroxyethyl methacrylate (HEMA), and polyethylene glycol dimethacrylate (PEGDM) were also combined to synthesize chemically photo-cross-linked hydrogels. PHEMA-based polymer and copolymers have been proven to be biocompatible and nonbiodegradable, and the resulting hydrogels show good swelling and oxygen permeability. Thus, PHEMA hydrogels have been modified and utilized in multiple tissue engineering applications, such as contact lens and artificial cornea, cartilage repair, and neural regeneration [154, 155].

Poly(Vinyl Alcohol) PVA is a widely explored synthetic polymer for hydrogel preparation [156] by either physically freeze-thawing [157, 158] or chemical cross-linking with monoaldehyde [159] or sebacoyl chloride [160]. PVA has pendant alcohol groups which is similar to PHEMA. PVA exhibits excellent biocompatibility, hydrophilicity, water absorption ability, sufficient mechanical properties, and capacity to form particles, films, and sponges. There are some undesired properties of PVA including poor thermal stability and nonbiodegradability, which requires modification to produce satisfactory properties. PVA can be conjugated with other biological factors for tissue engineering applications, such as copolymerization with PEG to produce biodegradable hydrogels [161] and modification with fibronectin to support cell adhesion [159].

Poly(Ethylene Glycol) PEG is a biocompatible material approved by the Food and Drug Administration (FDA) and has been widely used in biomedical fields [162]. PEG is a highly hydrophilic, inert, and antifouling polymer, which can be designed to incorporate a wealth of cross-linking functional groups. Various PEG derivatives have been used for hydrogel fabrication, including poly(ethylene glycol) diacrylate (PEGDA), PEGDM, poly(ethylene glycol) diacrylamide (PEGDAA), using a variety of mechanisms for polymer chain growth, like step polymerization, Michael addition, or radical polymerization [115, 163]. A variety of PEG-based hydrogels have been obtained using low molecular weight vinyl monomers (e.g. acrylates, methacrylates, or acrylamides) in the presence of photo-initiators or cross-linking agents [164]. The benefits of such polymerization are numerous, including the rapid gelation, well-characterized gelation kinetics, and feasibility of the initiation system with minimal cytotoxicity [165–167]. Nevertheless, one strict limitation regarding a photo-initiated system that restricts its clinical application is the capacity of light penetration into the body. Hubbell and coworkers fabricated PEG-based hydrogels via Michael addition using multi-thiol agents and multi-acrylate PEG compounds [168]. The gelation time can be modified by altering the concentration and pH of the hydrogel precursor solutions. PEG is a nondegradable material. Researchers can either take advantage of this feature and design special hydrogels that require long-term stability [169] or functionalize PEG with degradable moieties (e.g. incorporating poly(lactic acid) [PLA] to supply hydrolytic ester groups [170]) to create degradable networks.

Most recent studies demonstrate that PEG-based hydrogels possess physical and mechanical limitations that hinder their prospects for clinical translation, such as impractical gelation time, undesired or toxic cross-linking agents, uncontrolled swelling and degradation, and improper stiffness [171]. PEG also can be blended with PLGA, PLLA, and bioactive ligands to improve its mechanical properties, thermal sensitivity, and enzyme degradability.

Hyperbranched Polymer-Based Synthetic Hydrogels Hyperbranched polymers (HPs) are a type of highly branched or dendritic macromolecules with three-dimensional architecture [172, 173]. Their unique globular and dendritic structures endow them with superior characteristics such as abundant terminal functional groups, high solubility, and low viscosity. These features offer great potential of HPs in diverse fields of bioapplications including drug delivery, protein delivery, and gene transfection. Due to the high density of functional terminal groups, HPs are rather popular in the application of *in situ* forming hydrogels. The terminal functional groups and the backbones of the HPs can be modified affording various functions and properties by selecting proper synthesis approaches and monomers. These advantages pave the way for the establishment of injectable hydrogels with attractive properties, including excellent physicochemical properties, desirable degradability, and good biocompatibility as well as smart responsibility.

Up to now, various synthesis methods have been proposed to prepare HPs using commercial polymers. The most utilized approaches are "A2 + B3" polycondensation and radical copolymerization. Among diverse "A2 + B3" polycondensation,

Michael addition reaction between the amines and acrylates is appealing due to the relatively simple procedure that does not require protection and has no side products. However, only a few HPs were successfully obtained under very strict reaction conditions due to the limited monomer sources [174–176]. Another classical approach is the radical copolymerization of single vinyl monomer with a multivinyl monomers. By the introduction of a chain transfer agent, this polymerization can be used for the synthesis of various soluble highly branched polymers with better control. However, this approach only obtains HPs with poor yield and low branching degree with extremely broad molar mass distributions [177]. Wang and coworkers proposed the controlled free radical polymerization of divinyl monomers with kinetic and statistical control of the HPs structures. Using deactivation-enhanced atom transfer radical polymerization (DE-ATRP) [177–181] and reversible addition fragmentation chain transfer (RAFT) [182, 183] polymerization, the multivinyl polymerization achieved much higher monomer conversion and the gel point could be significantly delayed. The resulting hyperbranched polymers were used to form hydrogels [179, 184] or transfect genes into targeted cells (Figures 14.5 and 14.6) [176, 185–188]. For example, Wang and coworkers fabricated a thermoresponsive hyperbranched PEG-based copolymer with multi-acrylate functional groups from DE-ATRP that could cross-link by photopolymerization [179]. Temperature-responsive or thermoresponsive hydrogels undergo phase transition when the temperature increases above the lower critical solution temperature (LCST), which can be adjusted to below body temperature

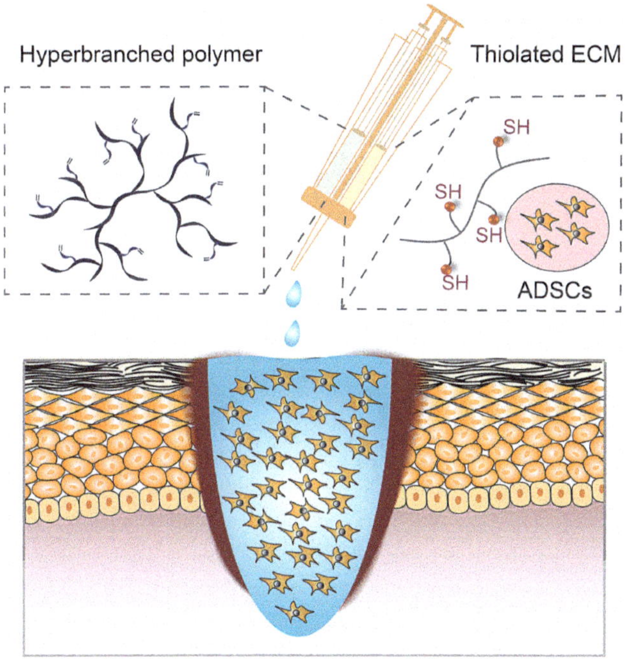

Figure 14.5 Schematic presentation of injectable hydrogel from hyperbranched polymers and thiolated ECM-based biopolymers as a system for stem cell delivery.

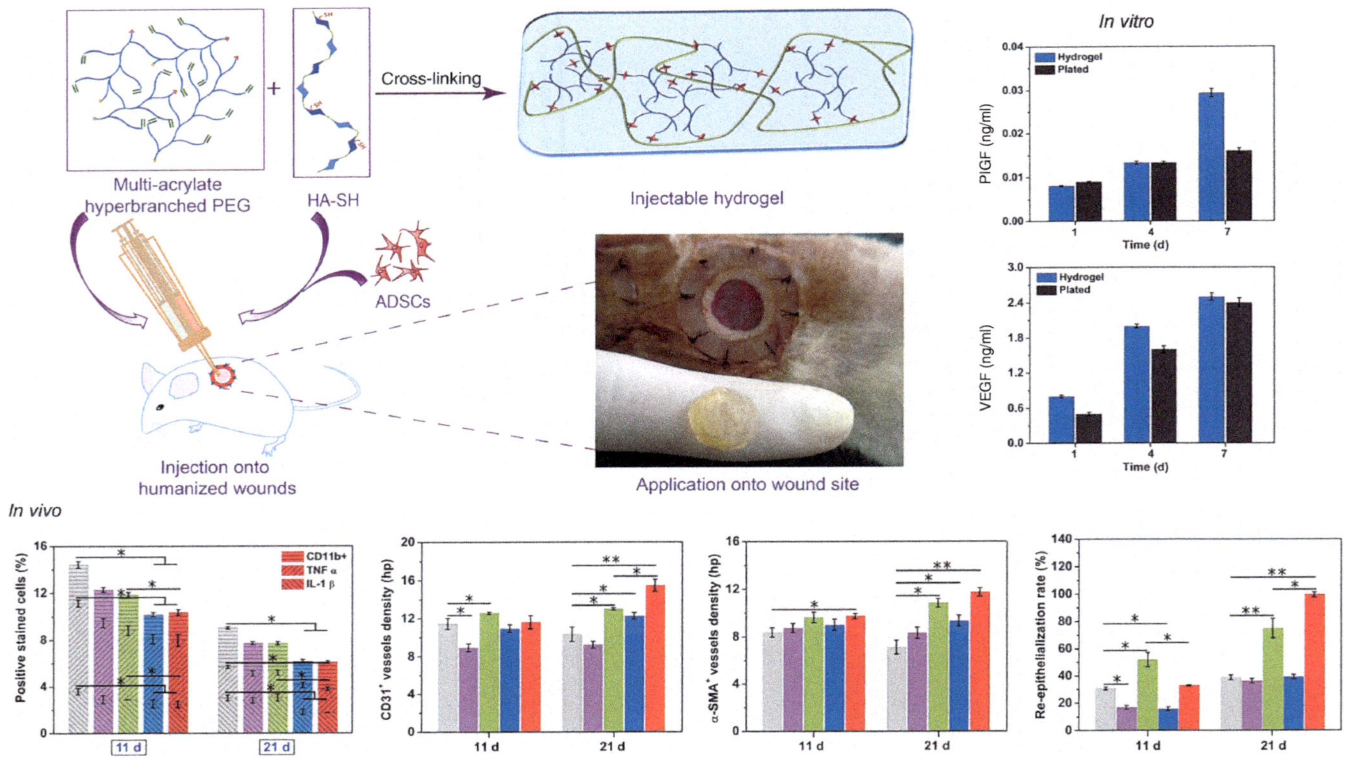

Figure 14.6 Summary of *in vitro* and *in vivo* studies of the *in situ* formed hydrogel prepared from a PEG-based hyperbranched polymer with thiolated hyaluronic acid. $^{*}p < 0.05$; $^{**}p < 0.01$. Source: Xu et al. [94]/with permission from Elsevier.

[189, 190]. Although significant progress has been achieved, several major challenges still exist, such as noxious and toxic reagents (e.g. copper catalyst in atom transfer radical polymerization (ATRP) and toxic chain transfer reagent for RAFT polymerization) and poor stability of thermoresponsive hydrogels.

14.3.1.3 Hybrid Injectable Hydrogels

Hydrogels based on the combination of biological macromolecules and synthetic polymers (so-called hybrid hydrogels [126, 127]) have drawn significant attention for biological and biomedical applications, because individual limitations of single material scaffolds (e.g. poor mechanical properties or lack of bioactivity or biomimetic features) are often overcome by the composite nature of the hybrid hydrogels, which present a wide range of mechanical and chemical features [118]. Several commonly used hybrid hydrogels are briefly presented below.

Interpenetrating Polymer Network (IPN) or Semi-IPN Interpenetrating polymer networking (IPN) is an approach in which hybrid hydrogels are generated by partially or fully interlacing (covalently or noncovalently) two or more polymer networks [191]. IPN hybrid hydrogels possess the properties that cannot be achieved by using a single polymer. For instance, PEG has been combined with collagen [192] or alginate [193] to fabricate IPN hydrogels in which the bioactivity of natural polymers is retained and the mechanical properties (such as hydrogel stiffness or toughness) can be improved. A semi-IPN structure was *in situ* developed following the previous progress of hyperbranched polymers by Wang and coworkers HPs using PEGDA, PEGMEMA, and (2-methoxyethoxy) ethyl methacrylate (MEO_2MA) via DE-ATRP can cross-link with a four-arm thiol functional cross-linker via thiol-ene Michael addition or physically and form semi-IPN hydrogel by mixing with HA macromolecule [180].

HA-Based Hybrid Hydrogels Because there are several reactive sites in the unmodified disaccharide unit of HA, chemical modification can be performed, thus, endowing HA derivatives with various properties. HA can be chemically modified with thiol, hydrazide, tyramine, and methacrylate groups to facilitate further hydrogel formation with specific cross-linkers via physical cross-linking, click chemistry, or radical polymerization [137]. For example, methacrylated HA macromers can combine with PEGDA and PEG-peptide macromers to produce stable hydrogels via photopolymerization [194]. Currently, there are several commercially available HA-based hybrid hydrogels for cell culture and regenerative medicine. HyStem™ HA-based hydrogels from BioTime is composed of thiol-modified HA, thiol-modified gelatin, and thiol-reactive cross-linker PEG-diacrylate [125]. The major drawbacks of such hydrogel products are relatively long gelation times and high cross-linker concentrations. Besides, it is hard for HyStem to balance the gelation time, hydrogel stiffness, and cellular response.

Hyperbranched Polymer-Based Hybrid Hydrogels As previously covered, HPs can generate injectable hydrogels using the UV photo-cross-linking method, while it might be limited by extra equipment requirements, clinical safety, and feasibility concerns. Thiol-ene click Michael addition has been recognized as a simple reaction that leads to ubiquitous implementation because of its high yield, removable and nontoxic byproducts, and rapid processing under mild reaction conditions [195–197]. Thus, Wang and coworkers further created *in situ* cross-linked hydrogels using hyperbranched PEG-based multi-acrylate macromers synthesized by ATRP or RAFT polymerization and thiolated HA or gelatin via Michael addition as a biocompatible cell culture niche [86, 198–200]. By altering the content of multifunctional groups that are essential for cross-linking, the hydrogel gelation time can be highly tuneable. Within an adequate gelation time, an injected mixture can stay in the position of interest and cell encapsulation can occur in a benign manner. Such hydrogel platforms have potential to address clinical needs for improved materials.

Based on this strategy, more work has been done for generation of injectable hybrid hydrogels as stem cell delivery platforms for tissue repair and regeneration by the Wang group [180, 198–204].

14.3.2 Injectable Hydrogels as Scaffolding for Stem Cells Delivery

As discussed above, although stem cell therapy holds great promise for the treatment of wounds, a complementary cell delivery niche is crucial to improve the performance of this therapy. Injectable hydrogels act as a scaffolding within which therapeutic cells (e.g. ADSCs) can be delivered to the defect site with moldable and minimal invasion and cell protection. In this microenvironment, the therapeutic cells can survive and perform their function. The injectable hydrogels that Wang group created have been proved to be reliable platform for 3D cell culture and stem delivery for wound healing (Figure 14.5). By altering the content of multifunctional groups that are essential for cross-linking, the hydrogel gelation time can be highly tuneable. Within an adequate gelation time, an injected mixture can stay in the position of interest and cell encapsulation can occur in a benign manner.

Wang and coworkers performed a study to examine the retention and function of ADSCs within an injectable hydrogel scaffold composed of hyperbranched PEG polymers and thiolated hyaluronic acid (HA-SH) [199]. The ADSCs were mixed and suspended within one of two precursor solutions. The viability of these cells was examined up to two weeks after these gels were formed. It was found that over 90% viability was observed after this period. Following their findings, Wang and coworkers had generated another ADSC-seeded hydrogel composed of hyperbranched PEG polymers and thiolated gelatin and assessed its wound healing ability in a murine wound model [200]. The hydrogels were formed within two minutes under physiological condition and with adjustable degradation and mechanical properties. The findings also demonstrated desired biocompatibility and enhanced stem cell properties of the hydrogels *in vitro*. Stem cell pluripotency and secretion profile were analyzed and data suggested that ADSCs encapsulated in the hydrogel maintained well-regenerative potential. By delivery of ADSCs to the murine skin wound model, the hydrogel provides a functional niche for stem cell retention and engraftment evidenced by a 14-day bioluminescence imaging of luciferase^{+} ADSCs. This platform was applied to a diabetic murine wound model, and high stem cell retention was detected in the more hostile wound environment [201]. In both studies, ADSC-hydrogel-based treatment decreases inflammatory cell infiltration, enhances neovascularization, and remarkably accelerates wound closure.

The Wang group has other studies that explored the potential of cell-seeded injectable hydrogel technology for chronic wound healing, like diabetic wounds. They developed an injectable hydrogel dressing from hyperbranched macromers using the kinetically controlled homopolymerization of PEGDA via a facile one-pot *in situ* RAFT polymerization and HA-SH (Figure 14.6) [94]. The advantages of this approach are (i) the elimination of the sophisticated and time-consuming synthesis procedure of RAFT agent, which requires toxic and noxious chemicals; (ii) the use of disulphiram (DS) as a biocompatible chain transfer agent reagent, which is as an old anti-alcoholic drug and recently has been reported as an anticancer drug [205]; and (iii) kinetically controlled polymerization of divinyl monomer for hyperbranched polymers using one-pot *in situ* RAFT polymerization. These new injectable hydrogels with stable mechanical properties, non-swelling, and antifouling properties were used to deliver ADSCs. Hydrogels with encapsulated ADSCs have demonstrated promising regenerative capabilities such as the maintenance of ADSC stemness and secretion abilities (PIGF, VEGF, and TGF-β) *in vitro*. The ADSC-embedded hydrogels were tested for the treatment of a diabetic wound in a splinted diabetic rat skin wound model, showing enhanced wound healing by inhibiting inflammation and promoting angiogenesis and reepithelialization.

Controlling the degradation rate in a way to match tissue regeneration is a challenging issue in the design of biomaterials for tissue repair and regeneration. Rapid degradation will not support sufficient tissue ingrowth and lead to fast release of encapsulated stem cells, whereas slow degradation will prevent proper tissue development. Linear poly(β-amino ester)s (PBAEs) developed by Langer and coworkers was obtained with a wide range of degradation rates (from hours to months) by applying diverse monomer sources [206]. By modifying the "A2+B4" Michael addition reaction, Wang and coworkers developed a series of hyperbranched poly(β-amino ester)s (HB-PBAEs) macromers (Figure 14.7) [203]. PEGDA monomers, with various number of PEG units and diamines with different hydrophobic chain lengths, were used for HB-PBAE macromer synthesis. The HP-PBAEs overcome the limitations of linear PBAEs such as fewer terminal functional groups and lower molecular weight leading to injectable hydrogels with low cross-linking density and weak mechanical properties. The HB-PBAEs have fast gelation with HA-SH via a "click" thiol-ene reaction. HB-PBAE–HA-SH hydrogels showed tuneable degradation profiles both *in vitro* and *in vivo*. The hydrogels with optimized degradation profiles encapsulating ADSCs were used to treat two different types of splinted excisional wounds – acute wounds with faster healing rates and diabetic wounds with slower healing and neo-tissue formation rates. The fast-degrading hydrogel showed accelerated wound closure in acute wounds, while the slow-degrading hydrogel exhibited better wound healing for diabetic wounds evidenced by inhibiting the prolonged inflammation, promoting vasculogenesis and reepithelialization. The results demonstrate that the new HB-PBAE-based hydrogel

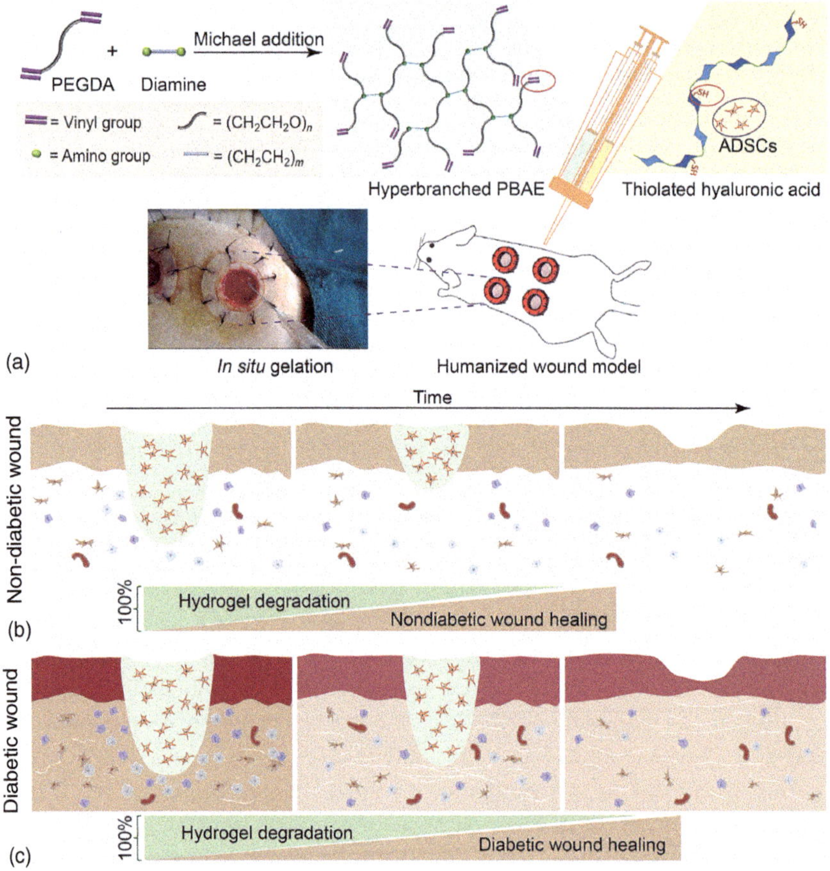

Figure 14.7 Schematic presentation of the formation of HB-PBAEs and proposed function of HB-PBAE/HA-SH hydrogels for modulating nondiabetic and diabetic wound healing. Crosslinking will happen once the groups of vinyl and thiol are reacting. Source: Xu, Q., et al. (2018), [203], Figure 01, Pg 08 / Royal Society of Chemistry / CC BY-NC 3.0.

in combination with ADSCs can be used as a well-controlled biodegradable skin substitute.

In another study, well-controlled "A2 + B4" Michael addition was used to synthesize a series of hyperbranched poly(β-hydrazide ester) macromers (HB-PBHE) with desired molecular weights (Figure 14.8) [204]. The macromer structure and functional groups (vinyl end groups and hydrazide contents) were confirmed. Due to the abundant vinyl end groups, HP-PBHEs can easily form hydrogels with HA-SH or upon UV irradiation under mild physiological conditions. HP-PBHEs and the resulting hydrogels with disulfide moieties possess significant antioxidative and radical scavenging abilities with a versatile tunable multi-responsive degradation property compared with the counterparts synthesized by an only dihydrazide monomer without disulfide bonds. The cell viability under a high ROS environment can be well maintained under the protection of disulfide containing hydrogels in *in vitro* experiments.

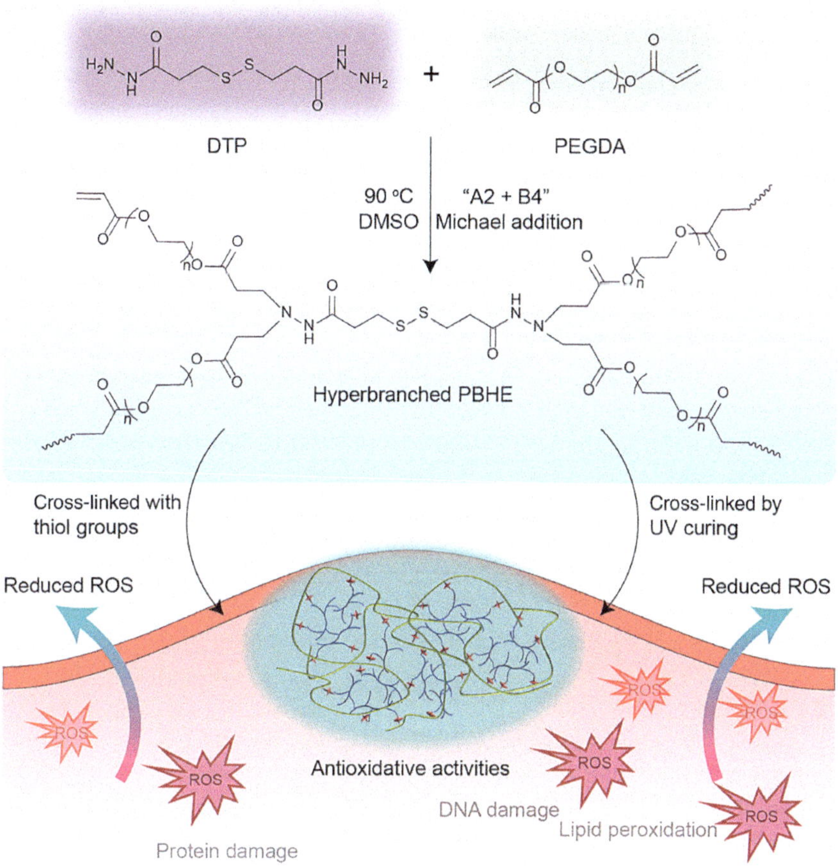

Figure 14.8 Preparation of HB-PBHE macromers and fabrication of antioxidative hydrogels [204].

References

1 Eming, S.A., Martin, P., and Tomic-Canic, M. (2014). Wound repair and regeneration: mechanisms, signaling, and translation. *Sci. Transl. Med.* 6: 265sr6.

2 Gurtner, G.C., Werner, S., Barrandon, Y., and Longaker, M.T. (2008). Wound repair and regeneration. *Nature* 453: 314–321.

3 Blais, M., Parenteau-Bariel, R., Cadau, S., and Berthod, F. (2013). Concise review: tissue-engineered skin and nerve regeneration in burn treatment. *Stem Cells Transl. Med.* 2: 545–551. https://doi.org/10.1002/sctm.17-0054.

4 ter Horst, B., Chouhan, G., Moiemen, N.S., and Grover, L.M. (2018). Advances in keratinocyte delivery in burn wound care. *Adv. Drug Delivery Rev.* 123: 18–32.

5 Rodgers, K. and Jadhav, S.S. (2018). The application of mesenchymal stem cells to treat thermal and radiation burns. *Adv. Drug Delivery Rev.* 123: 75–81.

6 Zulkowski, K. (2017). Understanding moisture-associated skin damage, medical adhesive-related skin injuries, and skin tears. *Adv. Skin Wound Care* 30: 372–378.

7 Castaño, O., Pérez-Amodio, S., Navarro-Requena, C. et al. (2018). Instructive microenvironments in skin wound healing: biomaterials as signal releasing platforms. *Adv. Drug Delivery Rev.* 129: 95–117.

8 Iismaa, S.E., Xenia, K., Nicks Amy, M. et al. (2018). Comparative regenerative mechanisms across different mammalian tissues. *npj Regener. Med.* 3: 1–20. https://doi.org/10.1038/s41536-018-0044-5.

9 Xue, M., Zhao, R., Lin, H., and Jackson, C. (2018). Delivery systems of current biologicals for the treatment of chronic cutaneous wounds and severe burns. *Adv. Drug Delivery Rev.* 129: 219–241.

10 Lin, Y.K., Chen, K.H., Ou, K.L., and Liu, M. (2011). Effects of different extracellular matrices and growth factor immobilization on biodegradability and biocompatibility of macroporous bacterial cellulose. *J. Bioact. Compat. Polym.* 26: 508–518.

11 Kim, B.S. et al. (2018). 3D cell printing of in vitro stabilized skin model and in vivo pre-vascularized skin patch using tissue-specific extracellular matrix bioink: a step towards advanced skin tissue engineering. *Biomaterials* 168: 38–53.

12 Barrientos, S., Stojadinovic, O., Golinko, M.S. et al. (2008). Growth factors and cytokines in wound healing. *Wound Repair Regener.* 16: 585–601.

13 Arandjelovic, P. and Kaur, P. (2014). The regenerative potential of epithelial stem cells in tissue repair. *Int. J. Biochem. Cell Biol.* 56: 107–110.

14 Hassan, W.U., Greiser, U., and Wang, W. (2014). Role of adipose-derived stem cells in wound healing. *Wound Repair Regener.* 22: 313–325.

15 Spiekman, M., Przybyt, E., Plantinga, J.A. et al. (2014). Adipose tissue-derived stromal cells inhibit TGF-β1-induced differentiation of human dermal fibroblasts and keloid scar-derived fibroblasts in a paracrine fashion. *Plast. Reconstr. Surg.* 134 (4): 699–712.

16 Sekhon, U.D.S. and Sen Gupta, A. (2017). Platelets and platelet-inspired biomaterials technologies in wound healing applications. *ACS Biomater. Sci. Eng.* 4: 1176–1192. https://doi.org/10.1021/acsbiomaterials.7b00013.

17 Rani, S. and Ritter, T. (2016). The exosome – a naturally secreted nanoparticle and its application to wound healing. *Adv. Mater.* 28: 5542–5552.

18 Lord, J.M. et al. (2014). The systemic immune response to trauma: an overview of pathophysiology and treatment. *Lancet* 384: 1455–1465.

19 Mendes, B.B. et al. (2018). Blood derivatives awaken in regenerative medicine strategies to modulate wound healing. *Adv. Drug Delivery Rev.* 129: 376–393. https://doi.org/10.1016/j.addr.2017.12.018.

20 Clark, R.A.F. (2006). Fibrin and wound healing. *Ann. N.Y. Acad. Sci.* 936: 355–367.

21 Serhan, C.N., Chiang, N., and Van Dyke, T.E. (2008). Resolving inflammation: dual anti-inflammatory and pro-resolution lipid mediators. *Nat. Rev. Immunol.* 8: 349–361.

22 Ruchaud-Sparagano, M.H., Mills, R., Scott, J., and Simpson, A.J. (2014). MPLA inhibits release of cytotoxic mediators from human neutrophils while preserving efficient bacterial killing. *Immunol. Cell Biol.* 92: 799–809.

23 Mittal, M., Siddiqui, M.R., Tran, K. et al. (2014). Reactive oxygen species in inflammation and tissue injury. *Antioxid. Redox Signaling* 20: 1126–1167.

24 Kolaczkowska, E. and Kubes, P. (2013). Neutrophil recruitment and function in health and inflammation. *Nat. Rev. Immunol.* 13: 159–175.

25 Cahill, T.J., Choudhury, R.P., and Riley, P.R. (2017). Heart regeneration and repair after myocardial infarction: translational opportunities for novel therapeutics. *Nat. Rev. Drug Discovery* 16: 699–717.

26 Veith, A.P., Henderson, K., Spencer, A. et al. (2018). Therapeutic strategies for enhancing angiogenesis in wound healing. *Adv. Drug Delivery Rev.* 146: 97–125.

27 Mitrousis, N., Fokina, A., and Shoichet, M.S. (2018). Biomaterials for cell transplantation. *Nat. Rev. Mater.* 3: 441–456. https://doi.org/10.1038/s41578-018-0057-0.

28 Lohmann, N. et al. (2017). Glycosaminoglycan-based hydrogels capture chemokines and rescue wound healing deficiency. *Sci. Transl. Med.* 9: eaai9044.

29 Tanno, H. et al. (2017). Invariant NKT cells promote skin wound healing by preventing a prolonged neutrophilic inflammatory response. *Wound Repair Regener.* 25: 805–815.

30 Li, J., Chen, J., and Kirsner, R. (2007). Pathophysiology of acute wound healing. *Clin. Dermatol.* 25: 9–18.

31 Spravchikov, N. et al. (2001). Glucose effects on skin keratinocytes implications for diabetes skin complications. *Diabetes* 50: 1627–1635.

32 Xu, K.-P., Li, Y., Ljubimov, A.V., and Yu, F.-S.X. (2009). High glucose suppresses epidermal growth factor receptor/phosphatidylinositol 3-kinase/Akt signaling pathway and attenuates corneal epithelial wound healing. *Diabetes* 58: 1077–1085.

33 Falanga, V. (2005). Wound healing and its impairment in the diabetic foot. *Lancet* 366: 1736–1743.

34 Wang, Y. et al. (2017). Burn injury: challenges and advances in burn wound healing, infection, pain and scarring. *Adv. Drug Delivery Rev.* 123: 3–17.

35 Liu, H., Yin, Y., and Yao, K. (2007). Construction of chitosan-gelatin-hyaluronic acid artificial skin in vitro. *J. Biomater. Appl.* 21: 413–430.

36 Browser, J. et al. (2011). Mesenchymal stem cell therapy and delivery systems in nonhealing wounds. *Adv. Skin Wound Care* 24: 337–342.

37 Singh, S., Young, A., and McNaught, C.E. (2017). The physiology of wound healing. *Surgery* 35: 473–477.

38 Zhang, X. et al. (2015). A systematic and quantitative method for wound-dressing evaluation. *Burn. Trauma* 3: 15.

39 Kim, J., Mirando, A.C., Popel, A.S., and Green, J.J. (2017). Gene delivery nanoparticles to modulate angiogenesis. *Adv. Drug Delivery Rev.* 119: 20–43.

40 Cao, L. et al. (2004). VEGF links hippocampal activity with neurogenesis, learning and memory. *Nat. Genet.* 36: 827–835.

41 Ofek, P., Tiram, G., and Satchi-Fainaro, R. (2017). Angiogenesis regulation by nanocarriers bearing RNA interference. *Adv. Drug Delivery Rev.* 119: 3–19.
42 Gonzalez-King, H. et al. (2017). Hypoxia inducible factor-1 a potentiates jagged 1-mediated angiogenesis by mesenchymal stem cell-derived exosomes. *Stem Cells* 35: 1747–1759.
43 Rafii, S., Butler, J.M., and Ding, B.S. (2016). Angiocrine functions of organ-specific endothelial cells. *Nature* 529: 316–325.
44 Okonkwo, U. and DiPietro, L. (2017). Diabetes and wound angiogenesis. *Int. J. Mol. Sci.* 18: 1419.
45 Lauer, G. et al. (2000). Expression and proteolysis of vascular endothelial growth factor is increased in chronic wounds. *J. Invest. Dermatol.* 115: 12–18.
46 Kolluru, G.K., Bir, S.C., and Kevil, C.G. (2012). Endothelial dysfunction and diabetes: effects on angiogenesis, vascular remodeling, and wound healing. *Int. J. Vasc. Med.* 2012: 1–30.
47 Dinh, T. et al. (2012). Mechanisms involved in the development and healing of diabetic foot ulceration. *Diabetes* 61: 2937–2947.
48 Ahmad, J. (2016). The diabetic foot. *Diabetes Metab. Syndr. Clin. Res. Rev.* 10: 48–60.
49 Longinotti, C. (2014). The use of hyaluronic acid based dressings to treat burns: a review. *Burn. Trauma* 2: 162.
50 Martin, P. (1997). Wound healing – aiming for perfect skin regeneration. *Science* 276: 75–81.
51 Penn, J.W., Grobbelaar, A.O., and Rolfe, K.J. (2012). The role of the TGF-β family in wound healing, burns and scarring: a review. *Int. J. Burns Trauma* 2: 18–28.
52 Wang, L. et al. (2017). Exosomes secreted by human adipose mesenchymal stem cells promote scarless cutaneous repair by regulating extracellular matrix remodelling. *Sci. Rep.* 7: 13321–13333. https://doi.org/10.1038/s41598-017-12919-x.
53 Gourdie, R.G., Dimmeler, S., and Kohl, P. (2016). Novel therapeutic strategies targeting fibroblasts and fibrosis in heart disease. *Nat. Rev. Drug Discovery* 15: 620–638.
54 Fang, S., Liu, H., and Xing, X. (2016). Umbilical cord-derived mesenchymal stem cell-derived exosomal MicroRNAs suppress myofibroblast differentiation by inhibiting the transforming growth factor-b/SMAD2 pathway during wound healing. *Stem Cells Tranls. Med.* 5 (10): 1–15.
55 Loots, M. (2002). Fibroblasts derived from chronic diabetic ulcers differ in their response to stimulation with EGF, IGF-I, bFGF and PDGF-AB compared to controls. *Eur. J. Cell Biol.* 81: 153–160.
56 Lerman, O.Z., Galiano, R.D., Armour, M. et al. (2003). Cellular dysfunction in the diabetic fibroblast: impairment in migration, vascular endothelial growth factor production, and response to hypoxia. *Am. J. Pathol.* 162: 303–312.
57 Diegelmann, R.F. and Evans, M.C. (2004). Wound healing: an overview of acute, fibrotic and delayed healing. *Front. Biosci.* 9: 283–289.

58 Reynolds, L.E. et al. (2005). Accelerated re-epithelialization in β3-integrin-deficient mice is associated with enhanced TGF-β1 signaling. *Nat. Med.* 11: 167–174.

59 Rousselle, P., Montmasson, M., and Garnier, C. (2018). Extracellular matrix contribution to skin wound re-epithelialization. *Matrix Biol.* 75–76: 12–26. https://doi.org/10.1016/j.matbio.2018.01.002.

60 Singer, A.J. and Clark, R.A.F. (1999). Cutaneous wound healing. *N. Engl. J. Med.* 341: 738–746.

61 Shirakata, Y. (2005). Heparin-binding EGF-like growth factor accelerates keratinocyte migration and skin wound healing. *J. Cell Sci.* 118: 2363–2370.

62 Stojadinovic, O. et al. (2005). Molecular pathogenesis of chronic wounds. *Am. J. Pathol.* 167: 59–69.

63 Brem, H. and Tomic-Canic, M. (2007). Cellular and molecular basis of wound healing in diabetes. *J. Clin. Invest.* 117: 1219–1222.

64 Zhang, B. et al. (2016). HucMSC exosome-delivered 14-3-3ζ orchestrates self-control of the Wnt response via modulation of YAP during cutaneous regeneration. *Stem Cells* 34: 2485–2500.

65 Lim, C.H. et al. (2018). Hedgehog stimulates hair follicle neogenesis by creating inductive dermis during murine skin wound healing. *Nat. Commun.* 9: 4903–4916. https://doi.org/10.1038/s41467-018-07142-9.

66 Peng, B., Chen, Y., and Leong, K.W. (2015). MicroRNA delivery for regenerative medicine. *Adv. Drug Delivery Rev.* 88: 108–122.

67 Hart, C. et al. (2004). Contribution of bone marrow–derived cells to skin: collagen deposition and wound repair. *Stem Cells* 22 (5): 580–589.

68 Ireton, J.E., Unger, J.G., and Rohrich, R.J. (2013). The role of wound healing and its everyday application in plastic surgery: a practical perspective and systematic review. *Plast. Reconstr. Surg. Glob. Open* 1: 1–10. https://doi.org/10.1097/GOX.0b013e31828ff9f4.

69 Buchstein, N. et al. (2009). Alternative proteolytic processing of hepatocyte growth factor during wound repair. *Am. J. Pathol.* 174: 2116–2128.

70 Werner, S., Krieg, T., and Smola, H. (2007). Keratinocyte-fibroblast interactions in wound healing. *J. Invest. Dermatol.* 127: 998–1008.

71 Chua, A.W.C. et al. (2016). Skin tissue engineering advances in severe burns: review and therapeutic applications. *Burns Trauma* 4: 14.

72 Phinney, D.G. and Pittenger, M.F. (2017). Concise review: MSC-derived exosomes for cell-free therapy. *Stem Cells* 35: 851–858.

73 Duelen, R. and Sampaolesi, M. (2017). Stem cell technology in cardiac regeneration: a pluripotent stem cell promise. *EBioMedicine* 16: 30–40.

74 Vizoso, F.J., Eiro, N., Cid, S. et al. (2017). Mesenchymal stem cell secretome: toward cell-free therapeutic strategies in regenerative medicine. *Int. J. Mol. Sci.* 18: 1852.

75 Fujita, Y. and Kawamoto, A. (2017). Stem cell-based peripheral vascular regeneration. *Adv. Drug Delivery Rev.* 120: 25–40.

76 Tran, C. and Damaser, M.S. (2015). Stem cells as drug delivery methods: application of stem cell secretome for regeneration. *Adv. Drug Delivery Rev.* 82, 83: 1–11.

77 Nakagawa, H., Akita, S., Fukui, M. et al. (2005). Human mesenchymal stem cells successfully improve skin-substitute wound healing. *Br. J. Dermatol.* 153: 29–36.

78 Phinney, D.G. and Prockop, D.J. (2007). Concise review: mesenchymal stem/multipotent stromal cells: the state of transdifferentiation and modes of tissue repair-current views. *Stem Cells* 25: 2896–2902.

79 Karp, J.M. and Leng Teo, G.S. (2009). Mesenchymal stem cell homing: the devil is in the details. *Cell Stem Cell* 4: 206–216.

80 Faroni, A., Mobasseri, S.A., Kingham, P.J., and Reid, A.J. (2015). Peripheral nerve regeneration: experimental strategies and future perspectives. *Adv. Drug Delivery Rev.* 82: 160–167.

81 Sakurada, K., McDonald, F.M., and Shimada, F. (2008). Regenerative medicine and stem cell based drug discovery. *Angew. Chem. Int. Ed.* 47: 5718–5738.

82 Wu, Y., Chen, L., Scott, P.G., and Tredget, E.E. (2007). Mesenchymal stem cells enhance wound healing through differentiation and angiogenesis. *Stem Cells* 25: 2648–2659.

83 Wu, Y., Zhao, R.C.H., and Tredget, E.E. (2010). Concise review: bone marrow-derived stem/progenitor cells in cutaneous repair and regeneration. *Stem Cells* 28: 905–915.

84 Madrigal, M., Rao, K.S., and Riordan, N.H. (2014). A review of therapeutic effects of mesenchymal stem cell secretions and induction of secretory modification by different culture methods. *J. Transl. Med.* 12: 1–14.

85 Kuo, Y.R. et al. (2011). Bone marrow-derived mesenchymal stem cells enhanced diabetic wound healing through recruitment of tissue regeneration in a rat model of streptozotocin-induced diabetes. *Plast. Reconstr. Surg.* 128: 872–880.

86 Dong, Y. et al. (2014). Performance of an in situ formed bioactive hydrogel dressing from a PEG-based hyperbranched multifunctional copolymer. *Acta Biomater.* 10: 2076–2085.

87 Crivelli, B. et al. (2017). Mesenchymal stem/stromal cell extracellular vesicles: from active principle to next generation drug delivery system. *J. Controlled Release* 262: 104–117.

88 Fini, M. et al. (2005). The healing of confined critical size cancellous defects in the presence of silk fibroin hydrogel. *Biomaterials* 26: 3527–3536.

89 Georgiou, M., Golding, J.P., Loughlin, A.J. et al. (2015). Engineered neural tissue with aligned, differentiated adipose-derived stem cells promotes peripheral nerve regeneration across a critical sized defect in rat sciatic nerve. *Biomaterials* 37: 242–251.

90 Toh, W.S., Lai, R.C., Hui, J.H.P., and Lim, S.K. (2017). MSC exosome as a cell-free MSC therapy for cartilage regeneration: implications for osteoarthritis treatment. *Semin. Cell Dev. Biol.* 67: 56–64.

91 Arno, A. et al. (2011). Stem cell therapy: a new treatment for burns? *Pharmaceuticals* 4: 1355–1380.

92 Rivera-Valdés, J.J. et al. (2017). Human adipose derived stem cells regress fibrosis in a chronic renal fibrotic model induced by adenine. *PLoS One* 12: 1–14. https://doi.org/10.1371/journal.pone.0187907.

93 Li, X. et al. (2018). Exosomes from adipose-derived stem cells overexpressing Nrf2 accelerate cutaneous wound healing by promoting vascularization in a diabetic foot ulcer rat model. *Exp. Mol. Med.* 50: 1–14.

94 Xu, Q. et al. (2018). A hybrid injectable hydrogel from hyperbranched PEG macromer as a stem cell delivery and retention platform for diabetic wound healing. *Acta Biomater.* 75: 63–74.

95 Zuk, P.A. et al. (2002). Human adipose tissue is a source of multipotent stem cells. *Mol. Biol. Cell* 13: 4279–4295.

96 Naderi, N. et al. (2017). The regenerative role of adipose-derived stem cells (ADSC) in plastic and reconstructive surgery. *Int. Wound J.* 14: 112–124.

97 Zhao, J., Hu, L., Liu, J. et al. (2013). The effects of cytokines in adipose stem cell-conditioned medium on the migration and proliferation of skin fibroblasts in vitro. *Biomed Res. Int.* 2013: 1–11.

98 Pu, C.M. et al. (2017). Adipose-derived stem cells protect skin flaps against ischemia/reperfusion injury via IL-6 expression. *J. Invest. Dermatol.* 137: 1353–1362.

99 Kato, Y. et al. (2015). Allogeneic transplantation of an adipose-derived stem cell sheet combined with artificial skin accelerates wound healing in a rat wound model of type 2 diabetes and obesity. *Diabetes* 64: 2723–2734.

100 Trottier, V., Marceau-Fortier, G., Germain, L. et al. (2008). IFATS collection: using human adipose-derived stem/stromal cells for the production of new skin substitutes. *Stem Cells* 26: 2713–2723.

101 Mooney, D.J. and Vandenburgh, H. (2008). Cell delivery mechanisms for tissue repair. *Cell Stem Cell* 2: 205–213.

102 Caló, E. and Khutoryanskiy, V.V. (2015). Biomedical applications of hydrogels: a review of patents and commercial products. *Eur. Polym. J.* 65: 252–267.

103 Fonder, M.A. et al. (2008). Treating the chronic wound: a practical approach to the care of nonhealing wounds and wound care dressings. *J. Am. Acad. Dermatol.* 58: 185–206.

104 Vowden, K. and Vowden, P. (2017). Wound dressings: principles and practice. *Surg.* 35: 489–494.

105 Schultz, G.S. et al. (2003). Wound bed preparation: a systematic approach to wound management. *Wound Repair Regener.* 11 (Suppl 1): S1–S28.

106 Madaghiele, M., Sannino, A., Ambrosio, L., and Demitri, C. (2014). Polymeric hydrogels for burn wound care: advanced skin wound dressings and regenerative templates. *Burns Trauma* 2: 153–161.

107 Kamoun, E.A., Kenawy, E.R.S., and Chen, X. (2017). A review on polymeric hydrogel membranes for wound dressing applications: PVA-based hydrogel dressings. *J. Adv. Res.* 8: 217–233.

108 Konieczynska, M.D. et al. (2016). On-demand dissolution of a dendritic hydrogel-based dressing for second-degree burn wounds through thiol–thioester exchange reaction. *Angew. Chem. Int. Ed.* 55: 9984–9987.

109 Langer, R. and Tirrell, D.A. (2004). Designing materials for biology and medicine. *Nature* 428: 487–492.

110 Li, Y., Rodrigues, J., and Tomás, H. (2012). Injectable and biodegradable hydrogels: gelation, biodegradation and biomedical applications. *Chem. Soc. Rev.* 41: 2193–2221.

111 Ko, D.Y., Shinde, U.P., Yeon, B., and Jeong, B. (2013). Recent progress of in situ formed gels for biomedical applications. *Prog. Polym. Sci.* 38: 672–701.

112 Dimatteo, R., Darling, N.J., and Segura, T. (2018). In situ forming injectable hydrogels for drug delivery and wound repair. *Adv. Drug Delivery Rev.* 127: 167–184.

113 Burdick, J.A., Mauck, R.L., and Gerecht, S. (2016). To serve and protect: hydrogels to improve stem cell-based therapies. *Cell Stem Cell* 18: 13–15.

114 Khademhosseini, A. and Langer, R. (2007). Microengineered hydrogels for tissue engineering. *Biomaterials* 28: 5087–5092.

115 Slaughter, B.B.V. et al. (2009). Hydrogels in regenerative medicine. *Adv. Mater.* 21: 3307–3329.

116 Huang, Q. et al. (2017). Hydrogel scaffolds for differentiation of adipose-derived stem cells. *Chem. Soc. Rev.* 46: 6255–6275.

117 Lutolf, M.P., Gilbert, P.M., and Blau, H.M. (2009). Designing materials to direct stem-cell fate. *Nature* 462: 433–441.

118 Pérez, R.A., Won, J.E., Knowles, J.C., and Kim, H.W. (2013). Naturally and synthetic smart composite biomaterials for tissue regeneration. *Adv. Drug Delivery Rev.* 65: 471–496.

119 Huebsch, N. et al. (2010). Harnessing traction-mediated manipulation of the cell/matrix interface to control stem-cell fate. *Nat. Mater.* 9: 518–526.

120 Vermonden, T., Censi, R., and Hennink, W.E. (2012). Hydrogels for protein delivery. *Chem. Rev.* 112: 2853–2888.

121 Censi, R., Di Martino, P., Vermonden, T., and Hennink, W.E. (2012). Hydrogels for protein delivery in tissue engineering. *J. Controlled Release* 161: 680–692.

122 Jones, A. and Vaughan, D. (2005). Hydrogel dressings in the management of a variety of wound types: a review. *J. Orthop. Nurs.* 9: S1–S11.

123 Madl, C.M., Heilshorn, S.C., and Blau, H.M. (2018). Bioengineering strategies to accelerate stem cell therapeutics. *Nature* 557: 335–342.

124 Yang, J.A., Yeom, J., Hwang, B.W. et al. (2014). In situ-forming injectable hydrogels for regenerative medicine. *Prog. Polym. Sci.* 39: 1973–1986.

125 Caliari, S.R. and Burdick, J.A. (2016). A practical guide to hydrogels for cell culture. *Nat. Methods* 13: 405–414.

126 Wang, C., Stewart, R.J., and KopeČek, J. (1999). Hybrid hydrogels assembled from synthetic polymers and coiled-coil protein domains. *Nature* 397: 417–420.

127 Kopeček, J. (2007). Hydrogel biomaterials: a smart future? *Biomaterials* 28: 5185–5192.

128 Rujitanaroj, P., Pimpha, N., and Supaphol, P. (2008). Wound-dressing materials with antibacterial activity from electrospun gelatin fiber mats containing silver nanoparticles. *Polymer* 49: 4723–4732.

129 Farris, S., Song, J., and Huang, Q. (2010). Alternative reaction mechanism for the cross-linking of gelatin with glutaraldehyde. *J. Agric. Food. Chem.* 58: 998–1003.
130 Ruszczak, Z. (2003). Effect of collagen matrices on dermal wound healing. *Adv. Drug Delivery Rev.* 55: 1595–1611.
131 Omobono, M.A. et al. (2015). Enhancing the stiffness of collagen hydrogels for delivery of encapsulated chondrocytes to articular lesions for cartilage regeneration. *J. Biomed. Mater. Res. Part A* 103: 1332–1338.
132 Wang, W., Sun, L., Zhang, P. et al. (2014). An anti-inflammatory cell-free collagen/resveratrol scaffold for repairing osteochondral defects in rabbits. *Acta Biomater.* 10: 4983–4995.
133 Gorgieva, S. and Kokol, V. (2011). Collagen- vs. gelatine-based biomaterials and their biocompatibility: review and perspectives. *Biomater. Appl. Nanomed.* 2011: 17–51. https://doi.org/10.5772/24118.
134 Fraser, J.R.E., Laurent, T.C., and Laurent, U.B.G. (1997). Hyaluronan: its nature, distribution, functions and turnover. *J. Intern. Med.* 242: 27–33.
135 Toole, B.P. (2001). Hyaluronan in morphogenesis. *Semin. Cell Dev. Biol.* 12: 79–87.
136 Necas, J., Bartosikova, L., Brauner, P., and Kolar, J. (2008). Hyaluronic acid (hyaluronan): a review. *Vet. Med.* 53: 397–411.
137 Burdick, J.A. and Prestwich, G.D. (2011). Hyaluronic acid hydrogels for biomedical applications. *Adv. Mater.* 23: 41–56.
138 Frenkel, J.S. (2014). The role of hyaluronan in wound healing. *Int. Wound J.* 11: 159–163.
139 Unterman, S.A. et al. (2012). Hyaluronic acid-binding scaffold for articular cartilage repair. *Tissue Eng. Part A* 18: 2497–2506.
140 Hwang, N.S., Varghese, S., Li, H., and Elisseeff, J. (2011). Regulation of osteogenic and chondrogenic differentiation of mesenchymal stem cells in PEG-ECM hydrogels. *Cell Tissue Res.* 344: 499–509.
141 Collins, M.N. and Birkinshaw, C. (2013). Hyaluronic acid based scaffolds for tissue engineering – a review. *Carbohydr. Polym.* 92: 1262–1279.
142 Fakhari, A. and Berkland, C. (2013). Applications and emerging trends of hyaluronic acid in tissue engineering, as a dermal filler and in osteoarthritis treatment. *Acta Biomater.* 9: 7081–7092.
143 Gerecht, S. et al. (2007). Hyaluronic acid hydrogel for controlled self-renewal and differentiation of human embryonic stem cells. *Proc. Natl. Acad. Sci. U.S.A.* 104: 11298–11303.
144 Segura, T. et al. (2005). Crosslinked hyaluronic acid hydrogels: a strategy to functionalize and pattern. *Biomaterials* 26: 359–371.
145 Xu, X., Jha, A.K., Harrington, D.A. et al. (2012). Hyaluronic acid-based hydrogels: from a natural polysaccharide to complex networks. *Soft Matter* 8: 3280–3294.
146 Heher, P., Mühleder, S., Mittermayr, R. et al. (2018). Fibrin-based delivery strategies for acute and chronic wound healing. *Adv. Drug Delivery Rev.* 129: 134–147.

147 Thompson, D.F., Letassy, N.A., and Thompson, G.D. (1988). Fibrin glue: a review of its preparation, efficacy, and adverse effects as a topical hemostat. *Drug Intell. Clin. Pharm.* 22: 946–952.

148 Branski, L.K. et al. (2011). Fibrin sealant improves graft adherence in a porcine full-thickness burn wound model. *Burns* 37: 1360–1366.

149 Knezevic, L. et al. (2017). Engineering blood and lymphatic microvascular networks in fibrin matrices. *Front. Bioeng. Biotechnol.* 5: 1–12.

150 Pill, K. et al. (2018). Microvascular networks from endothelial cells and mesenchymal stromal cells from adipose tissue and bone marrow: a comparison. *Front. Bioeng. Biotechnol.* 6: 156.

151 Bachmann, B. et al. (2018). Engineering of three-dimensional pre-vascular networks within fibrin hydrogel constructs by microfluidic control over reciprocal cell signaling. *Biomicrofluidics* 12: 042216.

152 Du, J. et al. (2017). Prompt peripheral nerve regeneration induced by a hierarchically aligned fibrin nanofiber hydrogel. *Acta Biomater.* 55: 296–309. https://doi.org/10.1016/j.actbio.2017.04.010.

153 Wichterle, O. and Lim, D. (1960). Hydrophilic gels for biological use. *Nature* 185: 117–118.

154 Kubinová, Š., Horák, D., and Syková, E. (2009). Cholesterol-modified superporous poly(2-hydroxyethyl methacrylate) scaffolds for tissue engineering. *Biomaterials* 30: 4601–4609.

155 Arslantunali, D., Budak, G., and Hasirci, V. (2014). Multiwalled CNT-pHEMA composite conduit for peripheral nerve repair. *J. Biomed. Mater. Res. Part A* 102: 828–841.

156 Drury, J.L. and Mooney, D.J. (2003). Hydrogels for tissue engineering: scaffold design variables and applications. *Biomaterials* 24: 4337–4351.

157 Cascone, M.G., Laus, M., Ricci, D., and Sbarbati Del Guerra, R. (1995). Evaluation of poly(vinyl alcohol) hydrogels as a component of hybrid artificial tissues. *J. Mater. Sci. Mater. Med.* 6: 71–75.

158 Hassan, C.M. and Peppas, N.A. (2000). Structure and morphology of freeze/thawed PVA hydrogels. *Macromolecules* 33: 2472–2479.

159 Nuttelman, C.R., Mortisen, D.J., Henry, S.M., and Anseth, K.S. (2001). Attachment of fibronectin to poly(vinyl alcohol) hydrogels promotes NIH3T3 cell adhesion, proliferation, and migration. *J. Biomed. Mater. Res. Part A* 57: 217–223.

160 Orienti, I., Treré, R., and Zecchi, V. (2001). Hydrogels formed by cross-linked polyvinylalcohol as colon-specific drug delivery systems. *Drug Dev. Ind. Pharm.* 27: 877–884.

161 Martens, P.J., Bryant, S.J., and Anseth, K.S. (2003). Tailoring the degradation of hydrogels formed from multivinyl poly(ethylene glycol) and poly(vinyl alcohol) macromers for cartilage tissue engineering. *Biomacromolecules* 4: 283–292.

162 Accardo, A. et al. (2018). Direct laser fabrication of free-standing PEGDA-hydrogel scaffolds for neuronal cell growth: engineering 3D biocompatible microenvironments. *Mater. Today* 21: 315–316.

163 Shu, X.Z., Liu, Y., Palumbo, F.S. et al. (2004). In situ crosslinkable hyaluronan hydrogels for tissue engineering. *Biomaterials* 25: 1339–1348.

164 Lin, C.-C. and Anseth, K.S. (2009). PEG hydrogels for the controlled release of biomolecules in regenerative medicine. *Pharm. Res.* 26: 631–643.

165 Park, H. et al. (2009). Effect of swelling ratio of injectable hydrogel composites on chondrogenic differentiation of encapsulated rabbit marrow mesenchymal stem cells in vitro. *Biomacromolecules* 10: 541–546.

166 Duan, S. (2005). Negative cooperative effect of cytotoxicity of a di-component initiating system for a novel injectable tissue engineering hydrogel. *Chin. Sci. Bull.* 50: 1093.

167 Ward, J.H. and Peppas, N.A. (2000). Kinetic gelation modeling of controlled radical polymerizations. *Macromolecules* 33: 5137–5142.

168 Wetering, P., Metters, A.T., Schoenmakers, R.G., and Hubbell, J.A. (2005). Poly(ethylene glycol) hydrogels formed by conjugate addition with controllable swelling, degradation, and release of pharmaceutically active proteins. *J. Controlled Release* 102: 619–627.

169 Dobner, S., Bezuidenhout, D., Govender, P. et al. (2009). A synthetic non-degradable polyethylene glycol hydrogel retards adverse post-infarct left ventricular remodeling. *J. Card. Fail.* 15: 629–636.

170 Wang, Y., Zhang, S., and Benoit, D.S.W. (2018). Degradable poly(ethylene glycol) (PEG)-based hydrogels for spatiotemporal control of siRNA/nanoparticle delivery. *J. Controlled Release* 287: 58–66.

171 Shea, T.M.O., Aimetti, A.A., Kim, E. et al. (2015). Synthesis and characterization of a library of in-situ curing, nonswelling ethoxylated polyol thiol-ene hydrogels for tailorable macromolecule delivery communication. *Adv. Mater.* 27: 65–72.

172 Zheng, Y., Li, S., Weng, Z., and Gao, C. (2015). Hyperbranched polymers: advances from synthesis to applications. *Chem. Soc. Rev.* 44: 4091–4130.

173 Wang, D., Zhao, T., Zhu, X. et al. (2015). Bioapplications of hyperbranched polymers. *Chem. Soc. Rev.* 44: 4023–4071.

174 Liu, Y. et al. (2003). Novel poly(amino ester)s obtained from Michael addition polymerizations of trifunctional amine monomers with diacrylates: safe and efficient DNA carriers. *Chem. Commun.* 20: 2630–2631. https://doi.org/10.1039/b309487a.

175 Lee, C.C., MacKay, J.A., Fréchet, J.M.J., and Szoka, F.C. (2005). Designing dendrimers for biological applications. *Nat. Biotechnol.* 23: 1517–1526.

176 Zhou, D. et al. (2016). The transition from linear to highly branched poly(β-amino ester)s: branching matters for gene delivery. *Sci. Adv.* 2: e1600102.

177 Zhao, T., Zheng, Y., Poly, J., and Wang, W. (2013). Controlled multi-vinyl monomer homopolymerization through vinyl oligomer combination as a universal approach to hyperbranched architectures. *Nat. Commun.* 4: 1873.

178 Wang, W. et al. (2007). Controlling chain growth: a new strategy to hyperbranched materials. *Macromolecules* 40: 7184–7194.

179 Dong, Y. et al. (2010). Dual stimuli responsive PEG based hyperbranched polymers. *Polym. Chem.* 1: 827–830.

180 Dong, Y. et al. (2012). Thermoresponsive hyperbranched copolymer with multi acrylate functionality for in situ cross-linkable hyaluronic acid composite semi-IPN hydrogel. *J. Mater. Sci. Mater. Med.* 23: 25–35.

181 Sigen, A. et al. (2017). Hyperbranched PEG-based multi-NHS polymer and bioconjugation with BSA. *Polym. Chem.* 8: 1283–1287.

182 Zheng, Y., Newland, B., Tai, H. et al. (2012). Single cyclized molecule structures from RAFT homopolymerization of multi-vinyl monomers. *Chem. Commun.* 48: 3085–3087.

183 Zhang, H. et al. (2015). On-demand and negative-thermo-swelling tissue adhesive based on highly branched ambivalent PEG–catechol copolymers. *J. Mater. Chem. B* 3: 6420–6428.

184 Tai, H., Tochwin, A., and Wang, W. (2013). Thermoresponsive hyperbranched polymers via in situ RAFT copolymerization of peg-based monomethacrylate and dimethacrylate monomers. *J. Polym. Sci. Part A Polym. Chem.* 51: 3751–3761.

185 Zhao, T. et al. (2014). Significance of branching for transfection: synthesis of highly branched degradable functional poly(dimethylaminoethyl methacrylate) by vinyl oligomer combination. *Angew. Chem. Int. Ed.* 53: 6095–6100.

186 Cutlar, L. et al. (2015). Highly branched poly(β-amino esters): synthesis and application in gene delivery. *Biomacromolecules* 16: 2609–2617.

187 Huang, J.-Y. et al. (2015). Tailoring highly branched poly(β-amino ester)s: a synthetic platform for epidermal gene therapy. *Chem. Commun.* 51: 8473–8476.

188 Zhou, D. et al. (2016). Highly branched poly(β-amino ester)s for skin gene therapy. *J. Controlled Release* 244: 336–346.

189 Ruel-Gariépy, E. and Leroux, J.C. (2004). In situ-forming hydrogels – review of temperature-sensitive systems. *Eur. J. Pharm. Biopharm.* 58: 409–426.

190 Klouda, L. and Mikos, A.G. (2008). Thermoresponsive hydrogels in biomedical applications. *Eur. J. Pharm. Biopharm.* 68: 34–45.

191 Soman, A., Mathew, F., Chacko, A.J. et al. (2014). Interpenetrating polymer network (Ipn) – hydrogels. *Pharma Innov. J.* 3: 59–66.

192 Munoz-Pinto, D.J., Jimenez-Vergara, A.C., Gharat, T.P., and Hahn, M.S. (2015). Characterization of sequential collagen-poly(ethylene glycol) diacrylate interpenetrating networks and initial assessment of their potential for vascular tissue engineering. *Biomaterials* 40: 32–42.

193 Hong, S. et al. (2015). 3D printing of highly stretchable and tough hydrogels into complex, cellularized structures. *Adv. Mater.* 27: 4035–4040.

194 Leach, J.B., Bivens, K.A., Collins, C.N., and Schmidt, C.E. (2004). Development of photocrosslinkable hyaluronic acid-polyethylene glycol-peptide composite hydrogels for soft tissue engineering. *J. Biomed. Mater. Res. Part A* 70A: 74–82.

195 Hoyle, C.E. and Bowman, C.N. (2010). Thiol-ene click chemistry. *Angew. Chem. Int. Ed.* 49: 1540–1573.

196 Kolb, H.C., Finn, M.G., and Sharpless, K.B. (2001). Click chemistry: diverse chemical function from a few good reactions. *Angew. Chem. Int. Ed.* 40: 2004–2021.

197 Nair, D.P. et al. (2014). The thiol-Michael addition click reaction: a powerful and widely used tool in materials chemistry. *Chem. Mater.* 26: 724–744.

198 Hassan, W., Dong, Y., and Wang, W. (2013). Encapsulation and 3D culture of human adipose-derived stem cells in an in-situ crosslinked hybrid hydrogel composed of PEG-based hyperbranched copolymer and hyaluronic acid. *Stem Cell Res. Ther.* 4: 32.

199 Dong, Y. et al. (2015). A rapid crosslinking injectable hydrogel for stem cell delivery, from multifunctional hyperbranched polymers via RAFT homopolymerization of PEGDA. *Polym. Chem.* 6: 6182–6192.

200 Dong, Y. et al. (2017). Injectable and tunable gelatin hydrogels enhance stem cell retention and improve cutaneous wound healing. *Adv. Funct. Mater.* 27: 1606619.

201 Dong, Y. et al. (2018). Acceleration of diabetic wound regeneration using an in situ–formed stem-cell-based skin substitute. *Adv. Healthc. Mater.* 17: 1–9. https://doi.org/10.1002/adhm.201800432.

202 Li, J. et al. (2018). Cartilage regeneration using arthroscopic flushing fluid-derived mesenchymal stem cells encapsulated in a one-step rapid cross-linked hydrogel. *Acta Biomater.* 79: 202–215.

203 Xu, Q. et al. (2018). Injectable hyperbranched poly(β-amino ester) hydrogels with on-demand degradation profiles to match wound healing processes. *Chem. Sci.* 9: 2179–2187.

204 Xu, Q. et al. (2018). Versatile hyperbranched poly(β-hydrazide ester) macromers as injectable antioxidative hydrogels. *ACS Appl. Mater. Interfaces.* 10: 39494–39504. https://doi.org/10.1021/acsami.8b15006.

205 Skrott, Z. et al. (2017). Alcohol-abuse drug disulfiram targets cancer via p97 segregase adaptor NPL4. *Nature* 552: 194–199.

206 Anderson, D.G. et al. (2006). A combinatorial library of photocrosslinkable and degradable materials. *Adv. Mater.* 18: 2614–2618.

Index

Multifunctional Hydrogels for Biomedical Applications, First Edition.
Edited by Ricardo A. Pires, Iva Pashkuleva, and Rui L. Reis.

n

o

p